D1255372

# DEMONSTRATIONS OF
# PHYSICAL SIGNS
## IN CLINICAL SURGERY

BY

## HAMILTON BAILEY, F.R.C.S.(Eng.), F.A.C.S., F.I.C.S., F.R.S.E.

*Surgeon, and Surgeon-in-charge of the Genito-urinary Department, Royal Northern Hospital, London;
Senior Surgeon, St. Vincent's Clinic and the Italian Hospital; Surgeon, Consolation Hospital,
Lambeth; General Surgeon, Metropolitan Ear, Nose, and Throat Hospital, London;
Consulting Surgeon, County Hospital, Chatham, Potter's Bar Hospital, and Clacton
Hospital; formerly External Examiner in Surgery, University of Bristol.*

### ELEVENTH EDITION

BALTIMORE:
THE WILLIAMS AND WILKINS CO.
1949

*First edition, August, 1927.*
*Reprinted, October, 1928.*
*Second edition, January, 1930.*
*Third edition, June, 1931.*
*Fourth edition, April, 1933.*
*Reprinted, May, 1934.*
*Fifth edition, October, 1935.*
*Reprinted, December, 1936.*
*Sixth edition, September, 1937.*
*Reprinted, August, 1938.*
*Seventh edition, January, 1940.*
*Reprinted, December, 1940.*
*Eighth edition, May, 1942.*
*Reprinted, December, 1942.*
*Ninth edition, March, 1944.*
*Reprinted, December, 1944.*
*Tenth edition, March, 1946.*
*Reprinted, November, 1947. (Special Export Edition.)*
*Eleventh edition, Pt. I, May, 1948.*
*Pt. II, August, 1948.*
*Pt. III, September, 1948.*
*Pt. IV, January, 1949.*

| | |
|---|---|
| *German First Edition* | 1939 |
| *,, Second Edition* | 1948 |
| *Turkish Edition* | 1943 |
| *Spanish Edition* | 1947 |
| *Bulgarian Edition* | 1948 |

*Italian Edition*
*Dutch Edition* } *in preparation*
*French Edition*

*Portuguese Edition*
*Chinese Edition*
*Finnish Edition* } *being negotiated*
*Greek Edition*

PRINTED IN GREAT BRITAIN BY JOHN WRIGHT AND SONS LTD.,
THE STONEBRIDGE PRESS, BRISTOL

The wards are the greatest of all research laboratories.

Sir Henry Wade    Ramon Guiteras Lecture  1932.

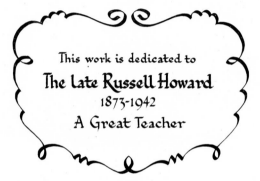

This work is dedicated to
The late Russell Howard
1873-1942
A Great Teacher

★

# PREFACE TO THE ELEVENTH EDITION

BEFORE the War, British colour blockmakers, defying Continental competition, turned out magnificent reproductions within a few weeks of receiving the original illustrations. During the War there were hardly any new apprentices to this trade, and because the apprenticeship is long and tedious, there have been comparatively few entries since the War. Consequently, the number of blockmakers has become depleted. When fewer men work shorter hours (some firms do not work at all on Saturdays) it is not surprising that the work for them to do accumulates. Foreign competition has ceased to exist. These factors have resulted in an unfortunate position (unfortunate for the reader, publisher, and author) whereby it seemed almost a condescension on the part of blockmakers to undertake their work. Should an order be accepted, a period of six months has often been required for its execution. In spite of the fact that cost has advanced nearly 100 per cent, certain faults in reproduction, such as incorrect skin tones, frequently result in further loss of time while the necessary adjustments are carried out. Further obstructions are encountered on all sides—in the delivery of paper, in printing, in book-binding, and so on.

In most trades concerned with production the Government has instituted a system of priorities, but the Ministry of Health has not succeeded in establishing any definite priority for medical literature. Although it is true that additional paper is licensed for export, and in special cases for editions of outstanding importance, the fact remains that medical students' text-books have in the main to take their turn in delivery of paper from the mills, printing, and binding, with manuals on greyhound racing and " How to Play Poker ".

Finding myself in a jungle of strangulating creepers, I determined to do my utmost to hasten snail-pace book production, an outcome of which is this paper-covered Part. As writing text-books is only a spare-time occupation of mine, had it not been for complete recreational sacrifices on the part of my wife, and the practical help of patients of mine in paper manufacturing, printing, and blockmaking businesses, I am sure the plan could not have materialized, for opposition to it was too great. It is my hope that readers, and especially reviewers, before they express disapproval of this break-away from long-established tradition, will weigh the advantages, which are apparent only in the light of understanding of economic conditions, with the disadvantages which are numerous and easily perceived. It is my belief that at any rate the members of the British Medical Students' Association, who have honoured me by making me one of their Vice-Presidents, will support me in this venture. Deeply conscious as I am of the debt I owe to the Profession, I have laboured assiduously to make the book more worthy than its predecessors of its continued popularity. Still adhering rigidly to the 20-year old conception that demonstrations of actual cases was what I wanted to convey, I have brought before the reader many new patients, but only after every technical detail, from the setting of the stage to the final proof of the illustration, has received my close attention. Time and again pictures that failed to pass a minimum standard of accuracy and artistry have been discarded at one or other stage of their metamorphosis.

Into the text I have grafted my accumulated clinical experience with special reference to imparting information to undergraduates and post-graduates in the wards and in the out-patient department. When I have not felt fully competent to speak from personal experience, I have studied the relevant literature and sought advice from those who are better able to assess the value of a particular physical sign than myself. Stimulating assistance in this direction has been afforded by my professional friends on both sides of the Atlantic, but to set out what I owe to them individually would fill many pages. Here and there it has been possible to accord a modicum of recognition for these services in the form of an appropriate footnote. Where this is not applicable, I can only refer the reader to the Table on p. ix. I am regretfully unable to indicate the actual illustrations of patients not my own in the tabulated list of my small army of indispensable helpers, owing to the fact that the illustrations of the final two parts are not yet correctly numbered.

HAMILTON BAILEY

86, *Brook Street,*
*London, W.* 1.

# FROM THE PREFACES TO PREVIOUS EDITIONS

THERE is a growing tendency to rely upon laboratory and other auxiliary reports for a diagnosis. A former chief, to whose clinical teaching I am for ever indebted, was wont to picture the modern graduate of medicine, when summoned to an urgent call, driving up to the patient's house followed by a pantechnicon containing a fully equipped X-ray installation, and a laboratory with a staff of assistants. Without these aids the future doctor would be unable to formulate a diagnosis. The history, and physical methods of examination, must always remain the main channels by which a diagnosis is made.

This work had its origin in a series of demonstrations given to students at the Liverpool Royal Infirmary, commencing in 1921. For some years I thought over the possibility of producing the substance of these demonstrations in book form, and in 1926 I finally set to work, Messrs. John Wright & Sons Ltd. producing the volume in 1927. I have to confess that in the beginning I wrote this, my first book to be published, quickly, and I wrote it because I wanted to get away from describing operative technique which, with my then unpractised pen, was becoming wearisome. I thought I would take a metaphoric holiday from the labours of compiling *Emergency Surgery*, so after the day's work at the hospital was over, I dictated the demonstrations without notes to my wife. Many of the photographs of the first edition were taken by one or other of us with a secondhand half-plate camera. A few of these pictures are still retained, for, in spite of many endeavours, they have yet to be bettered.

Individual physical signs are often known by the name of the person who first described them. In many respects this is an advantage, for an anatomico-pathological label is often cumbersome. On the other hand, an array of proper names is apt to bore the reader, especially if they do not conjure up personalities. By adding historical footnotes, not only is this objection overcome without lengthening the text, but due credit is given to those to whom we owe so much. If the reader is not interested in the matter, the footnotes can be disregarded.

The book has never presumed to be a complete treatise on clinical surgery ; its scope is clearly set out in Chapter I. I have always intended it to be what its name implies—demonstrations—hence the pictures.

# ACKNOWLEDGEMENTS

IN preparing the eleventh edition of this work I am deeply indebted to the undermentioned for various services intimately bound up with rendering the text and illustrations informative and accurate :—

## For Helpful Criticisms and Advice

J. ADAMS-RAY, M.D.  Surgeon-in-Chief, Out-Patient Department, Seraphimerhospital, Stockholm.
ANTHONY TURNER ANDREASEN, F.R.S.E., F.R.C.S.E.  Formerly Professor of Surgery, Calcutta.
FRANTISEK BAUER, M.D. (Prague), D.L.O. (Eng.).  Resident Surgical Officer, Huddersfield Royal Infirmary.
CHARLES ALLAN BIRCH, M.D. (Liverp.), F.R.C.P. (Lond.).  Medical Superintendent, Chase Farm Emergency Hospital, Enfield, Middlesex.
NORMAN B. CAPON, M.D. (Liverp.), F.R.C.P. (Lond.).  Professor of Child Health, University of Liverpool.
SOL M. COHEN, M.A. (Cape Town), F.R.C.S. (Eng.).  Surgeon, Southern Hospital, Dartford, Kent.
WARREN H. COLE, M.D., F.A.C.S.  Professor of Surgery, University of Illinois, Chicago.
HAROLD DODD, Ch.M. (Liverp.), F.R.C.S. (Eng.).  Surgeon, King George's Hospital, Ilford, Essex.
B. A. G. A. EDELSTON, M.D. (Edin.).  Folkestone.
ERNEST FREDERICK FINCH, M.D., M.S. (Lond.), F.R.C.S. (Eng.).  Emeritus Professor of Surgery, University of Sheffield.
FREDERICK PATRICK FITZGERALD, M.B., Ch.B., B.A.O., F.R.C.S.I.  Surgeon to the Orthopædic Department, Royal Northern Hospital, London.
WILLIAM BASHALL GABRIEL, M.S. (Lond.), F.R.C.S. (Eng.).  Surgeon, Royal Northern Hospital, London.
ROBERT MCNEILL LOVE, M.S. (Lond.), F.R.C.S. (Eng.).  Surgeon, Royal Northern Hospital, London.
T. P. MCMURRAY, C.B.E., M.Ch. (Belf.), F.R.C.S.E.  Professor of Orthopædic Surgery, University of Liverpool.
CLIFFORD NAUNTON MORGAN, M.B., B.S. (Lond.), F.R.C.S. (Eng.).  Assistant Surgeon, St. Bartholomew's Hospital, London.
PETER PRINGLE, LL.B. (Lond.), M.R.C.S. (Eng.), L.R.C.P. (Lond.), D.I.H.  Chief Medical Officer, British Electricity Authority.
LAMBERT ROGERS, M.Sc. (Wales), F.R.C.S. (Eng.), F.R.C.S.E., F.A.C.S., F.R.A.C.S.  Professor of Surgery, University of Wales.
CHARLES ROPER, M.D. (Cantab.).  Chatham.
BENJAMIN WILLIAM RYCROFT, O.B.E., M.D. (St. And.), F.R.C.S. (Eng.), D.O.M.S.  Surgeon, Royal Eye Hospital, London.
IAN SCOTT SMILLIE, Ch.M. (Edin.), F.R.C.S.E.  Lecturer in Orthopædic Surgery, University of St. Andrews.
ERICH HUGO STRACH, M.D. (Prague).  Orthopædic Registrar, Royal Albert Edward Infirmary, Wigan.
STANLEY WAY, M.R.C.S. (Eng.), L.R.C.P. (Lond.), M.R.C.O.G.  Associate Surgeon, Department of Gynæcology, Royal Victoria Infirmary, Newcastle-upon-Tyne.
ROBERT MILNES WALKER, M.S. (Lond.), F.R.C.S. (Eng.).  Professor of Surgery, University of Bristol.
EUGENE WOLFF, M.B., B.S. (Lond.), F.R.C.S. (Eng.).  Ophthalmic Surgeon, Royal Northern Hospital, London.

## For Presentation of Clinical Illustrations

RICHARD SIDNEY ALLISON, M.D. (Belf.), F.R.C.P. (Lond.).  Physician-with-Charge of Out-Patients, Royal Victoria Hospital, Belfast.
FRANTISEK BAUER, M.D. (Prague), D.L.O. (Eng.).  Resident Surgical Officer, Huddersfield Royal Infirmary.
THOMAS ADRIEN BOUCHIER-HAYES, M.B., B.Ch., B.A.O., F.R.C.S.I.  Assistant Surgeon, Richmond Hospital, Dublin.
REGINALD HAROLD BOYD, M.B., Ch.B. (N.Z.), F.R.C.S.E.  Consulting Venereologist, Essex County Council.
SIR HUGH CAIRNS, K.B.E., M.B., B.S. (Adelaide), F.R.C.S. (Eng.).  Nuffield Professor of Surgery, University of Oxford.
JOHN A. COBB, M.B., B.S., F.R.C.S. (Eng.), F.R.S.E.  Surgeon, Ear, Nose and Throat Department, Royal Infirmary, Sheffield.
The late LIEUT. SAMUEL MORRIS GREEN, M.B., Ch.B. (Liverp.).  R.A.M.C.
SOL M. COHEN, M.A. (Cape Town), F.R.C.S. (Eng.).  Surgeon, Southern Hospital, Dartford, Kent.
WARREN H. COLE, M.D., F.A.C.S.  Professor of Surgery, University of Illinois, Chicago.
C. C. COLEMAN, M.D., F.A.C.S.  Professor of Neurological Surgery, Richmond, Virginia.
MAX CUTLER, M.D. (Maryland), F.A.C.S.  Surgeon, Mary Reese Hospital, Chicago.
Messrs. PARKE DAVIS AND CO. LTD.
FREDERICK PATRICK FITZGERALD, M.B., Ch.B., B.A.O., F.R.C.S.I.  Surgeon to the Orthopædic Department, Royal Northern Hospital, London.
MURRAY THOMSON GREIG, B.Sc. (N.Z.), F.R.C.S. (Eng.), New Zealand.

### For Presentation of Clinical Illustrations—continued

LOUIS CONSTANT DANIEL HERMITTE, *M.B., Ch.B. (Edin.).* Pathologist and Bacteriologist, Royal Infirmary, Sheffield.
ALBERT ERNEST HODGSON, *M.D. (Edin.).* Lecturer in Infectious Diseases, University of Liverpool.
BASIL STANLEY KENT, *M.B., B.S. (Lond.), D.A. (Eng.).* Eastbourne.
CECIL PATRICK MALLEY, *M.B., B.Ch., B.A.O., F.R.C.S. (Eng.).* Surgeon, Metropolitan Ear, Nose and Throat Hospital, London.
The late JOHN THOMSON, *M.D., F.R.C.P. (Edin.).* Physician, Royal Edinburgh Hospital for Sick Children.
SIR CECIL WAKELEY K.B.E., C.B., *F.R.S.E., D.Sc. (Lond.), F.R.C.S. (Eng.), F.A.C.S., F.R.A.C.S.* Editor, British Journal of Surgery.

### For Drawings and Coloration

Mr. TOM ARMES
Mr. TOM FISHER
Dr. GUY MACKARNESS

Miss BROWN-KELLY
Miss HELEN LORRAINE (U.S.A.)
Mr. A. K. MAXWELL
Miss VERA MOREL (U.S.A.)

Dr. MARJORIE CRUMP
Dr. CRANSTON LOW
Miss MARGARET McLARTY

### For taking Photographs

Mr. G. A. CLOUD
JOHN EAST *M.B., F.R.C.S. (Eng.)*
Miss MARJORY H. SHAW

Dr. E. C. W. COOKE
Mr. F. R. NEWENS
Mr. D. STEVENSON CLARK

Mr. HUBERT DAVEY
Mr. THOMAS A. NICHOLSON

### For taking Radiographs

Miss K. C. CLARK, F.S.R.

### For Organizing Out-patients for Clinical Photographs

Sister PAULINE, C.B.E., *S.R.N., S.C.M., C.S.M.M.G.* Theatre Sister, St. Vincent's Clinic, London.
Sister E. WEAVER *S.R.N.* Sister-in-Charge of the Out-Patient Department, Royal Northern Hospital, London.
Sister M. NAYLOR, *S.R.N.* Out-Patient Sister, County Hospital, Chatham.

### For Verification of Anatomical Data

LEICESTER ATKINSON, *F.R.C.S. (Eng.).* Surgical Registrar, Middlesex Hospital, London.
ALLAN CLAIN, *M.B., Ch.B. (Cape).*
THOMAS NICOL, *F.R.S.E., D.Sc. (Lond.), M.D., F.R.C.S.E.* Professor of Anatomy, King's College Hospital, London.

### For Verification of Historical Footnotes

WALTER REGINALD BETT, *M.R.C.S. (Eng.), L.R.C.P. (Lond.), F.R.S.L.*
WILLIAM JOHN BISHOP, *F.L.A.* Librarian, Wellcome Historical Medical Museum.
THOMAS JOHN SHIELDS, *F.L.A.* Librarian, British Medical Association.

### For Compiling the Glossary

JAMES HENDERSON BROWN, Medical Student, Edinburgh University.
JOHN SPENCE MEIGHAN, *B.Sc., M.B., Ch.B. (Glas.).*

### For Reading the Proofs

DENIS NEVILLE BARON, *M.B., B.S. (Lond.).* Flight Lieutenant, R.A.F.V.R.
WALTER REGINALD BETT, *M.R.C.S. (Eng.), L.R.C.P. (Lond.), F.R.S.L.*
JOHN RAWSON ELDER, *M.B., Ch.B. (N.Z.), F.R.C.S.E.* Chief Assistant in Surgery, Hillingdon County Hospital, Uxbridge, Middlesex.
NORMAN OTWAY KNIGHT GIBBON, *M.B., Ch.B. (Liverp.), F.R.C.S.E.* Senior Registrar, Royal Infirmary, Liverpool.
EDGAR A. KAUFFMANN, *B.A. (Cantab.),* Medical Student, Middlesex Hospital.
WILLIAM DANIEL LOVELOCK-JONES, *B.Sc. (Wales), M.B., Ch.B., F.R.C.S.E.* Medical Superintendent, St. Mary's Emergency Hospital, Amersham, Bucks.
ALEX. D. ROBERTSON, Medical Student, Edinburgh University.
BENJAMIN MEYER STEEN, *L.R.C.P., L.R.C.S. (Edin.).*
KEITH WESTLAKE, *B.A. (Cantab.),* Medical Student, Middlesex Hospital.

# CONTENTS

# DEMONSTRATIONS OF PHYSICAL SIGNS IN CLINICAL SURGERY

*CHAPTER I*

## INTRODUCTORY

THE making of a surgical diagnosis resolves itself into seven stages—usually not more than three or four of these will be found necessary.

1. A history is taken and a general observation of the patient is made.

2. Physical signs are elicited.

3. A mental process on the part of the surgeon, whereby 1 and 2 are sifted and correlated, and a logical conclusion is drawn.

4. A differential diagnosis is entertained : this is also a mental process—largely one of exclusion, but reinforced, when possible, by further physical signs.

5. Confirmatory scientific tests—usually performed by a colleague—e.g., radiological, chemical, bacteriological, and histological examinations.

6. The more accessible parts of the interior are rendered visible by ingeniously constructed tubes, such as the cystoscope, sigmoidoscope, œsophagoscope, gastroscope, and bronchoscope.

7. A biopsy or an exploratory operation is performed.

If a diagnosis is still found wanting after the seven stages have been exploited, there remains but one court of appeal—the post-mortem room.

The seven stages may be termed the ' surgical crescendo '. *It is mainly with the second stage and the latter part of the fourth that this book is concerned.*

" Data, give me data ! " expostulated Sherlock Holmes. In the demonstrations that follow I have striven to train the student to elicit and assemble data upon which to formulate a reasoned diagnosis.

" If it is a question of doubt in diagnosis, you may often observe that one man solves the doubt when the others could not, and the way in which one man happened to solve it is this : he applied to the diagnosis of the case some method of examination which the others have not applied."     C. B. LOCKWOOD, *Clinical Surgery.*

**Armamentarium.**—A few simple instruments are necessary ; their cost is small. Practically all the apparatus employed in the descriptions that accompany this work are shown in *Fig.* 1. The boot-maker's size-stick is not mentioned specifically in the text, but it is a useful means of measuring not only the foot, but other parts of the body, especially when we are comparing one side with the other.

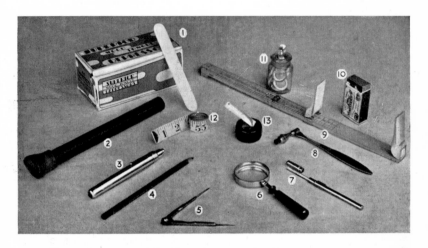

*Fig.* 1.—Apparatus used for diagnostic purposes in this book. 1, Wooden tongue depressor ; 2, Author's transilluminoscope ; 3, Electric pocket torch ; 4, Indelible pencil ; 5, Dividers ; 6, Magnifying glass ; 7, Clinical thermometer ; 8, Patella hammer ; 9, Boot-maker's size-stick ; 10, Box of wooden matches ; 11, Finger stalls ; 12, Linen tape measure ; 13, Metal tape measure.

To become a competent up-to-date clinician, the student and the practitioner must become familiar with the use of a rectal, vaginal, and nasal speculum, together with the auriscope, laryngoscope, and ophthalmoscope. In spite of requests to do so, I have made no attempt to demonstrate the use of these important aids to diagnosis because : (1) I consider that this is beyond the scope of physical signs ; (2) consideration of this aspect of clinical surgery would greatly increase the size of the book ; and, perhaps most important of all, (3) I am still in need of further instruction in the use of some of these instruments myself.

CHARLES BARRETT LOCKWOOD, 1856–1914, *Surgeon, St. Bartholomew's Hospital, London.*

## CHAPTER II

## SOME BASIC PHYSICAL SIGNS

BEFORE we commence the subject of physical signs, let us, as it were, tune up by harping for a moment on that fundamental principle of clinical surgery—*comparison*. When it is possible to compare an

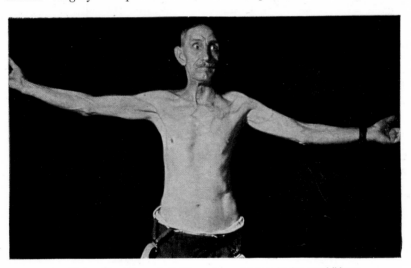

Fig. 2.—The left arm is slightly swollen and enlarged veins are visible on that side. Case of spontaneous thrombosis of the axillary vein. An example of the value of comparison.

injured or diseased member or side with the corresponding normal member or side (*Fig.* 2), the opportunity should be seized greedily. Throughout the book it is assumed that this principle will be observed studiously by the reader.

## THE LOCATION OF PAIN

Whenever pain is a feature of the case, it is an excellent practice to instruct the patient to point to the site of the pain. More often than not he will indicate an area vaguely, or commence to rub the part. Ask him to place one finger on the spot where the pain is felt most (*Fig.* 3).

I make great use of the pointing test, and often go further and insist on the patient palpating the area himself in order to find out if there is a tender place ; only after the patient has completed *his* physical examination do I commence mine.

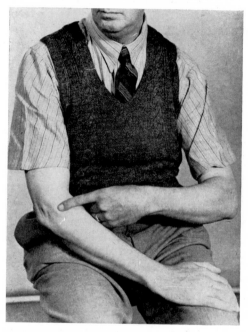

Fig. 3.—Patient pointing to the site of the pain.   Case of tennis elbow.

The possibility of pain being *referred* should be to the fore in the clinician's mind.   Notable examples (*Fig.* 4) are the initial pain of acute appendicitis, which is referred to the umbilicus (*see* Chapter XXIII), left shoulder-pain from subdiaphragmatic irritation (*see* Chapters XXIII and XXIV), pain in the knee referred from the hip (*see* Chapter XXVII), and pain from the tongue referred to the ear (*see* Chapter VI).

## LOCAL  TEMPERATURE

A sign of great value in early cases of inflammation is increased heat of the affected part.   A good method of testing for

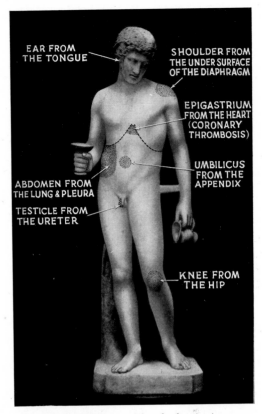

*Fig.* 4.—Leading examples of referred pain.

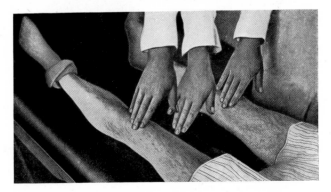

*Fig.* 5.—Testing local temperature in the case of the knee-joint. The hand is passed rapidly from the non-affected to the affected side and back again.

this, but one that requires a little practice, is to pass the hand rapidly from the non-affected to the affected area, and back again. *Fig.* 5 shows such a manœuvre being carried out in the case of a knee-joint.

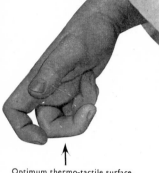

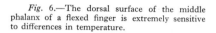

Optimum thermo-tactile surface.

Sir Thomas Lewis advised that before attempting to detect differences of skin temperature, the observer should

*Fig.* 6.—The dorsal surface of the middle phalanx of a flexed finger is extremely sensitive to differences in temperature.

ascertain that his own hand is warm by placing it against his neck. Sir Thomas recommended that the dorsal, rather than the palmar, surface of the hand should be used, and the best testing surface for delicate observations is the dorsal surface of the middle phalanx of the flexed finger (*Fig.* 6).

## PITTING ON PRESSURE

In order to confirm a suspicion of œdema, pressure is exerted by the thumb or finger in the case of a massive infiltration (e.g., of the legs) (*Fig.* 7), while in a comparatively localized swelling the index finger should always be employed. Pressure is maintained for 10 to 15

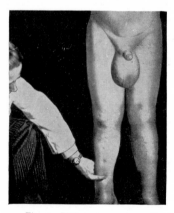

*Fig.* 7.—Pitting on pressure. Case of œdema due to a failing heart. The patient was sent to hospital as a case of extravasation of urine. Note the œdematous scrotum.

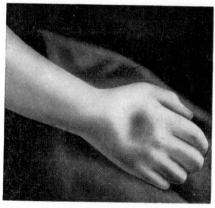

*Fig.* 8.—Pit on pressure on the back of an œdematous hand. Case of thrombosis of axillary vein.

SIR THOMAS LEWIS, 1881–1945, *Physician-in-Charge of Department of Clinical Research, University College Hospital, London.*

seconds. Should the sign be positive, a pit will be seen at the spot where the pressure was exerted (*Fig.* 8). When visible depression is doubtful, the palmar surfaces of the fingers are passed over the area, for minor degrees of pitting are sometimes better felt than seen. If the area is tender (e.g., inflammatory œdema), the index finger is used, and increasing pressure is exerted slowly.

Palpable œdema occurs when the excess of fluid increases the lymph volume by 8 per cent. The interpretation of the sign is that the tissues are infiltrated with fluid. " Œdema gives rise to a soft pitting, while if pus be present, induration can always be felt. If this fact is borne in mind, many embarrassing mistakes will be avoided " (Kanavel).

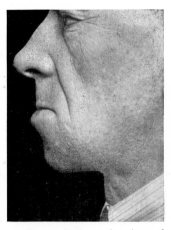

*Fig.* 9.—Angioneurotic œdema of the lower lip. At the height of an attack, before this photograph could be taken the lip was nearly double this size.

Œdema of subcutaneous tissues may be due to a variety of causes, among which are an outpouring of lymph associated with inflammation, blocking of lymphatic vessels by carcinoma cells or by filaria, a deficient peripheral circulation, e.g., a failing heart, an overdose of intravenous fluid, extravasation of urine, and vitamin starvation (e.g., that associated with beri-beri : I have seen it follow starvation consequent upon a duodenal fistula). Perhaps the most perplexing form is angioneurotic œdema (*Fig.* 9). The œdema can be in front of one's very eyes and disappear before the students can be summoned from a near-by refectory to observe it.

## ELICITATION OF FLUCTUATION

Fluctuation is the most elementary, and probably the oldest, physical sign in surgery. Yet how frequently one sees this test attempted in such a manner as to render the result absolutely valueless ! The technique was described by Howard Marsh thus :—

" Fingers straight, a little flexed upon the metacarpals ; the number of fingers depends upon the size of the swelling—usually the index finger of each hand is sufficient."

Always test for fluctuation in two planes at right angles to each other. To illustrate the necessity of this basic principle, the familiar experiment of fluctuation across the normal thigh may be taken. Fluctuation through the quadriceps, or any other muscle, can be elicited in a transverse direction ; if, however, the experiment is

ALLEN BUCKNER KANAVEL, 1874–1938, *Professor of Surgery, Northwestern University, Chicago.*
FREDERICK HOWARD MARSH, 1839–1915, *Surgeon, St. Bartholomew's Hospital, London.*

repeated in the longitudinal axis of the limb, the sign of fluctuation will be absent (*Fig.* 10).

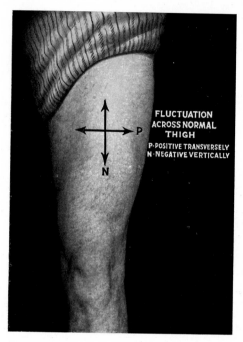

FLUCTUATION
ACROSS NORMAL
THIGH
P-POSITIVE TRANSVERSELY
N-NEGATIVE VERTICALLY

*Fig.* 10.—Showing the necessity of always trying fluctuation in two planes at right angles to each another.

We will proceed to examine a swelling of moderate size for fluctuation. The pulp of the tip of the right forefinger is placed half-way between the centre and the periphery of the swelling. This is the ' watching finger ', *and it is kept motionless throughout the procedure* (*Fig.* 11). The left forefinger is now placed upon a point at an equal distance from the centre, diagonally opposite the first. This is the ' displacing finger '. If the ' watching finger ' is displaced by the pressure exerted by the ' displacing finger ' *in both axes of the swelling*, then fluctuation is present, and we know that the swelling in question contains fluid.

There is a second method of eliciting the sign which is suited particularly to small swellings. The technique is illustrated in *Fig.* 12. The two fingers of the left hand are the ' watching fingers ' and should be kept motionless. This procedure also must be tried in

two planes at right angles to one another before the sign is pronounced positive. Some authorities consider that the second method
is so reliable that it should be the standard method for use in all cases.
The first method has served me well, and on this account I retain it.

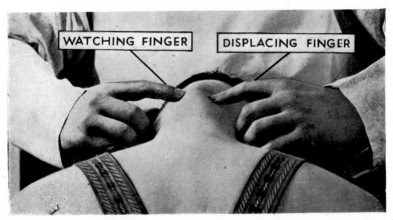

*Fig.* 11.—Standard method of testing for fluctuation. Case of tuberculous abscess connected
with the third cervical vertebra.

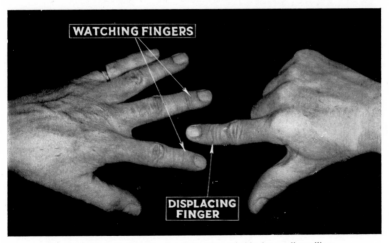

*Fig.* 12.—Method of testing for fluctuation suitable for small swellings.

When a swelling is mobile in a soft surrounding medium (e.g., a
cyst of the breast), it is necessary, before testing for fluctuation, to
have the lump ' fixed ' by an onlooker (*Fig.* 13).

Other examples of fluctuation are shown in *Figs.* 14 and 15.

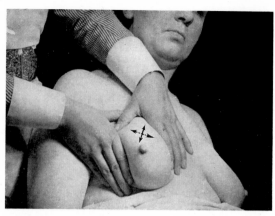

*Fig.* 13.—Testing for fluctuation in a movable lump. The lump must first be fixed by an assistant. When this has been done, fluctuation can be sought for in the usual way.

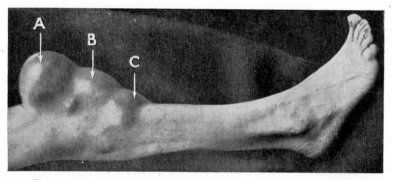

*Fig.* 14.—Fluctuation could be demonstrated from A to B but not from B to C. This proved that the swelling A–B was a distended prepatellar bursa and the swelling C a distended infrapatellar bursa, which, as is well known, has no communication with the former.

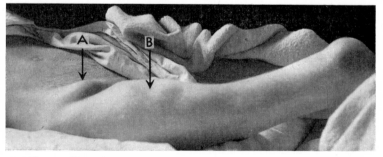

*Fig.* 15.—Fluctuation could be demonstrated from above to below Poupart's ligament (A–B) in this case of psoas abscess.

Does a lipoma fluctuate? This is a vexed question, and one that puzzles the student considerably. It can be stated emphatically that many lipomata *do* fluctuate. Fluctuation spells fluid; fat *is* fluid at body temperature. Lipomata superficial to the deep fascia (the usual situation) are an elementary clinical problem, because their *lobulation* can be made out. A lipoma beneath the fascia is often exceedingly difficult to diagnose, because fluctuation can be elicited, and the overlying fascia masks its lobulation. (*Fig.* 16.)

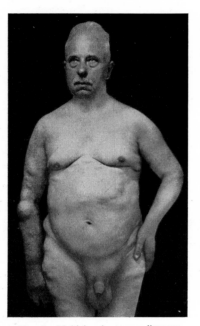

Adenomata of the thyroid are paradoxical so far as the sign of fluctuation is concerned. " The solid adenomata feel cystic, and the cystic adenomata feel solid " (Sir James Walton). The explanation is simple. In a cystadenoma of the thyroid the cyst is usually very tense, and is situated in a semi-solid medium (the thyroid tissue with its colloid vesicles), whilst the ' solid ' adenoma is but an aggregation of tiny cysts—the colloid-filled spaces that constitute the neoplasm.

The sign of fluctuation is unreliable in a swelling with a diameter of less than three-quarters of an inch. In such cases Paget's

*Fig.* 16.—Multiple subcutaneous lipomata (Dercum's disease).

test may be tried. *Paget's test* : A solid is most hard in its centre, whereas a cyst is least hard in its centre.

## TRANSLUCENCY

The electric torch has materially aided the routine application of this very useful sign, which, if positive, often sheds light upon the nature of a swelling (*Fig.* 17).

There is one trap which must be borne in mind constantly, and that is ' *normal skin illumination* ' (*Fig.* 18). Unfortunately, it is not possible always to work with a lamp of exactly the same candle-power. It therefore behoves us always to make a point of trying out what is

FRANCIS XAVIER DERCUM, 1856–1931, *Professor of Neurology, Jefferson Medical College, Philadelphia.*
SIR JAMES WALTON, *Contemporary Consulting Surgeon, London Hospital.*
SIR JAMES PAGET, 1814–1899, *Surgeon, St. Bartholomew's Hospital, London.*

the ' normal skin illumination ' for the lamp.   If this precaution is
neglected, this very valuable and absolute sign becomes unreliable.
In a strong light, especially in the summer sunlight, the sign should

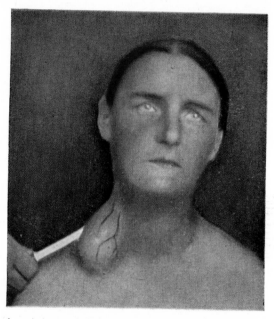

*Fig.* 17.—A cystic hygroma.   The only brilliantly translucent swelling of the neck.

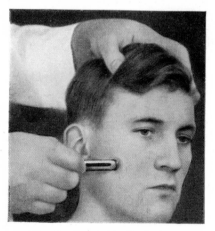

*Fig.* 18.—Normal skin illumination.

be elicited in the shade of a screen. In doubtful cases the room must be darkened, or, if possible, the patient taken to a dark room.

## CREPITUS

There are several varieties of crepitus, each being a sign of fundamental diagnostic importance.

**Bone Crepitus.**—An attempt to elicit this sign should only be made when facilities for an early X-ray examination are not available. Great circumspection and gentleness are required. On movement of the part coarse grating is so characteristic as to make the diagnosis unmistakable. The crepitus of a separated epiphysis is similar, but softer.

**Joint Crepitus.**—The joint is moved with one hand while the other hand is laid upon the joint (*Fig.* 19).

When present, joint crepitations are unmistakable. They are divided into :—

1. Fine crepitations, which are present in many sub-acute and chronic joint affections........................——>

2. Coarse crepitations, which usually signify osteo-arthritis.......................................——>

3. A ' click ' which, if a constant feature, may be a significant sign of a displaced cartilage or a loose body——>

**Crepitus of Tenosynovitis** is found over an inflamed tendon-sheath when effusion has taken place into the sheath. An excellent example is traumatic synovitis occurring in an extensor tendon-sheath of the forearm. The hand is laid upon the arm above the wrist, and the patient is instructed to open and close his hand (*Fig.* 20). The site of election for a traumatic tenosynovitis is the point where the extensor pollicis brevis and abductor pollicis longus cross the extensores carpi radialis longus and brevis (*Fig.* 20, inset). This region should be sought and examined with care, particularly in cases of obscure pain near the wrist.

**The Crepitus of Surgical Emphysema.**—From a clinical stand-point surgical emphysema, a condition in which gas is present in the subcutaneous tissues, can be divided into three varieties. In all of them a peculiar crackling sensation is imparted to the examining fingers.

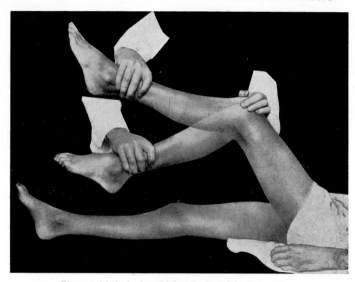

*Fig.* 19.—Method of examining the knee-joint for crepitus.

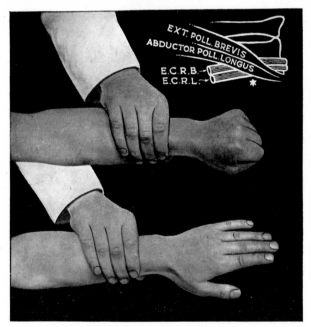

*Fig.* 20.—Testing for crepitus in suspected tenosynovitis. The site of election of traumatic tenosynovitis is depicted above the asterisk of the inset.

E.C.R.B. = Extensor carpi radialis brevis.

E.C.R.L. = Extensor carpi radialis longus.

When one places the fingers fan-wise on the affected area and exerts light pressure, a sensation similar to that of likewise palpating a horse-hair mattress is experienced (Dooley).

1. *Traumatic.*—Is seen most commonly as a complication of fractured ribs. A broken rib penetrates the lung, and air extravasates into the subcutaneous tissues. Surgical emphysema sometimes extends widely. I have seen a case in which the crepitus could be elicited from the angle of the jaw to the scrotum. It is important to inquire where the swelling commenced. If it began on one side of the face it is possible that there is a fracture of some part of the wall of the corresponding nasal fossa, and air has been forced into the sub-cutaneous tissues by the patient blowing his nose. In such circum-stances there is no need to presume that a chest lesion is the cause of the emphysema (Phillips). Other sources of traumatic air extra-vasation into the subcutaneous tissues are a breach of continuity of the larynx (usually due to an accident) and a fractured skull implicating an air sinus such as a frontal sinus.

2. *Infective.*—Crepitus similar to the above is found in gas gangrene, but the patient always exhibits other signs of that condition.

3. *Extraneous.*—Subcutaneous effusions of blood are wont to produce physical conditions which give a positive surgical emphysema sign. Typical surgical emphysema is sometimes found after saline has been administered by the subcutaneous route, but a more common source of perplexity to the uninitiated is when air becomes imprisoned during the closure of an operation wound. Several times I have been called because the house surgeon has elicited subcutaneous crepitus and has thought that gas gangrene had developed in the wound which, except for crepitus in the subcutis around it, showed nothing amiss and the patient's condition gave rise to no anxiety.

## THE PULSE

Details of examination of the pulse are dealt with thoroughly in medical works. A few points of especial surgical importance are noted here.

1. Always regard with a certain amount of suspicion the pulse reading of a patient *immediately* after he has entered hospital, when he is likely to be excited and nervous. A reading twenty minutes later is more likely to register accurately what we desire to know.

DENIS DOOLEY, *Contemporary Senior Resident Medical Officer, Charing Cross Hospital. London.*
JAMES PHILLIPS, *Contemporary Consulting Surgeon, Royal Infirmary, Bradford.*

### The Normal Pulse Reading

| Age in years | | | Pulse-rate per minute |
|---|---|---|---|
| Fœtus | .. | .. | .. 140 |
| 0– 1 | .. | .. | .. 135 |
| 1– 2 | .. | .. | .. 120 |
| 3– 4 | .. | .. | .. 110 |
| 5– 9 | .. | .. | .. 90 |
| 9–11 | .. | .. | .. 85 |
| 12–17 | .. | .. | .. 80 |
| Adult | .. | .. | .. 72 |

2. Remember that the *normal* pulse-rate varies with age. This is most important, especially when one is dealing with children. It is futile to count the pulse-rate of a baby if you do not know what the normal reading should be ! I have found students, and not a few post-graduates, who were quite unpossessed of this knowledge.

3. A few perfectly healthy individuals have a much slower pulse-rate (bradycardia*) than is set out in the standard table.

4. Frequent pulse-readings are of considerable assistance in the diagnosis of internal hæmorrhage. By a frequent pulse-reading I do not mean a four-hourly chart, but an hourly, or even half-hourly, record. This record can be kept on a separate piece of paper, as below, or it can be charted in red ink above the temperature chart.

| 3.30 p.m. | 82 | (On admission) |
|---|---|---|
| 4. 0 p.m. | 80 | — |
| 4.30 p.m. | 88 | — |
| 5. 0 p.m. | 90 | — |
| 5.30 p.m. | 108 | * |

' Operation decided upon (case of ruptured spleen).

There are good reasons for revising the British system of charting graphically only the temperature. It is to be hoped that the instantly comprehended picture of temperature, pulse and respirations, all graphically recorded in differential standard colours on the same chart, will soon become a national routine.

5. Oft-repeated pulse-readings are of paramount importance in the management of cases of head injury. A gradual slowing of, or a rise in, the pulse-rate is of such diagnostic importance in early cases that it is advisable to make a routine practice of a half-hourly pulse chart.

---

\* *Bradycardia.* Greek, βραδύς = slow.

6. If the pulse cannot be felt, try the other wrist; occasionally an anomaly of the radial artery makes even a full pulse difficult or impossible to feel. Should one be unsuccessful in feeling the pulse at either wrist, try the brachial or carotid arteries. When the pulse is too rapid to be counted (over 150 beats per minute) a stethoscope applied to the precordial area will usually enable the heart-beats to be counted. If, in spite of treatment for an hour, the pulse at the wrist remains too weak to be felt or too rapid to be counted, no matter how bright the patient may appear he almost always dies. (*See also* FEELING THE PULSE IN THE LOWER EXTREMITY, Chapter XXIII.)

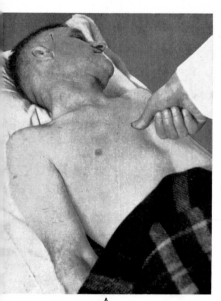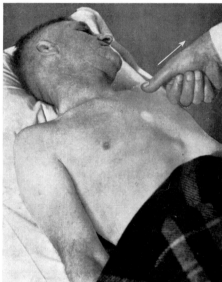

A         B

*Fig.* 21.—In shock, the skin remains blanched for a split second longer than normal.

7. The pulse-rate as a sign of shock is notoriously unreliable. An estimation of the blood-pressure is the best measurement we have at present, but this, again, is not always to be trusted. Every morsel of clinical evidence that can be gleaned by physical signs is of value. A reduced rate of blood-flow through the skin can be made apparent, with practice, by the following method: Press the thumb against the sternum and hold it there (*Fig.* 21 A). Then remove it quickly (*Fig.* 21 B). Normally the time required for the blanched area to turn pink is less than a second; in cases of early shock the reaction is noticeably longer (P. B. Price).

2

PHILIP BARTON PRICE, *Contemporary Assistant Surgeon, Johns Hopkins Hospital, Baltimore, U.S.A.*

## OBSERVING NORMAL AND ABNORMAL SUPERFICIAL VEINS

So simple is it that there are many Naamans ; yet to be enabled to assess the venous pressure, and thereby reap a harvest of highly

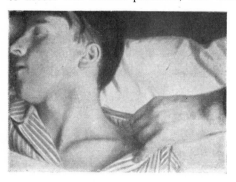

important clinical data, it is only necessary to retract the attire that hides the root of the patient's neck (*Fig. 22*).

**The External Jugular Vein.**—When the venous pressure is within normal limits, with the head resting upon a pillow, the external jugular vein is either not visible, or visible only for a short distance above the clavicle (Sir Thomas Lewis). If the venous pressure is

Fig. 22.—Retracting the nightdress in order to display the external jugular vein should become a clinical habit. In patients who are undergoing continuous intravenous therapy the external jugular vein should be kept uncovered for all to see.

raised, as in myocardial failure or anoxæmia, the external jugular vein will indicate it. *Engorgement of the external jugular vein is the earliest and best sign that a patient is receiving too much fluid intravenously.*

Bilateral enlargement of the external jugular vein is seen in singers, due to continued endeavour to reach the top note. If the enlargement is unilateral (*Fig. 23*) it may be due to the vein being partially occluded in the supraclavicular fossa by enlarged lymphatic glands, a neoplasm or a subclavian aneurysm.

**Enlarged Veins over the Thoracic Inlet** are sometimes the key to the diagnosis of a retrosternal goitre (*see* Chapter XII).

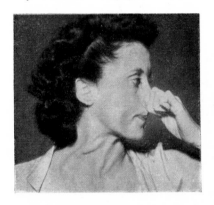

Fig. 23.—Great enlargement of the right external jugular vein made evident by the patient blowing her nose. The patient had a small adenoma of the thyroid, but this seemed to be insufficient to account for the condition.

**A Series of Superficial Venules over the Costal Margin** (*Fig. 24, A*) is often seen. Whatever may be said to the contrary, I am quite sure they are without any clinical significance.

NAAMAN, " Captain of the host of the King of Syria ", was cured of his leprosy by Elisha, who told him to wash in Jordan seven times. Of this advice Naaman was at first scornful because of its simplicity. (2 Kings v.)

SIR THOMAS LEWIS, 1881–1945, *Physician-in-charge of Department of Clinical Research, University College Hospital, London.*

**The Caput Medusæ** (*Fig.* 24,B).—Radiating veins issuing from the umbilicus can be taken as positive evidence of obstruction to the portal venous system.

**Inguino-axillary Veins** (*Fig.* 24,C).— If there is an obvious superficial venous communication between the axilla and

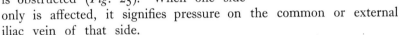

Fig. 24.—A symposium of enlarged superficial veins of the trunk. A, superficial venules over the costal margin ; B, Caput Medusæ ; C, inguino-axillary.

Scarpa's triangle on both sides, it is evidence that the inferior vena cava is obstructed (*Fig.* 25). When one side only is affected, it signifies pressure on the common or external iliac vein of that side.

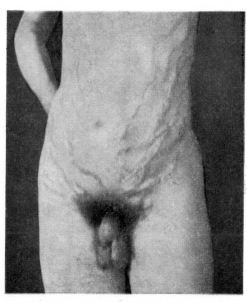

Fig. 25.—Enlargement of the superficial epigastric and circumflex iliac veins. Case of thrombosis of the inferior vena cava.

In any situation, dilated veins coursing over a deep-seated neoplasm are often noticeable.

For **Varicose Veins** *see* Chapter XXXIII.

MEDUSA, *one of the three Gorgons whose fine hair was turned into snakes* (*Greek mythology*).
ANTONIO SCARPA, 1747–1832, *Professor of Surgery, Modena, and Professor of Anatomy, Pavia, Italy.*

## VOMIT

One meets people who, after inspecting a dish containing vomit, wisely pronounce that it is ' anæsthetic vomit ', ' peritonitis vomit ', and so on.    Personally, I am able to recognize only :—

1. The vomit of ingested material.    Such vomit is acid in reaction.
2. Vomit containing blood : (a) Containing a varying percentage of recently shed blood ;  (b) Containing blood-clot ;  (c) Containing altered blood and blood-clot.
3. Vomit containing bile.
4. ' Fæcal ' vomit.
5. Vomit containing fæces.
6. A peculiar vomit associated with acute dilatation of the stomach.

Far be it from me to under-estimate the value of inspecting the vomitus ;  but it is necessary to emphasize that in most instances it is asking too much to expect to formulate a diagnosis by its aid alone.

Sometimes there is a doubt whether the specimen contains blood or dark bile.    Dilute it with water.    If it is bile a green tinge will become apparent.

Vomit containing old blood-clot that has become disintegrated has aptly been called ' coffee-grounds ' vomit.    Unfortunately the term is much abused, and it is not uncommon to find every dark vomit reported as ' coffee-grounds '.    Here again, dilution with water will sometimes clear up the nature of a doubtful specimen.

It should be borne in mind that red wine or medicine containing iron may give rise to a ' coffee-grounds ' appearance of the vomit.

' Fæcal ' vomiting is found in late intestinal obstruction.    It is distinguished from other vomits, not by its appearance, but by its odour.    Vomited tea may *look* like fæcal vomit.

Vomit containing formed fæces is seen rarely, and must signify that there is a communication between the transverse colon and the stomach, unless the patient is a coprophagist.

The peculiar vomit associated with acute dilatation of the stomach is considered fully in Chapter XXV.

The witnessing of the act of vomiting is of some value in obtaining data upon which to base a diagnosis ;  for instance, it may be noted that the vomitus is ejected forcibly, as in the projectile vomiting of infantile pyloric stenosis, or that it is effortless and comes up in mouthfuls, as in established peritonitis.

## FÆCES

Inspection of the fæces sometimes provides an important clue to the diagnosis. Totally unreliable is the much quoted pipe-stem stool supposed to occur in stenosis, particularly carcinomatous strictures of the rectum. Various characteristic stools are illustrated in *Figs.* 26–31.

### CHARACTERISTIC STOOLS

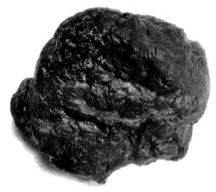

*Fig.* 26.—Melæna stool. Bleeding duodenal ulcer.

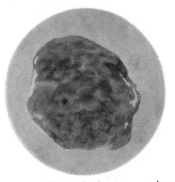

*Fig.* 27.—Blood-stained mucus passed per rectum by a patient with amœbic dysentery.

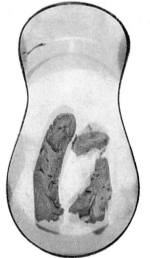

*Fig.* 28.—Clay-coloured stool. Complete obstruction to the common bile-duct by carcinoma of the pancreas.

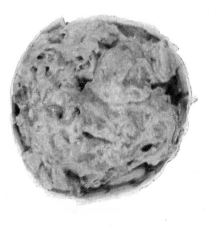

*Fig.* 29.—Stone in common bile-duct causing partial obstruction of the duct.

★ *Melæna.*  Greek, μέλαινα, fem. of μέλας = black.

## CHARACTERISTIC STOOLS—*continued*

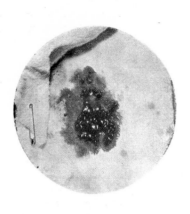

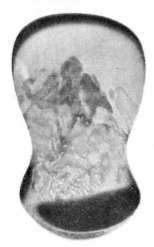

Fig. 30.— 'Red-currant jelly' stool of intussusception.

*Fig.* 31.—Ulcerative colitis. Note the blood-stained mucus clinging to the bed-pan.

### HICCUP

Hiccup is sometimes of considerable surgical significance. Occurring in the course of peritonitis, repeated hiccup often means that the diaphragmatic peritoneum has become inflamed. Hiccup is a fairly regular accompaniment of advanced uræmia—even one diaphragmatic contracture may give the clinician a lead. On hearing the characteristic sound he should ask the patient to protrude his tongue. If the tongue feels less moist than normal there is a strong probability that further investigation will prove that the blood-urea is high.

### THE TONGUE IN RELATION TO THE PATIENT'S GENERAL CONDITION

The tongue is a well-known indicator of the patient's general condition; the astute clinician of days gone by never omitted its careful scrutiny. The very way in which the patient responds to the request ' put out your tongue ' may give some valuable information; there is no mistaking protrusion of a tongue that has been practised in front of a mirror by a hypochondriacal patient.

A coated tongue, as everyone knows, is indicative of constipation or a gastro-intestinal upset, and the tongue is rarely clean in cases of inflammatory intra-abdominal lesions. So it comes about that a coated tongue is some confirmatory evidence of appendicitis.

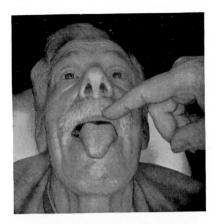

*Fig.* 32.—Testing for dryness of the tongue. Case of retention with overflow due to an enlarged prostate.

However, a coated tongue is often seen in habitual smokers and mouth-breathers.

A smooth, red tongue is frequently seen in cases of

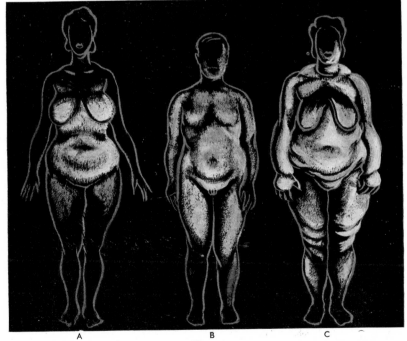

A         B         C

*Fig.* 33.

(A) *Pituitary obesity* is limited to the trunk. The arms and the legs below the knee are often shapely, and even delicate.

(B) *Adiposo-genitalis* (Fröhlich). The typical " brewer's drayman " appearance is unmistakable. Much fat in the region of the mons veneris and around the pelvic girdle suggests this syndrome.

(C) *Hypothyroid obesity* is generalized. Frequently there are pads of fat on the dorsum of the hands and in the supraclavicular fossæ. (*After Kotz and Parker.*)

ALFRED FRÖHLICH, *Contemporary. Formerly Professor of Experimental Pathology, Vienna. Now living in the U.S.A.*

prolonged suppuration, and it is occasionally referred to as ' the hectic tongue '.

In surgical practice it is the relative dryness of the tongue that makes it a most vulnerable indicator. In intestinal obstruction, uræmia, and dehydration from any cause, the tongue is dry and brown.

*In intestinal obstruction* a dry, brown tongue is of grave omen.

*In uræmia* the tongue is dry, and moderate degrees of this dryness can be determined only by touching the protruding tongue with the finger (*Fig.* 32).

(For examination of the diseased tongue *see* Chapter XI.)

## GENERAL BUILD OF THE PATIENT

That a patient has recently lost weight is suggested by his clothes, particularly the waist of his trousers, being too commodious. Obesity usually has no particular significance, but the clinician should cultivate the habit of endeavouring to segregate those of the grossly fat whose adiposity is due to endocrine disharmony. In this connexion *Fig.* 33 is helpful.

## INCIDENTAL OBSERVATION OF THE FACE AND HANDS

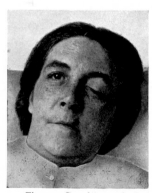

*Fig.* 34.—Complete ptosis (3rd nerve paralysis) should immediately suggest cerebrospinal syphilis. This patient's Wassermann reaction was strongly positive.

" You are looking better " ; even a layman can discern signs in the face that portray improvement in a patient's condition. There is no doubt that the experienced clinician subconsciously makes more use of observing the facies than he is inclined to realize.

A glance at the face of a patient who has been seen before will often indicate (without the aid of other methods of examination) whether the condition from which he is suffering is responding to treatment. Important as is this relative assessment, we are concerned here particularly with the first glance at the face of a patient seen for the first time (*Fig.* 34).

The general diagnostic importance of the facies is enormous, but unfortunately much that can be learned therefrom cannot be put into words.

AUGUST VON WASSERMANN, 1866–1925, *Director of the Institute for Experimental Therapy, Berlin.*

The eyes—those windows of the mind*—tell much (*Fig.* 35). Even the way the patient looks at you while he recounts his history may reveal sincerity or shiftiness. Slight bulging of the eyeballs,

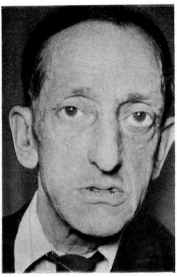

Fig. 35.—Arcus senilis in a patient 44 years of age. He complained of pain in the calf on walking (intermittent claudication). His eyes reveal premature senility.

especially if combined with a nervous manner, should foretell the necessity of excluding hyperthyroidism in due course. Pin-point pupils, or at least small pupils (*Fig.* 36), suggest tabes dorsalis or

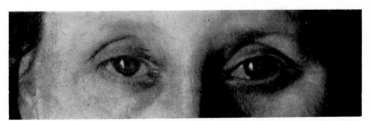

Fig. 36.—Pin-point pupils were noticed as this patient was giving her history of " being unable to hold her water ". The pupils gave the Argyll Robertson reaction. Knee-jerks were absent. Diagnosis—incontinence of urine due to tabes dorsalis.

narcotic drug addiction. A yellow tinge of the conjunctivæ, unnoticed by others, may be apparent in good daylight to a trained observer.

* " Mistress, look on me ; Behold the window of my heart, mine eye." Shakespeare, *Love's Labour Lost*, V. 2. 848.

In the heyday of life possibly there is some foundation for the popular idea that bagginess under the eyes is a sign of debauchery ; more often it is of ominous clinical significance (*Figs.* 37 and 38).

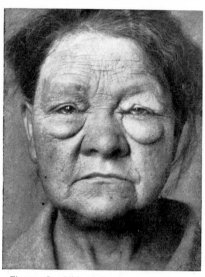

Fig. 37.—In addition to bagginess under the eyes, very dry skin.   Myxœdema.

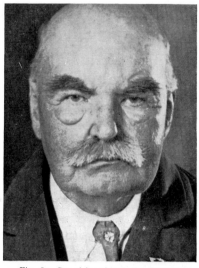

Fig. 38.—Complains of frequency and dysuria. Bagginess under the eyes suggested nephritis. Urine loaded with albumin without macroscopical evidence of pus.

Persons with acne rosacea go through life branded as secret drinkers. The ' port-light ' (red) nosed are very much maligned

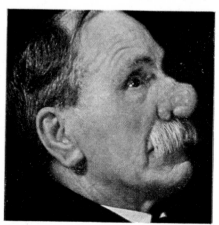

Fig. 39.—Rhinophyma.

individuals ; even their more tolerant friends are wrong again when they say it must be due to indigestion. For years I have been dealing with patients with serious indigestion ; they are no more afflicted with a ' port-light ' than the rest of humanity. I have marvelled that a teetotaller with what is known as ' bottle-nose ' (*Fig.* 39) has not been driven to seek surgical relief earlier.

" Is he weather-beaten, or is it a faint cyanotic tinge ? "
We look at the nail-beds to determine this point.   The patient
has a bulldog jaw and heavy features, suggesting acromegaly
(*Fig.* 40).   He is requested to hold up his hands ; spade-like hands
(*Fig.* 41) confirm the suspicion.   Regarding the hands one does not
need the mysteries of palmistry to read in them something of the

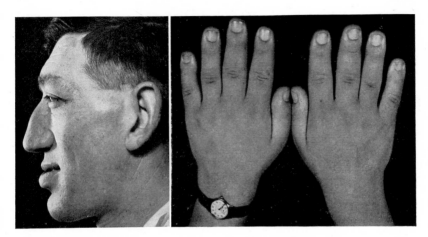

*Fig.* 40.—' Lantern jaw ' acromegaly.     *Fig.* 41.—Spade-like hands belonging to patient shown in
*Fig.* 40.

past, a great deal of the present, and even a little of the future.   In
them is written the record of age and sex ; of occupation and habits ;
of skill or ineptitude ; of hard work or indolence (Cutler).

So much for a superficial introduction to an important and
fascinating study, proficiency in which the clinician should strive to
acquire.

Condict Walker Cutler, Jun., *Contemporary Associate Surgeon, Roosevelt Hospital, New York City.*

*CHAPTER III*

## SOME GENERAL PRINCIPLES IN THE EXAMINATION OF JOINTS

**Gait** may be an aid to diagnosis.

1. The shuffle with everted toes of a person with extreme flat-foot is so characteristic as to be depicted on the music halls.

2. The waddle of a case of bilateral congenital dislocation of the hip cannot fail to attract attention, and the limp in unilateral cases is fairly characteristic (*Fig.* 42).

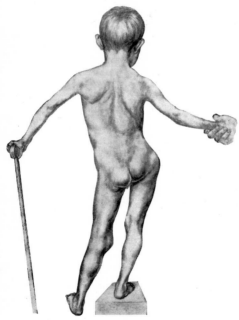 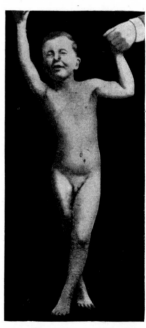

Fig. 42.—Unilateral congenital dislocation of the hip. (*After Sultan.*)

Fig. 43.—The 'scissors gait' of spastic paraplegia (Little's disease). (*Dercum.*)

3. The toddle of a patient with paralysis agitans is hurried because the centre of gravity is too far forward, and he is trying to keep up with it.

4. A short leg gives the patient a limp that can be recognized easily.

5. As the patient walks, a stiff knee causes the affected leg to be swung outwards or else the shoulder to be shrugged.

6. The patient with a dropped foot scrapes his toe along the ground. An examination of his boot will reveal that the toe of the sole is worn thin.

7. The ataxic gait of tabes. The patient keeps his feet widely apart, lifts them abnormally high, and bangs the heel violently on to the ground.

8. A high-stepping gait is seen in some neurasthenic states, strychnine poisoning, and foot-drop from any cause.

9. The scissors gait of spastic diplegia (Little's disease) (*Fig.* 43) is a sign of considerable importance. Progression is accomplished by a series of circular steps.

10. The gait in cerebellar tumour. The patient walks as though endeavouring to maintain his equilibrium on a rolling ship, to which may be added the further similarity of a sudden lurch, usually to the side of the lesion (Campbell Thomson).

11. Intermittent claudication, or intermittent limping, is a premonitory sign of impending gangrene. A muscle in activity requires more blood than a muscle at rest, and consequently, when a patient with endarteritis begins to walk, if the demand of the muscles for more blood cannot be met by the hardened artery, the muscles go into cramp, and the patient thus limps intermittently; often he comes to a complete standstill. An intelligent patient frequently says, "I can only walk (say) 400 yards without stopping."

## ROUTINE
## EXAMINATION OF A JOINT

*Observe the Position of the Affected Limb.*—A recently inflamed joint takes up the position of greatest ease. In the case of the knee, elbow, and wrist joints, the patient keeps the joint in semiflexion. In the case of a recently inflamed hipjoint, he maintains it not only in semiflexion, but in abduction and external rotation as well (*Fig.* 44), for this is the position of greatest

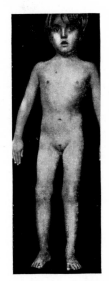

*Fig.* 44.—Position adopted in early tuberculosis of the right hipjoint; the position of greatest ease.

capacity of this joint. In other words this is the position of greatest ease.

The ankle-joint, when inflamed, is kept more or less at a right angle, with perhaps a slight inclination to plantar flexion.

*Compare the Joint with that of the Opposite Side.*—The joint may be obviously larger than its fellow, but wasting of adjacent musculature can exaggerate the discrepancy. See that sufficient of the patient's anatomy is displayed to enable you to compare the limbs with special reference to muscular symmetry.

When a joint is inflamed, wasting of neighbouring muscles occurs, even after a comparatively short time, e.g., a week or ten days. Such wasting affects certain groups of muscles in a constant and

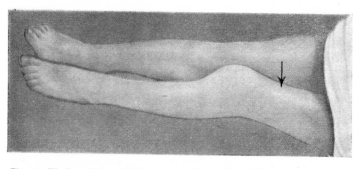

*Fig.* 45.—Wasting of the quadriceps in a case of tuberculosis of the knee. This case also demonstrates why bygone clinicians called this condition ' tumor albus ' (white swelling.)

characteristic distribution ; for instance, the quadriceps when the knee-joint is involved (*Fig.* 45), and the deltoid in the case of the shoulder. Minor degrees of muscular wasting can be determined only by taking accurate measurement at identical points on each side and having both limbs in identical positions. For this purpose the metal tape measure shown in *Fig.* 1 is better than one made of linen, for it obviates errors due to ' drag '.

*The Pointing Test.*—If pain is a leading symptom, ask the patient to point with one finger to the site of the pain.

*Palpation.*—When a joint has been recently injured or is acutely inflamed, physical examination must be conducted with great circumspection. In other circumstances we can proceed as follows :—

The surface of the joint is palpated and any special points of tenderness noted. Next, the joint is moved. Commencing cautiously, we put the joint through its full range of movement, if this is feasible and does not cause pain. Limitation of all movements of a joint indicates *arthritis* of that joint. Restriction of certain movements only, suggests *an extra-articular lesion.* When the movements are free and painless up to a point, and from thenceforth are limited and accompanied by pain, *intra-articular adhesions* are the probable cause. A particular movement only may be so involved.

*Joint Crepitus.*—The technique of eliciting joint crepitus is dealt with on p. 13.

**Auscultation,** combined with passive movement of a joint, may reveal a very early stage of roughness or grating not recognizable by other means. In the earliest stages, fine hair-like crepitations are heard, especially at the end of complete flexion and extension.

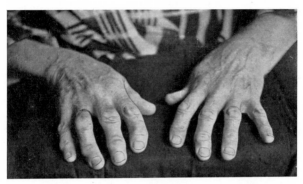

Fig. 46.—Heberden's nodes are usually an accompaniment of arthritis deformans of the aged, as in this case, but the nodes are sometimes seen in younger individuals with psoriasis, and more rarely still following local trauma.

Sites of auscultation should be chosen that are as free as possible from hair. The following are the best situations for applying the stethoscope : (1) Over the flexor surface of the wrist ; (2) Over the superior radio-ulnar joint ; (3) In front of the shoulder ; (4) Over the mandibular joint in women, but a little in front of it in men ; (5) Over the most prominent part of the internal condyle of the femur. (Walters.)

If, from physical signs, a diagnosis of subacute or chronic arthritis has been made, and there is no history of an accident, then :—

    1. Examine the other joints (*Fig.* 46).

    2. Test the urine (two-glass test, *see* Chapter XXI). If possible, supplement by prostatic massage (*see* Chapter XXII). This will help to eliminate gonorrhœa as the cause.

WILLIAM HEBERDEN, 1710–1801, *Physician to George III and to the illustrious writer, Dr. Samuel Johnson.*
CHARLES F. WALTERS, 1875–1944, *Surgeon, Royal Infirmary, Bristol.*

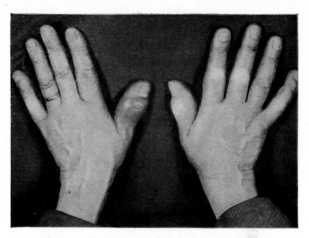

Fig. 47.—Gouty arthritis with an acute exacerbation.

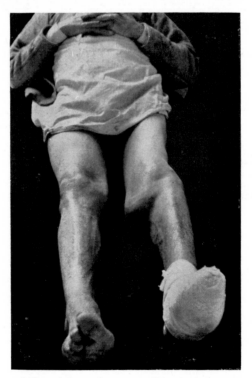

Fig. 48.—A case of Charcot's knee.  Spontaneous dislocation has occurred.  There is also a large perforating ulcer of the foot which is covered by the dressing.

3. Examine the gums for pyorrhœa and the tonsils.   Do not jump to any conclusions concerning the findings.

Methods of examining individual joints are considered in more detail later in this book.   Here will be included a few points of general diagnostic importance.

1. Gout is now rare in Britain, and it does not always attack the big toe joint (*Fig.* 47).   It is easily mistaken for acute bacterial arthritis.

2. A symptomless symmetrical synovitis suggests syphilis.

3. A painless flail joint, often associated with effusion, should bring to mind neuropathy (Charcot's arthritis) (*Fig.* 48).   Do not miss it by forgetting to test the tendon-jerks and the reaction of the pupils.   If the latter findings do not agree with the former, take

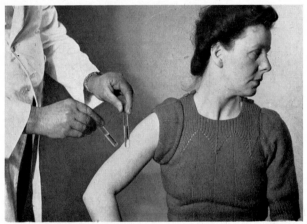

*Fig.* 49.—Testing for appreciation of temperature.   One test-tube is filled with hot, and the other with cold, water.

two test-tubes, fill one with hot water and one with cold, and test for the appreciation of temperature by the limbs (*Fig.* 49).   Temperature appreciation is lost in syringomyelia.   Further tests are made in the laboratory (Wassermann reaction, Kahn test, and blood-coagulation time) and by radiography.

4. Most important of all, in every unexplained monarticular arthritis suspect tuberculosis until it has been proved to be otherwise. The somewhat spindle-shaped nature of certain tuberculous joints, with the pulpy thickening of the synovial membrane, the raised temperature over the joint, especially after exercises, the muscular wasting that is usually present, all serve to distinguish tuberculous disease from traumatic synovitis (Timbrell Fisher).

3

JEAN-MARTIN CHARCOT, 1825–1893, *Physician, Hôpital Salpêtrière, Paris.*

AUGUST VON WASSERMANN, 1866–1925, *Director of the Institute for Experimental Therapy, Berlin.*

REUBEN L. KAHN, *Contemporary Bacteriologist, University of Michigan, U.S.A.*

A. TIMBRELL FISHER, *Contemporary Orthopædic Surgeon, St. John's Clinic, London.*

## CHAPTER IV

## LOCALIZED SWELLINGS

### The Diagnosis of a Lump.—

*Step* 1.—The first essential procedure is to leave no stone unturned in the endeavour to make certain in what *anatomical plane* the lump is situated. Ask yourself, " Is it in the skin (*Figs.* 50 and 56), subcutaneous tissue (*Fig.* 53), muscle (*Figs.* 51 and 52), tendon, nerve (*Fig.* 54), or bone (*Fig.* 55) ; or is it attached to some particular organ ? "

*Step* 2.—Determine the physical characteristics of the lump, such as whether it is cystic or solid, regular or irregular, hard or otherwise.

*Step* 3.—Having finished the examination of the case, if the diagnosis is still to seek, run through the following little catechism to yourself :—

1. Is the lump congenital ? If not—
2. Is it traumatic ?
3. Is it inflammatory ? If so, is it acute or chronic ?
4. Is it neoplastic ? If so, is it benign or malignant ? If malignant, is it primary or secondary ?
5. If it is none of these, a degeneration is about the only thing left.

Of the multitudinous variety of lumps that are presented to the surgical clinician for diagnosis, the simplest is the sebaceous cyst. Manifestly the swelling is *in* the skin. Because the swelling is often comparatively small it is not always possible to be certain whether it is cystic. Elementary as is the diagnosis, when a sebaceous cyst occurs in an unusual situation it is surprising how often the lump is misdiagnosed. Sometimes an obvious punctum (*Fig.* 56) settles the diagnosis without any further ado.

Throughout the demonstrations that follow, reference will be made to the diagnosis of lumps in various regions and particular organs, but before leaving this important subject it is necessary to demonstrate some physical signs of general application.

## SOME LUMPS FOR DIAGNOSIS

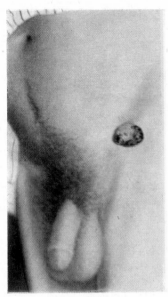

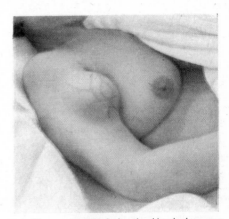

*Fig.* 51.—Not attached to the skin, the lump can be moved freely on the humerus. When the biceps muscle contracts the lump moves with the muscle. With the biceps contracted the mobility of the tumour decreases. Diagnosis : Sarcoma of the biceps muscle.

*Fig.* 50.—Pedunculated papilloma. Slowly increasing in size for fifteen years, it finally outgrew its vascular supply and it has become gangrenous.

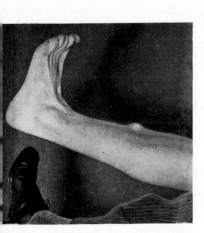

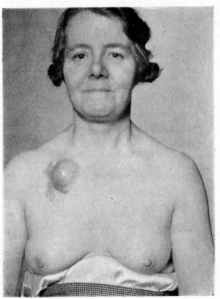

*Fig.* 52.—When the patient dorsiflexes his foot, the lump appears. When he plantar-flexes it, it disappears. Case of hernia of a portion of the tibialis anticus through the deep fascia, remotely following a pitchfork wound.

*Fig.* 53.—The patient stated that a lump had been removed three months previously, but had returned. The lump is in the subcutaneous tissue. Case of recurrent fibroid of Paget (a relatively benign form of fibrosarcoma).

SIR JAMES PAGET, 1814–1899, *Surgeon, St. Bartholomew's Hospital, London.*

## SOME LUMPS FOR DIAGNOSIS

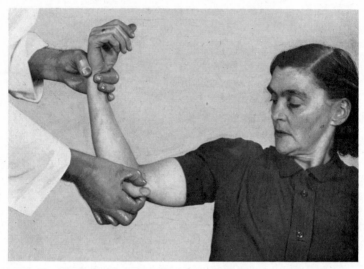

*Fig.* 54.—The swelling can be moved freely from side to side, but not upwards or downwards. When it is pressed, the patient experiences sharp pain shooting into the hand. Tumour of the sheath of the ulnar nerve.

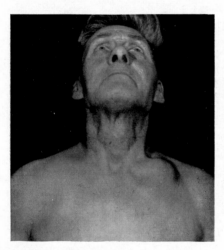

*Fig.* 55.—The left clavicle is expanded ; the swelling appeared in a matter of weeks. It would be quite correct to make a diagnosis of ' probably malignant disease of bone ', but is it primary or secondary ? *See* Chapter XXX.

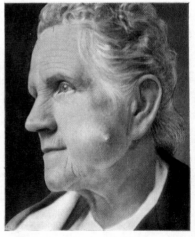

*Fig.* 56.—Owing to its large size, it is impossible to verify that the cystic swelling arises in the skin, but the obvious punctum leaves no doubt concerning the diagnosis—sebaceous cyst.

**Hydatid Thrill.**—Three fingers are placed on the swelling, the middle one being pressed firmly, and the lateral ones lightly. Then the middle finger is percussed firmly, and, after each stroke, the percussing finger is allowed to rest momentarily (*Fig.* 57). The ' hydatid thrill ' is an after-thrill, which is felt by the adjacent two fingers.

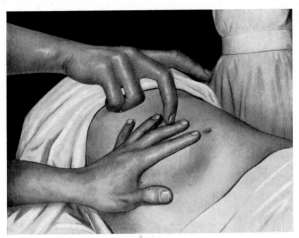

*Fig.* 57.—Testing for a hydatid thrill.

**The Sign of an Aneurysm** (*Differential Diagnosis of a Pulsating Swelling*).—It is often a perplexing problem to decide whether the pulsation of a swelling is *transmitted* from a neighbouring artery or whether the swelling itself is pulsating.

Great help can be obtained by fixing two match-stalks with plasticine on to the skin overlying the swelling.

If the pulsation is transmitted, the movements of the matches during each throb of the pulse are as shown in *Fig.* 58. It will be observed that they remain parallel with each other. On the other hand, if the swelling is truly expansile, the excursions of the indicators are as shown in *Fig.* 59.

It may be possible to compress the main artery above the swelling. In the case of an aneurysm (*Fig.* 60) pulsations cease and the swelling decreases in size. Usually reliable, these signs are vitiated by considerable clot formation within the aneurysm.

It should always be remembered that a very rapidly growing vascular neoplasm, particularly a bone sarcoma, often pulsates very

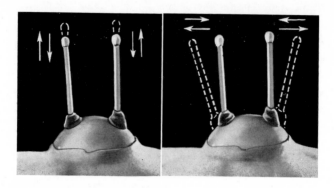

*Fig.* 58.—Transmitted  pulsation.     *Fig.* 59.—Expansile  impulse.  The
sign of an aneurysm.

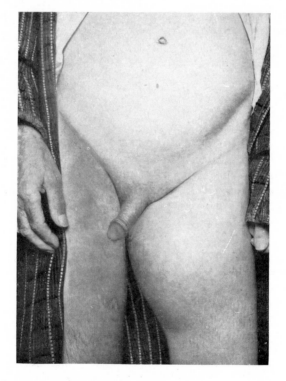

*Fig.* 60.—Aneurysm  of  the  femoral  artery.   Expansile  impulse  present.

obviously. " A swelling which has most of the characteristics of, but is not, an aneurysm, is a sarcoma." (Rutherford Morison.)

**The Sign of Emptying.**—When the swelling is compressed it diminishes in size considerably or disappears ; when the pressure is released, it refills slowly (*Fig.* 61). This is *the* sign of a cavernous hæmangioma (*Fig.* 62), but it is also present in lymphangiomata, and certain meningoceles, particularly those with a very narrow neck.

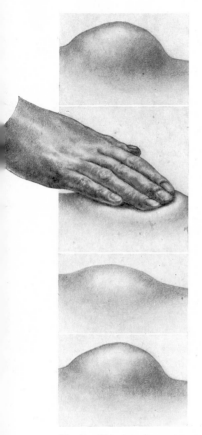

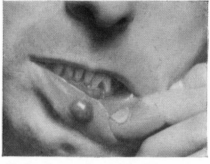

*Fig.* 62.—Cavernous hæmangioma of the lower lip.

On a miniature scale, the sign of emptying is useful in the diagnosis of capillary nævi, which blanch when the skin about them is put on the stretch. In this way tiny capillary nævi can be distinguished from Campbell de Morgan spots. The latter are raspberry red, and do not show the sign of emptying. The spots, by the way, are of no clinical significance. They were at one time thought to suggest carcinoma.

*Fig.* 61.—The sign of emptying.

## ON ' SPOT ' DIAGNOSIS (*Syn.* ' Snap Diagnosis ')

As a rule, lightning diagnoses are to be disparaged ; often dramatic, they may prove dangerous. More reliance can be placed

JAMES RUTHERFORD MORISON, 1853-1939, *Professor of Surgery, University of Durham, Newcastle-upon-Tyne.*
CAMPBELL DE MORGAN, 1811-1876, *Surgeon, Middlesex Hospital, London.*

upon a conclusion based on data gleaned from touch as well as sight (*Fig.* 63). However, there are clinical conditions that should be apparent to the diagnostician almost immediately. Take, for instance, diffuse neurofibromatosis (*Fig.* 64). If a student palpates one nodule, ponders, and then commences examining another of these subcutaneous swellings, it usually transpires that he is not cognisant of this clinical entity. There are a number of lumps

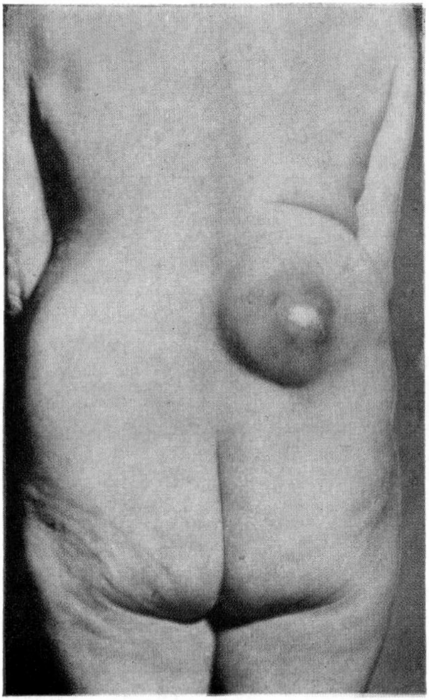

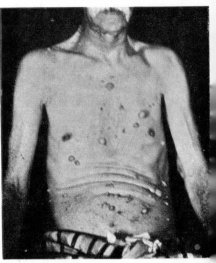

*Fig.* 63.—Students who examined this patient concluded that the swelling was an abscess, but it is not tender, the periphery feels 'wooden' and lacks superficial œdema. It is doubtful whether the sign of local heat is present. Case of sarcoma springing from the erector spinæ.

*Fig.* 64.—When diffuse neurofibromatosis is associated with cutaneous pigmentation and the presence of multiple sessile and pedunculated tumours on the skin, the condition is known as von Recklinghausen's disease, or molluscum fibrosum.★

that can be only one thing, and if the clinician is familiar with the condition, an absolute diagnosis is forthcoming almost immediately. Naturally their number increases with experience. The foundation of 'spot' diagnosis is to have encountered several exactly similar cases previously. *Figs.* 65–69 illustrate some clinical entities, which, once seen, can be diagnosed at almost lightning speed.

---

★ *Molluscum fibrosum.*   Latin, *molluscus*, from *mollis* = soft.

FRIEDRICH DANIEL VON RECKLINGHAUSEN, 1833–1910, *Professor of Pathology, Strassbourg.*

## 'SPOT' DIAGNOSIS

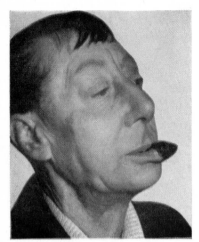

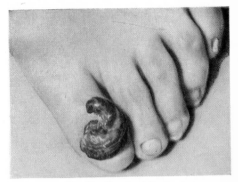

*Fig.* 66.—Onychogryphosis.

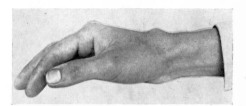

*Fig.* 65.—A sebaceous horn growing from the skin of the lower lip.

*Fig.* 67.—Simple ganglion of the dorsum of the wrist.

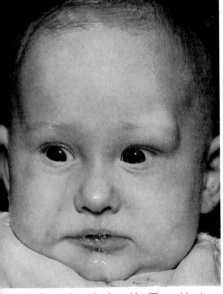

*Fig.* 68.—External angular dermoid. The position is so constant that it allows of 'spot' diagnosis.

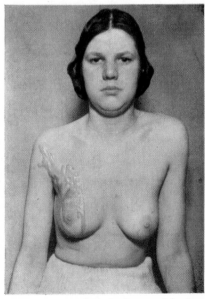

*Fig.* 69.—Keloid developing in a scar following a burn.

*Onychogryphosis.* Greek, ὄνυξ = nail + γρύπωσις = curving.

## CHAPTER V

### SIGNS OF LOCAL INFLAMMATION
### ULCERS AND SINUSES

THAT redness, swelling, heat, and tenderness, to which may be added loss of function, are the cardinal signs of inflammation was first expounded by Celsus.

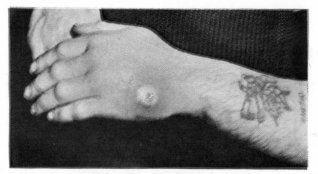

*Fig.* 70.—Typical early carbuncle.

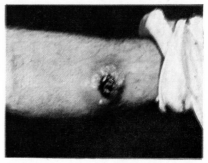

*Fig.* 71.—Cutaneous anthrax. Outstanding clinical features are a circumscribed vesiculated lesion, relatively little pain, and an absence of pus.

No better demonstration of these signs can be given than in the case of a simple boil. Where a boil ends and a carbuncle (*Fig.* 70) begins is nebulous, but there is no mistaking a fully

AULUS AURELIUS CORNELIUS CELSUS (1st *Century, A.D.*), *Roman encyclopædist, and medical author.*

developed example of the latter. That the urine must be tested for sugar in cases of carbuncle and multiple boils cannot be repeated too often. Notwithstanding this injunction, it should be remembered that sugar is sometimes present in the urine of patients with multiple boils, not because the patients are diabetic, but because of the toxæmia. Boils and carbuncles of the face have a sinister reputation. A virulent boil of the face may be mistaken for anthrax. Even in cases where the black central scab and surrounding vesicles make the diagnosis of anthrax (*Fig.* 71) practically certain, confirmation by bacteriological examination of the serum from a vesicle is essential.

## ACUTE LYMPHANGITIS

Superficial lymphatic vessels can be seen as one or more red lines coursing up the limb (*Fig.* 72) to the regional lymphatic

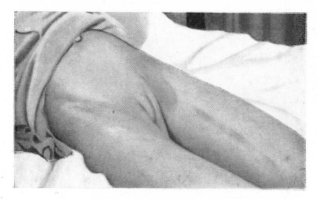

*Fig.* 72.—Acute lymphangitis with subcutaneous cellulitis over the inguinal lymph-nodes.

nodes, which are usually enlarged and tender. Sometimes the initial lesion is so minute that it cannot be found even after a careful search.

## PHLEBITIS

Phlebitis and thrombosis occurring in deep veins have to be recognized by their effects, for there may be no physical signs of the condition itself. Phlebitis of superficial veins is easily recognized, and because thrombosis and phlebitis go hand in hand (thrombophlebitis) the veins feel like tender, hard cords. Varicose veins are frequently the seat of phlebitis (*Fig.* 73).

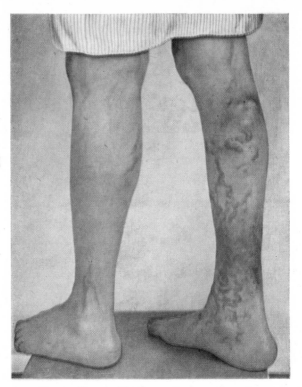

*Fig.* 73.—Thrombophlebitis occurring in varicose veins.

## CELLULITIS

The part affected is swollen, tense, and tender.    Later it becomes red, shiny, and boggy (*Fig.* 74).    Look for a wound, blister, or abrasion where organisms could have gained entrance.    Examine the regional lymphatic nodes for enlargement.    After the local examination has been concluded, take the patient's temperature.

In the case of a child, where no obvious abrasion exists in the immediate vicinity, bear in mind Rutherford Morison's aphorism : " Cellulitis occurring in children is never primary in the cellular tissues, but secondary to an underlying bone infection."

From the point of view of differential diagnosis, early cellulitis may be said to have :—

1. *No edge.*                     3. *No pus.*
2. *No fluctuation.*        4. *No limit.*

JAMES RUTHERFORD MORISON, 1853–1939, *Professor of Surgery, University of Durham, Newcastle-upon-Tyne.*

**Cellulitis of the Face** is sometimes difficult to distinguish from erysipelas (*Fig.* 75). In this connexion, Milian's ear sign may prove helpful.

*Milian's Ear Sign.*—As facial erysipelas spreads, it involves the ear because it is a cuticular lymphangitis. On the other hand, all subcutaneous inflammations stop short of the pinna because of close adhesion of the skin to the cartilage.

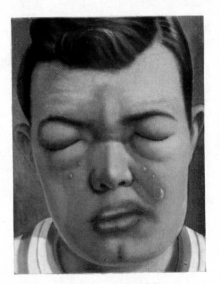

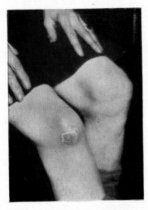

Fig. 74.—Subcutaneous cellulitis spreading from an infected prepatellar bursa.

*Fig.* 75.—Erysipelas of face.

**Cellulitis of the Orbit** (*Fig.* 76) gives rise to proptosis, œdema of the eyelids, and œdema of the conjunctiva (chemosis). It must be distinguished from thrombophlebitis of the cavernous sinus (*see Fig.* 176). In thrombophlebitis of the cavernous sinus the patient's general condition is always extremely grave, while in orbital cellulitis the local signs usually predominate.

**Ludwig's Angina** is cellulitis occurring under the deep cervical fascia. In many instances of this condition the floor of the mouth becomes œdematous ; in *Fig.* 77 the tongue can be seen displaced upwards by the swelling and œdema. On several occasions I have seen signs identical with Ludwig's angina follow the impaction of a salivary calculus in Wharton's duct ; when one is examining a case of brawny œdema of the neck it is well worth palpating the floor of the mouth for a calculus (*see* p. 67).

GASTON MILIAN, 1871–1945, *Dermatologist, Hôpital Saint-Louis, Paris.*
WILHELM VON LUDWIG, 1790–1865, *Professor of Surgery and Midwifery, Tübingen, Württemberg, Germany.*
THOMAS WHARTON, 1614–1673, *Physician, St. Thomas's Hospital, London.*

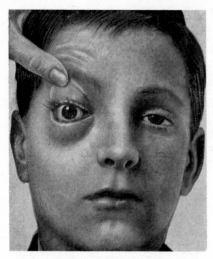

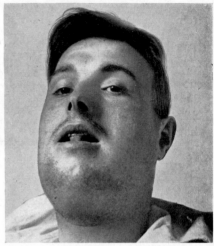

*Fig.* 76.—Orbital cellulitis. Owing to the œdema of the eyelids the proptosed globe is not apparent unless the eyelid is opened forcibly.

*Fig.* 77.—Ludwig's angina. The swelling in the submental region, and the inability to close the mouth owing to œdema of the tongue and floor of the mouth, can be seen.

## ULCERS

When one is examining an ulcer particular attention should be paid to the following points :—

*The Shape.*—Is it round, oval, irregular, or serpiginous\* ?

*The Edge.*—This may be sloping downwards towards the crater, undermined, punched out, or everted.

*The Floor.*—The most typical is the slough in a gummatous ulcer, which looks like wet wash-leather.

*The Base.*—Whether indurated or attached to deeper structures.

*The Surrounding Tissues.*—Look for signs of inflammation, pigmentation, or varicosity.

After an ulcer has been examined it is essential to consider next its lymphatic drainage and the nodes connected therewith. Sometimes these are obviously involved ; more often a systematic and painstaking examination by palpation is required.

---

\* *Serpiginous,* creeping like a serpent. Healing in one place while extending in another.

As is shown diagrammatically in the following sketches ulcers are of four main varieties :—

1. A tertiary syphilitic ulcer is punched out – ⟶
2. The so-called septic ulcer has sloping edges – ⟶
3. The tuberculous ulcer is characterized by under-mined edges – – – – – – – – – – – – – – – – ⟶
4. A carcinomatous ulcer has everted edges which to the palpating fingers feel hard – – – – – – – – ⟶

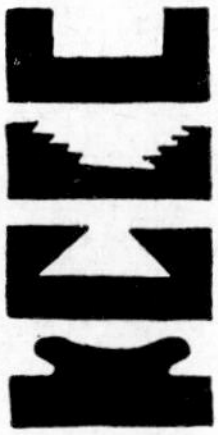

*The Hunterian chancre* (primary syphilitic sore) (*Fig.* 78) is a true ulcer. It is usually oval, has sloping edges, and exudes a discharge that is often blood-stained. When first inspected it is often covered by a crust, removal of which reveals the base covered with pink granulations. To the palpating fingers the ulcer is hard ; even when the lesion

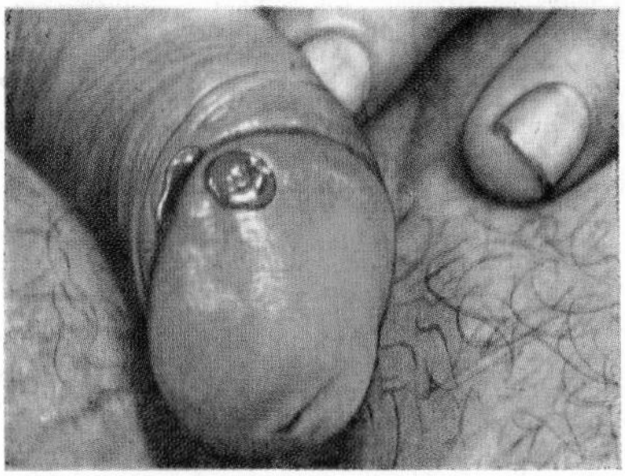

*Fig.* 78.—Hunterian chancre.

is palpated through the prepuce the hardness is apparent—it has been likened to the sensation of feeling a buried button.

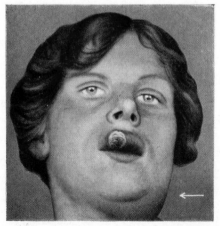

Fig. 79.—Primary chancre of the upper lip. Note the great enlargement of the submental and submaxillary lymphatic nodes, which is characteristic.

JOHN HUNTER, 1728–1793, *Surgeon, St. George's Hospital, London.*

The lymph-nodes of the groin can be felt slightly enlarged; 'shotty' is the term that has been given to them. By 'shotty' we understand that the nodes are hard and small. This is very different from the extravagant enlarge-

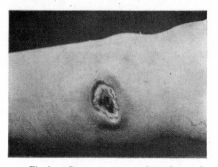

Fig. 80.—Cutaneous gumma situated over the middle two-fourths of the tibia—a characteristic situation. Compare the varicose ulcer (*Fig.* 83).

ment of the regional lymphatic nodes that occurs when a primary sore is extragenital (*Fig.* 79).

*A gummatous ulcer* is unquestionably punched out and painless (*Fig.* 80). The wash-leather base may contain one or more 'islands' of normal tissue that have escaped the gummatous necrosis. In passing it may be mentioned that wash-leather sloughs occur in tissue undergoing radium necrosis.

A healed gumma gives a circular 'tissue-paper' scar, which is strong evidence of a previous syphilitic infection.

The punched-out appearance (*Fig.* 81) so characteristic of gummata is seen sometimes in varicose ulcers (*see Fig.* 83) and often in trophic ulcers, particularly perforating ulcer of the foot (*see Fig.* 82), which is associated with tabes dorsalis and other diseases of the central nervous system.

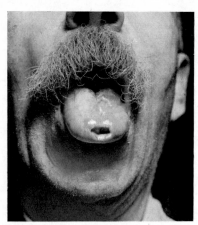

Fig. 81.—Gumma of tongue.

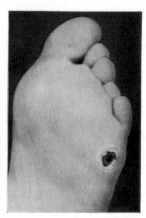

Fig. 82.—Perforating ulcer of the foot in a case of tabes dorsalis. Perforating ulcers are usually 'punched out'.

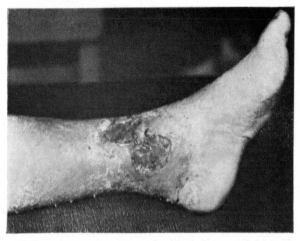

*Fig.* 83.—Varicose ulcers are apt to appear in pigmented areas, and they tend to 'ride the vein'. They are almost confined to the lower quarter of the leg.

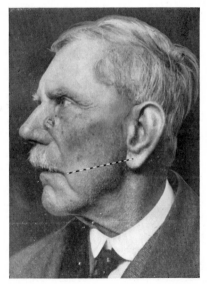

*Fig.* 84.—A rodent ulcer usually occurs above an imaginary line joining the angle of the mouth and the lobule of the ear.

4

*A tuberculous ulcer* nearly always has undermined edges. So far as I am aware, this characteristic is shared only by some bedsores. Tuberculous ulcers are usually painful.

*A carcinomatous ulcer* can hardly be mistaken, especially after the eversion and the induration of the edge of the ulcer have been observed.

With *rodent ulcers*,★ particularly early ones, these features of malignancy are not nearly so obvious. The fact that a rodent ulcer is usually situated above a line joining the angle of the mouth with the external auditory meatus (*Fig.* 84) should put the clinician on his guard. Its outline is circular, its edge, if not everted, is definitely raised, and this heaped-up edge often shows nodules possessing a peculiar pearl-like lustre. Minute venules in the edge of the ulcer are characteristic.

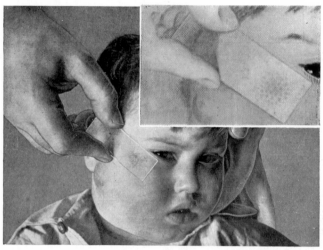

*Fig.* 85.—The ' apple-jelly ' test for lupus. Inset shows ' nodules ' which become apparent on pressure.

When *lupus vulgaris*† (cutaneous tuberculosis) as a cause of cutaneous ulceration is suspected, take a glass slide (or a glass tongue depressor) and press it firmly over the lesion (*Fig.* 85). Pressure removes the surrounding hyperæmia, and apple-jelly-like nodules become apparent (*Fig.* 85, inset). When performed in daylight, this test is most reliable.

---

★ *Rodent ulcer*, so called because it gnaws the tissues (even bone) like a rat.

† *Lupus vulgaris*. Latin, *Lupus* = a wolf. *Vulgaris* = ordinary. " Lupus is a malignant ulcer . . . and it is very hungry like unto a wolf." (Philip Barrow, *Method of Physicke*, 1590.)

## SINUSES AND FISTULÆ

A *fistula* implies a tunnel connecting two epithelial surfaces, whereas a *sinus* is a blind track opening on to the skin or a mucous surface. Several references to fistulæ and sinuses in particular situations will be made later in the book.

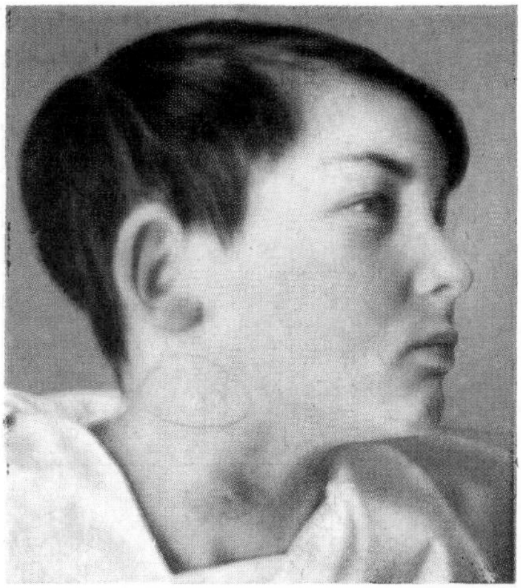

Fig. 86.—Sinus connected with suppurating tuberculous lymph-nodes. In this case the affected nodes are in the upper third of the neck, and the sinus opens in the lower third.

The opening of a sinus may be situated at a considerable distance from the underlying pathological lesion. (*Fig.* 86 illustrates a case in point.)

A point of great clinical significance is exuberant granulation tissue ('proud flesh') around the orifice (*Figs.* 87, 88). Almost without exception, this signifies that necrosis of bone is proceeding in the depths of the sinus. The cause of exuberant granulations is a foreign body—any

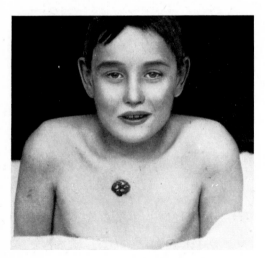

Fig. 87. — Exuberant granulation tissue around a sinus. Case of osteomyelitis of the sternum.

foreign body—dead bone being the commonest.

Probing of sinuses should, on the whole, be condemned during clinical examination; it should be done in an operating theatre. If necessary, an exception may be made in the case of bone necrosis, for probing is a valuable method of ascertaining whether a sequestrum is loose. The sterile probe comes in contact with hard, bare bone. Bareness alone does not mean that it is dead ; the sensation of dead bone is

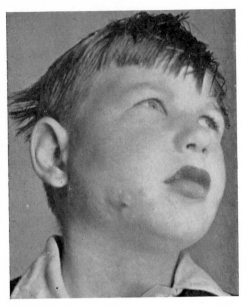

Fig. 88.—Sinus overlying the mandible. The patient has a carious molar tooth. The sinus soon healed after dental extraction.

that there is nothing whatsoever between the probe and the bone. If the bone is bare but alive, the impression is that there is a film of soft material (granulations) between the probe and the bone. If dead bone be loose, pressure with the probe may cause it to move (Robert Milne).

Multiple indurated sinuses, especially about the lower jaw and neck, suggest actinomycosis (*Fig.* 89). Express a little of

Fig. 89.—Actinomycosis of the neck. Pus expressed from one of the sinuses showed cayenne-pepper granules (the little dots within the drop of pus shown in the inset, which is actual size).

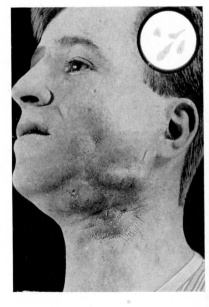

the pus into a test-tube half-full of water. Cork the tube and shake vigorously. If cayenne-pepper granules (*Fig.* 89, inset), so characteristic of actinomycosis, are present, they will soon sink to the bottom of the test-tube.

ROBERT MILNE, *Contemporary Consulting Orthopædic Surgeon, London Hospital.*

## CHAPTER VI

## THE MOUTH

THE multiplication of instruments and apparatus designed to reveal hidden pathological conditions sometimes makes the practitioner lament that he lacks facilities for special examination. In the case of the mouth this is certainly not true. Seated in his consulting room, armed with little more than an electric torch and a spatula, he can, if he will, become a master of intrabuccal living pathology and diagnosis, for his opportunities are unrivalled.

For use in an examination of the mouth, wooden spatulæ, which are bought ready sterilized in boxes, are to be preferred. After being used once the spatula is thrown away.

## EXAMINATION OF THE LIPS AND THE BUCCAL ORIFICE

Abnormalities of the buccal orifice are usually obvious. If a hare-lip is present the clinician will inspect at once the roof of the mouth to satisfy himself concerning the integrity of the palate (*see* p. 65).

White linear scars radiating from the corners of the mouth (rhagades*) suggest congenital syphilis, and should be sufficient to initiate a search for other stigmata. A median crack in the lower lip is common in cold weather. In some individuals the crack becomes chronically inflamed and bleeds readily.

To examine a swelling or ulcer, the lip must be everted in order that its mucous surface can be inspected properly (*Fig.* 90). The examination of the lip is concluded by

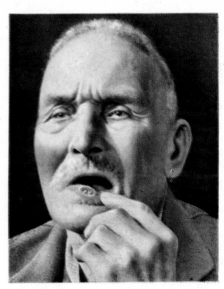

*Fig.* 90.—Carcinoma of the lip in an elderly retired agricultural labourer.

* *Rhagades.* Greek, ῥαγάς, pl. ῥαγαδες = a crack.

palpation of the cervical lymphatic nodes, and particular attention is paid to the submental group, which are often not easy to feel when only moderately enlarged. It is also worth while to search for enlargement of that inconstant bucco-facial lymph-node (*see* p. 84) in these cases.

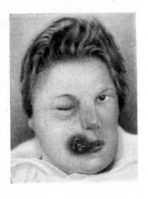

*Fig.* 91.—Carbuncle of upper lip. Œdema sufficient to close the eyelids of the corresponding side is a danger signal (*see* text).

The most dangerous situation in the body for a carbuncle is the upper lip (*Fig.* 91). A complication that frequently heralds the oncoming of fatal pyæmia is thrombo-phlebitis of the cavernous sinus (*see* p. 99). A sign that foretells impending danger is spreading œdema from the lip to the inner canthus, and this is usually found in the presence of suffusion of the corresponding eyelid.

## EXAMINATION OF THE TEETH

The teeth are inspected. The task of remembering when normal eruption occurs is aided considerably by the diagrams here shown (*Fig.* 92). It is stated that absence of the lateral incisors (not a very common abnormality) in a mother predisposes to a cleft palate in her child. I have not been able to confirm this observation.

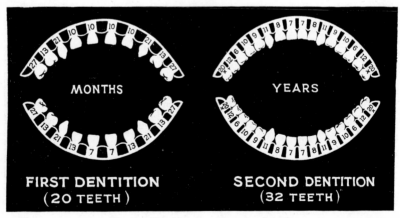

*Fig.* 92.—The date of eruption of each tooth.

If the case is one of a swelling in the jaw, careful attention to the dental formula may throw light upon the diagnosis. If a missing tooth cannot be accounted for in any other way, it is fairly good evidence that the swelling is an odontome (*Fig.* 93), a diagnosis that can be confirmed readily by radiography.

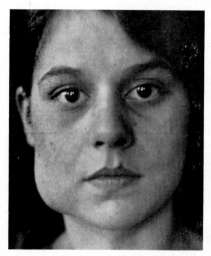

*Fig.* 93.—A missing tooth clinched a clinical diagnosis of odontome, which was later confirmed by X rays.

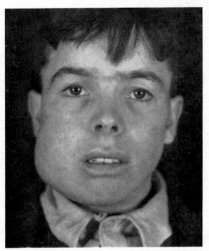

*Fig.* 94.—Fœtor, local tenderness and some degree of trismus make the diagnosis of dento-alveolar abscess certain.

In a gastric case, examination of the teeth should never be omitted. If the patient wears a denture, insist upon its being removed before proceeding with the examination. Note particularly whether there are sufficient molars in opposition to carry out mastication efficiently.

**Hutchinson's Teeth** are good confirmatory evidence of congenital syphilis. " It is, if taken alone, by far the most valuable of the signs by which we recognize in adolescents the effect of inherited syphilis " (Sir Jonathan Hutchinson). The teeth of the second dentition alone are affected, and it is only the upper central incisors that afford indisputable evidence of congenital syphilis. These teeth are smaller than normal. They are peg-topped—that is, broader

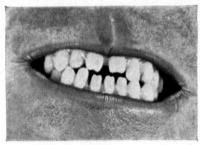

*Fig.* 95.—Hutchinson's teeth.

towards the gum than at their free edge, and notched (*Fig.* 95).  Sometimes these teeth are yellowish in colour and marked by transverse
ridges, but I have often noted that Hutchinson's teeth, while retaining
the peg-top and the notch, are highly polished, white, and unridged.

**Moon's Teeth** are occasionally helpful in the diagnosis of congenital syphilis ; they are dome-topped (top near gum) first molars.

### EXAMINATION OF THE GUMS

In order to examine the gums the lips must be everted fully.  In
pyorrhœa the periodontal membrane has given way.  The gums have
receded, consequently the teeth appear long.  If the gums are pressed
they bleed readily ; some-
times a bead of pus exudes.

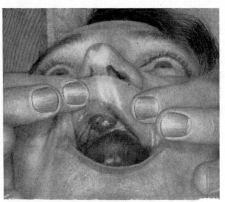

Fig. 96.—Everting the lips to examine the
gums.  In this case hyperplasia of the gum due
to an ill-fitting denture is present.

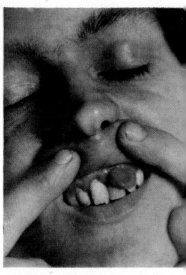

Fig. 97.—A granulomatous epulis.

As is well known, bleeding
gums are a leading sign in scurvy
and in other conditions due to lack
of vitamin C.  What is not so well
known and is quite as important,
is that bleeding gums occur in uræmia.  The gums are not as spongy
as in scurvy : in fact they may look nearly normal (F. J. Wright).

If the patient wears a denture, examine the gums with special
reference to the plate, which is removed for the purpose.  Among
conditions directly due to an ill-fitting denture is what is known as
a ' prosthetic ' ulcer.  Another condition due to the irritation of the
dental plate is hyperplasia of the gum (*Fig.* 96), a swelling that closely
simulates a granulomatous epulis (*Fig.* 97).

HENRY MOON, 1845–1892, *Dental Surgeon, Guy's Hospital, London.*
FREDRICK JAMES WRIGHT, *Contemporary Medical Officer, Colonial Medical Service, Nairobi, Kenya
    Colony.*

**The Lead Line.**—This sign should be looked for in patients who work with lead, e.g., painters. The 'blue line' if inspected closely will be seen to consist of a series of grey-black dots situated about 1 mm. from the free margin of the gum. They are best seen with the aid of a magnifying glass.

Almost identical with the lead line are the bismuth (*Fig.* 98) and mercury lines. When the last two come into the diagnostic arena, some discreet inquiries should be made as to whether

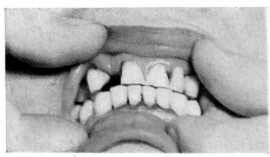

*Fig.* 98.—Bismuth line in a patient undergoing anti-syphilitic treatment.

the patient has been receiving treatment for venereal disease. In former days, the free use of Bipp* in a wound had to be taken into consideration. These 'metal' lines seldom occur unless there is considerable pre-existing parodontal infection.

## EXAMINATION OF THE TONSILS

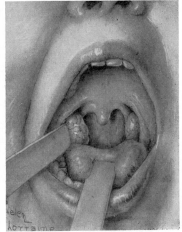

*Fig.* 99.—By pressure against the anterior pillar of the fauces an apparently small buried tonsil may be everted from its bed. At the same time crypts are opened and their contents squeezed out (after Irwin Moore).

The tongue is depressed with a spatula, and, while the patient says 'Ah', the tonsils are inspected with the aid of a torch. To decide whether the tonsils are normal in size and healthy, enlarged or diseased, it is necessary for them to be displayed. The best method is to depress the tongue with one spatula while the tip of a second spatula gently compresses the anterior pillar of the fauces (*Fig.* 99). This everts the tonsil from its bed. Increasing pressure will expose and open the crypts, and their contents may be discharged (Irwin Moore).

---

* *Bipp* = Bismuth Iodoform Paraffin Paste.

IRWIN MOORE, *Contemporary Consulting Surgeon, Metropolitan Ear, Nose, and Throat Hospital, London.*

**Peritonsillar Abscess** (*Quinsy*).—The patient enters the consulting room with a handkerchief in his hand and the head held forwards

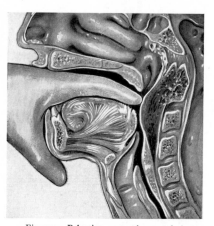

and upwards. He talks as though he had a hot potato in his mouth, and makes frequent, painful swallowing movements (Ovens). When asked where the pain is, the patient usually points to the region of the tonsillar lymph-node (*see* p. 103). Some degree of trismus may make the examination difficult. Usually the abscess is mainly in front. The soft palate on that side is bulging and œdematous. The anterior pillar of the fauces is red and swollen.

*Fig.* 100.—Palpating a retropharyngeal abscess through the open mouth. In this case (an adolescent) the abscess is secondary to spinal caries. Suppurating retropharyngeal lymph-nodes are also a cause of this condition.

More rarely the abscess is behind the tonsil, which is pushed forward. It is, in fact, a parapharyngeal abscess.

**Retropharyngeal Abscess.**—The patient is usually an infant.

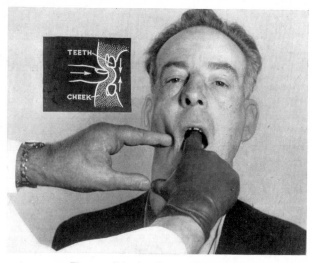

*Fig.* 101.—Palpating the root of the tongue.

Gerald Hugh Campbell Ovens, *Contemporary Surgeon, King Edward Hospital, Ealing, London.*

By depressing its tongue, and examining the back of the throat in a good light, the posterior pharyngeal wall is seen protruding. Pharyngeal palpation (*Fig.* 100) may be necessary.

*Method of palpating the pharynx, choanæ\*, and the back of the tongue.*—Ask the patient to open the mouth widely. Holding all the fingers straight and stiff, press the finger-tips firmly into the cheek (*Fig.* 101) in such a way that they intervene between the teeth (*Fig.* 101, inset). Should the patient ' bite ', he will bite his cheek and not your palpating right index finger. By employing this manœuvre, Logan Turner taught his students how to confirm the presence of adenoids. In the absence of adenoid vegetations, the roof of the normal nasopharynx feels smooth.

A more comfortable method for all concerned is to provide a tablet of a surface anæsthetic, e.g., amethocaine, for the patient to suck ten minutes before the examination. It requires energy and keenness to have these tablets to hand when they are required, for the occasion to use them is comparatively infrequent.

## EXAMINATION OF THE TONGUE

Ask the patient to put out his tongue, and note whether the organ is protruded in the middle line. If it is deviated, do not jump to a conclusion, for often a patient will deliberately rotate his tongue because he is trying to show you something on one side of it (*Fig.* 102). Ask the patient to put

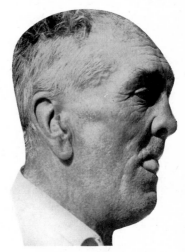

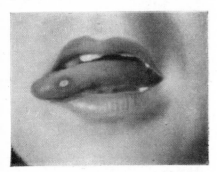

Fig. 102.—Peptic or dyspeptic ulcer of the tongue.

Fig. 103.—Ankyloglossia. The patient is protruding his tongue to the fullest extent.

his tongue straight out as far as he can. We are now able to judge whether there really is any pathological anchoring of the musculature (ankyloglossia) (*Fig.* 103).

---

\* *Choanæ* (posterior nares). Greek, χοάνη = a funnel.

ARTHUR LOGAN TURNER, 1865–1939, *Surgeon, Ear and Throat Department, Edinburgh Royal Infirmary.*

In the general examination by inspection, a particular point to look for is indentation of the tip and sides of the tongue. Indentations indicate that the organ is swollen and marked by the teeth. Next, pay particular attention to the dorsum, which is, of course, normally covered by the filiform and fungiform papillæ (*Figs.* 104, 105). If the tongue is fissured, do not jump to the conclusion that the condition is necessarily syphilitic. *Congenital fissured tongue* (*Fig.* 106) is not a very uncommon condition ; it is believed to be the result of tongue-sucking in early childhood (John Thomson). Note that the fissures are mainly transverse, while in syphilitic glossitis the fissuring

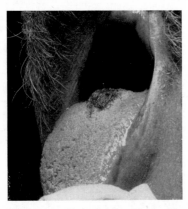

Fig. 104.—Black or hairy tongue. The filiform papillæ are much lengthened and covered with a black or brown fur. The cause of the condition is disputed.

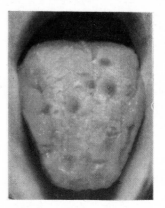

Fig. 105.—Venous hæmangiomata of the tongue. The patient complained of blood-stained saliva.

is predominantly longitudinal (*Fig.* 107). In *chronic superficial glossitis* the normal surface of the dorsum of the tongue is lost (*Fig.* 108). When the condition is advanced we see the classical picture most graphically described by Butlin—" the tongue looks as though it had been covered with white paint that had hardened, dried, and cracked ". In early doubtful cases of chronic superficial glossitis press a glass slide on the surface of the tongue ; viewed in this manner, thickened epithelium will appear more obvious. In advanced cases palpate each diseased area carefully ; induration in one of these is sufficient to warrant the assumption that malignant change has occurred. Leukoplakia of the tongue (*Fig.* 109) is a precarcinomatous condition.

Continuing the routine examination of the tongue : ask the patient to rotate the tongue upwards towards the roof of his mouth.

JOHN THOMSON, 1856–1926, *Physician, Hospital for Sick Children, Edinburgh.*
SIR HENRY TRENTHAM BUTLIN, 1845–1912, *Surgeon, St. Bartholomew's Hospital, London.*

This reveals the under-surface of the tongue and the floor of the mouth.

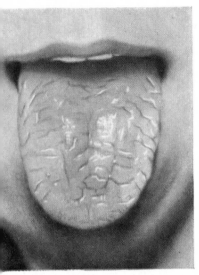

Fig. 106.—Congenital fissuring of the tongue. The fissures are mainly transverse.

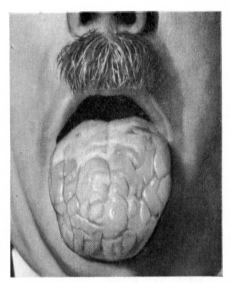

Fig. 107.—Syphilitic glossitis. The fissures are mainly longitudinal.

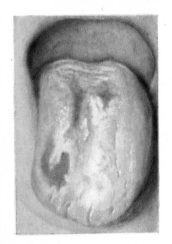

Fig. 108.—Early chronic superficial glossitis.

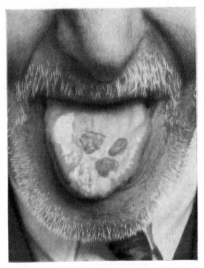

Fig. 109.—Leukoplakia glossitis.

**An Ulcer is Present on the Tongue.**—Before proceeding further, take a swab and dry the tongue thoroughly. The characters of the ulcer are then studied (*see* p. 47). In the case of an ulcer on the side, or slightly on the under-surface of the tongue, pay particular attention to the possibility of a decayed or broken tooth or an irregularity on a denture being the causative agent. A *dental ulcer* (*Fig.* 110) is often the precursor of a *carcinomatous ulcer* (*Fig.* 111). Palpation of the tongue is carried out with a gloved finger, and while the

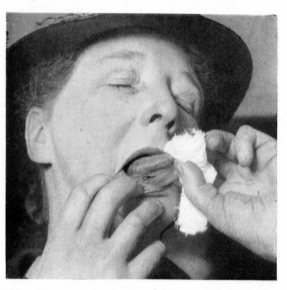

Fig. 110.—Dental ulcer. In its early stages it is often somewhat elongated.

manœuvre is in progress the tip of the tongue may be held in a swab in order to steady the organ ; this, however, is by no means always necessary.

If there is no obvious lesion to palpate, the finger is passed gently over the whole of the tongue and the floor of the mouth.

Palpation of the back of the tongue causes retching, which can be prevented only by the use of a local anæsthetic. The method of palpating the back of the tongue described on p. 59 is extremely valuable ; occasionally, by this manœuvre a lesion is discovered that otherwise would be missed.

It must be remembered that often lingual pain is referred to the ear, and patients with an advanced carcinoma of the tongue sometimes present themselves with a wad of cotton-wool in one ear, complaining solely of earache. The explanation of this phenomenon is that the lingual nerve has become involved and the pain is referred to the auriculo-temporal nerve. No examination of the tongue, mouth and pharynx is complete without the systematic palpation of the cervical lymphatic nodes (*see* p. 102).

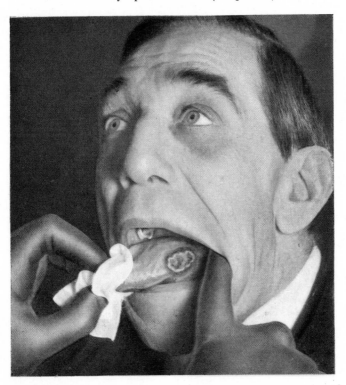

*Fig.* 111.—Carcinoma secondary to a dental ulcer.

## EXAMINATION OF THE FLOOR OF THE MOUTH

Ask the patient to put the tip of the tongue on the roof of the mouth and to bend the head slightly forward. Most people understand these instructions, but a few of the less intelligent patients seem quite unable to control the movements of the tongue, and this makes the examination difficult.

A *ranula* can be recognized at once as a patently translucent cystic swelling often of a bluish tinge (*Fig.* 112), situated on one side of the frænum, though on occasions it extends under the frænum to the opposite side.     Often Wharton's duct can be seen traversing the

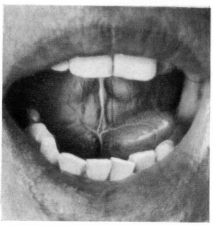

Fig. 112.—A ranula is invariably translucent.

dome of the cyst.     Ranulæ are not always simple and may extend into the depths of the neck ; therefore carefully palpate under the jaw for an extension of the swelling, and complete the examination by a bidigital palpation with one finger in the mouth and one beneath the jaw (*see Fig. 69, p. 120*).

*Sublingual dermoid cysts* can be either median or lateral (*Fig.* 113), and either above or below the mylohyoid.     When above the mylohyoid, the opaque white cyst is discernible through the normal mucous membrane ; the opacity differs completely from the transparency of a ranula.

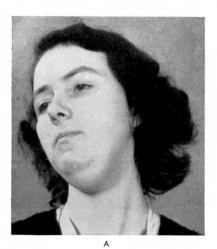

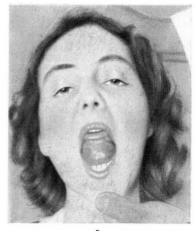

A                                                                         B

Fig. 113.—Median sublingual dermoid cyst.  A, The swelling beneath the chin ;
B, The swelling in the floor of the mouth.

In all cases the neck must be examined, and the swelling palpated bimanually (*see Fig.* 69).

When the cyst is median, and below the mylohyoid, consider its possible relationship to the thyroglossal tract (*see* p. 120).

When the floor of the mouth is examined for an *ulcer*, inspect after drying with a swab. Unless the ulcer is situated near the middle line it cannot be seen. Palpate the floor of the mouth very thoroughly, sliding the finger well back into the lateral sublingual sulcus. When this manœuvre causes pain, and blood is seen on the examining finger, we cannot persist in the examination ; but, other things being equal, it is highly suggestive of a carcinoma lurking within the depths of the sulcus.

The floor of the mouth will be considered further in the examination of the submaxillary salivary gland (*see* p. 67).

## EXAMINATION OF THE PALATE

Examination of the palate is an instance where physical examination is facilitated by an infant crying. The more the child cries the better the view obtained. If a cleft is present, determine its extent, whether it involves the hard or the soft palate, or both. That the more mature patient has a hole or cleft in the palate can be suspected when he addresses you in that peculiar explosive nasal voice which accompanies a leakage of the sound waves into the nasal cavity.

**Inspection of Palate.—** Ask the patient to tilt his head slightly backwards and to open his mouth to its fullest extent. If the light is good, the whole of the palate can be observed,

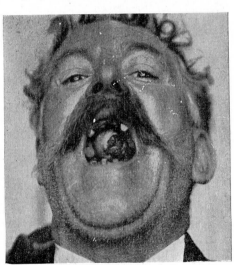

Fig. 114.—Dermoid cyst of the palate, present for many years. A malignant change has lately occurred in its wall.

and any abnormality detected at once (*Fig.* 114). The height of the palatal arch varies with individuals, a very high palate being caused by nasal obstruction (adenoids, deviated nasal septum) which leads to

5

mouth breathing. In the narrow ' gothic '* type of palate the teeth are crowded. A hole in the middle of the soft palate (*Fig.* 115) is good presumptive evidence of previous syphilis (gumma). However, it is sometimes unwise to jump to conclusions ; when an operation for closure of a cleft palate has been only partially successful, a hole may

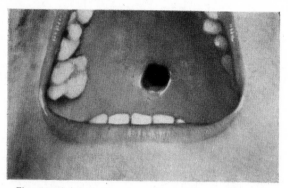

*Fig.* 115.—A hole in the palate.   Wassermann strongly positive.

be left in the middle line at the junction of the hard and the soft palate, and in the past such a case has beguiled a series of candidates for higher examinations.

To touch the soft palate causes the normal patient to gag. The neurasthenic patient allows the clinician to stroke his soft palate with impunity, and this knowledge may be used on occasions with advantage (*see* Chapter XXXIV).

*See also* EXAMINATION OF THE MAXILLA, p. 74.

---

* Gothic arch—a pointed arch characteristic of the architecture in Western Europe during the later Middle Ages.

AUGUST VON WASSERMANN, 1866–1925, *Director of the Institute for Experimental Therapy, Berlin .*

## CHAPTER VII

# THE SALIVARY GLANDS

## EXAMINATION OF THE SUBMAXILLARY SALIVARY GLANDS

ENLARGEMENT of the submaxillary salivary gland causes a swelling beneath the angle of the jaw (*Fig.* 116). When the patient volunteers the information that the swelling appears only before or during meals, send for a lemon* and ask him to suck a little of the juice. An interesting and diagnostic phenomenon may be witnessed (*Fig.* 117) which is proof positive that Wharton's duct is obstructed.

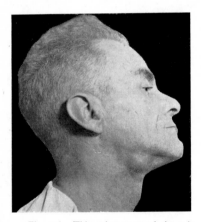

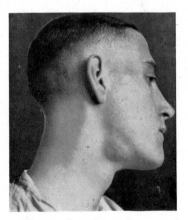

*Fig.* 116.—This enlargement of the sub-maxillary salivary gland, present for many months, did not vary in size. Case of mixed tumour.

*Fig.* 117.—Intermittent enlargement of the submaxillary salivary gland. It became evident after the patient had sucked a lemon. Case of a stone in the posterior third of Wharton's duct.

**Inspection of the Floor of the Mouth.**—The orifices of Wharton's ducts are inspected with the aid of a pocket torch, and the two sides compared. In a number of cases of salivary calculus some aberration is visible on the affected side. When secondary infection has supervened the ampulla is likely to be inflamed; sometimes pus can be seen exuding from the duct. Occasionally a stone impacted in the ampulla will be observed (*Fig.* 118).

---

* Lemon essence is just as good. I keep a bottle of it in my clinic.

THOMAS WHARTON, 1614–1673, *Physician, St. Thomas's Hospital, London.*

A dry swab is inserted under the tongue, and some lemon-juice is placed upon the dorsum. The patient is then asked to keep the swab in place with his finger while he moves the tongue about so as to taste the juice.

He is then instructed to open the mouth widely, and to raise the tip of the tongue towards the roof of the mouth. The swab is removed and, quickly, the (dried) floor of the mouth inspected with the

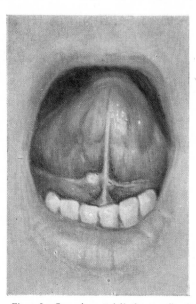

*Fig.* 118.—Stone impacted in the ampulla of Wharton's duct.

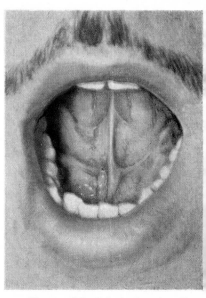

*Fig.* 119.—Saliva is flowing from the orifice of Wharton's duct on the right side, but on the left there is no secretion, for the posterior part of the duct is blocked by a calculus.

aid of a pocket-torch. Normally, saliva can be seen flowing, occasionally being ejected, from Wharton's ducts. In cases of obstruction by a calculus there will be little or no secretion from the affected side (*Fig.* 119). If doubt exists as to whether the duct on one side is functioning, a pledget of gauze is held over the orifice that is pouring forth secretion while the doubtful side is re-inspected. Steady pressure applied in the submaxillary triangle over the gland may produce a secretion or a purulent exudate in cases where the duct is partially occluded.

**Palpation of the Submaxillary Salivary Gland.**—As the submaxillary gland is composed of two portions, a larger (cervical) beneath, and a smaller (buccal) above, the mylohyoid muscle, there can be but one efficient method of examining the whole gland, and that is by bimanual palpation (*Fig.* 120).

If it can be ascertained that there are contiguous intrabuccal and cervical swellings, this is good evidence that the swelling in question is an enlarged submaxillary *salivary* gland.

When only a cervical portion is palpable, enlarged lymphatic nodes (*Fig.* 121) are the probable cause. Often such nodes are intimately blended with the capsule of the salivary gland. An enlarged facial lymphatic node (*Fig.* 122) is a clinical entity capable of segregation.

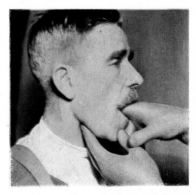

*Fig.* 120.—Bimanual palpation of the submaxillary salivary gland.

**A Method of Palpating Wharton's Duct.**—The patient's head is flexed and inclined somewhat to the affected side, in order to relax the musculature. The index finger is inserted into the mouth, the pulp of the finger being placed upon the internal surface of the alveolus. The finger is passed backwards, following the alveolus until its posterior extremity is reached. The tip of the finger is insinuated

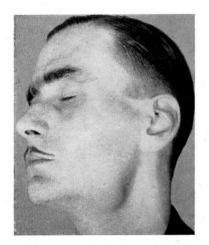

*Fig.* 121. — Tuberculous submaxillary lymphadenitis. The swelling does not vary in size and on bimanual palpation there is no contiguous swelling in the floor of the mouth.

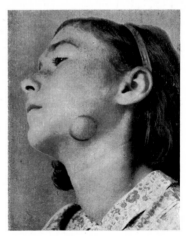

*Fig.* 122.—An enlarged facial lymphatic node. There is a constant lymph node in juxtaposition to the facial artery as it winds around the mandible.

between the alveolus just behind the last molar tooth and the side of the posterior third of the tongue, and rotated through a right angle, so that the pulp of the finger is directed downwards. In conjunction with the fingers of the other hand beneath the jaw, the whole course of Wharton's duct is palpated for a calculus, from behind forward. In about one out of four patients this manœuvre brings on retching, but even in this event the valuable information required is elicited before any severe discomfort is experienced.

## EXAMINATION OF THE PAROTID GLAND

**Inspection.**—Characteristic of a general enlargement of a parotid salivary gland—e.g., parotitis (*Fig.* 123)—is a swelling in front of the tragus that extends downwards and backwards, filling up the normal depression situated below and in front of the lobule of the ear (*Fig.* 124).

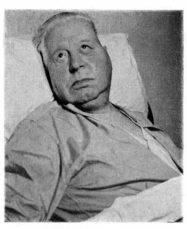

Fig. 123.—Acute suppurative parotitis. The whole of the parotid gland is enlarged.

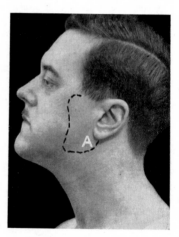

Fig. 124.—The extent of a general enlargement of the parotid salivary gland. Obliteration of the normal depression (A) behind the angle of the jaw is characteristic.

**Palpation** should be carried out as follows :—

1. Examine the main body of the gland ; the anterior limit is difficult to define precisely, but if the patient clenches his teeth, the masseter is thrown into relief, and the gland lies over the posterior aspect of the muscle.

2. Palpate the glenoid prolongation ; if there is a fullness there, be assured that it is continuous with the main body of the gland.

3. Inspect the orifice of Stensen's duct. This is done by retracting the cheek with a spatula (*Fig.* 125). The orifice of the duct lies opposite the second upper molar tooth. In suppurative parotitis, gentle pressure exerted over the gland from without often causes a gush of purulent saliva, and the diagnosis, which up to that time has been in doubt, becomes indisputable. Even when pus is absent the orifice of the duct may show evidence of inflammation. In doubtful minor degrees of inflammation the orifice should be compared with that of the opposite side.

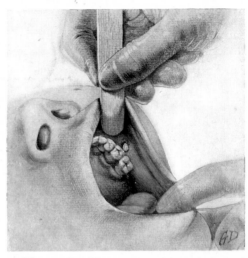

Fig. 125.—Examining the orifice of Stensen's duct. A gush of purulent saliva is seen being ejected in this case of subacute parotitis.

The course of Stensen's duct should be palpated for a calculus in suggestive cases. Stensen's duct lies about one finger's breadth below the zygoma. The anterior part of the duct can be palpated satisfactorily between the finger and thumb, the finger being in the mouth (*Fig.* 126); but the major part of the duct is rendered inaccessible to the examining fingers by the intervention of the strong masseter muscle with its tendinous intersections.

*Bilateral enlargement* of the parotid glands is not always due to mumps ; cases of acute, subacute, and chronic parotitis due to bacteria occur. In chronic parotitis the swelling is almost, if not entirely, painless.

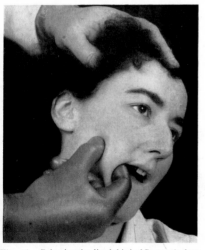

Fig. 126.—Palpating the distal third of Stensen's duct.

Niels Stensen, 1638–1686, *Professor of Anatomy. Copenhagen ; later Bishop, Titiopolis, Greece.*

*Unilateral enlargement* of the parotid gland is not necessarily due to a calculus ; indeed, in my experience recurrent subacute and chronic bacterial parotitis are more common causes than is a calculus.

A little known, but not very uncommon, condition that causes much diagnostic confusion is congenital parotid sialectasis.* Recurrent attacks of painful swelling of the parotid gland occur. The condition is usually unilateral (*Fig.* 127), but bilateral cases are encountered.

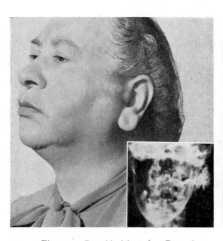

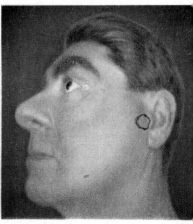

Fig. 127.—Parotid sialectasis. Recurring attacks of painful swelling of the parotid gland have occurred for many years. Inset : sialogram of this case, showing greatly distended ducts and alveoli.

Fig. 128.—Pre-auricular adenitis. The primary focus is an infected abrasion near the lateral canthus.

The differential diagnosis between an inflammatory swelling of the parotid gland and pre-auricular lymphadenitis (*Fig.* 128) is sometimes difficult. In pre-auricular lymphadenitis the swelling is likely to be confined to the region immediately in front of the tragus. The normal depression (A) (*see Fig.* 124) is not obliterated in pre-auricular adenitis.

In pre-auricular adenitis, a primary focus must be sought. Usually this is to be found in the region of the eyebrow, the lids, or the conjunctiva of the same side. More rarely it is situated within the external auditory meatus.

**Tumours of the Parotid Gland.**—Mixed parotid tumours are peculiar in remaining benign for months or often years and then undergoing a malignant change. It is, of course, possible for a

---

* *Sialectasis.*  Dilatation of the ducts and alveoli of the (parotid) salivary gland. Likened to *bronchiectasis* of the lung.

neoplasm to arise in any part of the parotid gland ; nevertheless, most mixed parotid tumours have their beginning in a comparatively circumscribed area—a little in front of and above the angle of the jaw (*Fig.* 129). So constant is this finding that it may be described as the typical location of this neoplasm.

The only other common starting point (and it is very much less common than the foregoing) is in the region immediately in front of the tragus. Here the differential diagnosis between an enlarged

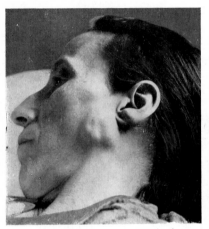

Fig. 129.—Mixed parotid tumour in the most characteristic situation.

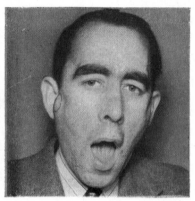

Fig. 130.—Early mixed parotid tumour situated immediately in front of the tragus.

pre-auricular lymphatic node and a mixed parotid tumour is, at the first examination, impossible, unless some cause for an enlarged lymphatic node can be discovered. The patient illustrated in *Fig.* 130 had a firm, rounded, solid swelling immediately in front of the tragus. He said that it had been present for six weeks. When the patient opened his mouth the swelling was thrown into prominence by the condyle of the jaw, not that this has any diagnostic significance, but it did enable one to palpate the swelling more thoroughly. The swelling proved to be a mixed parotid tumour.

By testing the mobility of a parotid tumour, endeavour to find out if it is still innocent. In this connexion it must be emphasized that an examination of a case of parotid tumour is not complete without testing the functional integrity of the seventh cranial nerve. An examination of the cervical lymphatic nodes is also indicated ; metastases occur only in advanced cases.

## CHAPTER VIII

## THE FACE AND JAWS

### EXAMINATION OF THE MAXILLA

THE anterior surface is most obviously available for examination, but we must go further and remember that the maxilla has five surfaces.

1. *The posterior surface* can be dismissed at once; forming as it does the anterior boundary of that deep recess, the sphenomaxillary

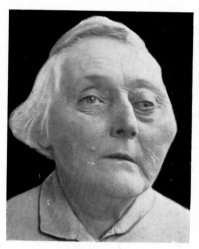

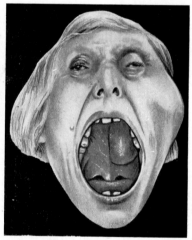

Fig. 131.—Malignant upper jaw. In addition to expanding the antero-external surface of the maxilla, the growth has displaced the orbital contents.

Fig. 132.—Examining the upper jaw. The inferior surface of the maxilla is the hard palate. In this case of sarcoma of the upper jaw the corresponding side of the hard palate was involved.

(pterygo-palatine) fossa, no part of the body is more completely beyond the reach of clinical methods.

2. *The superior surface* helps to form the floor of the orbit; therefore the levels of the inferior orbital margins are compared carefully. Extreme bulging of the floor of the orbit causes proptosis (*Fig.* 131). A glance at each profile of the patient is taken in order that the protuberance of the eyeballs may be compared.

3. *The antero-external surface* is palpated. While this is being done, note if there is any sign of overflow of tears (epiphora) on the affected side, and question the patient about this. The naso-lacrimal duct may become involved early in malignant disease of the maxilla.

4. Much of the upper jaw is available for examination through the mouth.

*a.* Examine the teeth and compare the dental formulæ; missing teeth must be accounted for—careful attention to this has often elucidated diagnosis, e.g., in odontomata.

*b.* The *inferior surface* of the maxilla forms the major part of the hard palate. In certain cases of malignant upper jaw, the swelling can be seen sharply defined by the raphe (*Fig.* 132).

*c.* A large part of the anterior surface is beneath the cheek, and

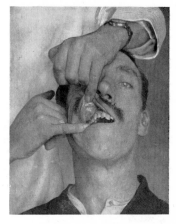

Fig. 133.—Examining the buccal aspect of the upper jaw.

without the intervention of the cheek (*Fig.* 133) much more can be made out than by external palpation. Pass the index finger between the cheek and the jaw. With the thumb outside, and the finger still inside, the zygomatic process should be palpated.

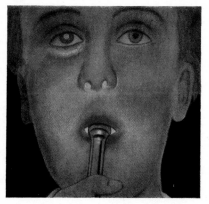

Fig. 134.—Dark-room transillumination of the maxillary antra. In this case the left side fails to illuminate, and suggests an infected antrum.

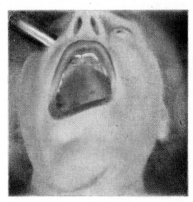

Fig. 135.—In ordinary clinical practice transillumination of the antra by this method is more serviceable. It can be carried out effectively in a *darkened* room.

5. By occluding the nares one at a time and asking the patient to blow through the nose, some rough idea of the *medial surface* of the maxilla may be obtained.    If the nostril on the affected side is *not*

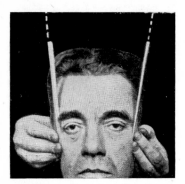

*Fig.* 136.—Rockey's method of determining the presence of a depressed fracture of the malar bone or zygomatic arch.

blocked, we know at least that the medial wall of the maxilla is not bulging to any great extent.    If there should be unilateral nasal obstruction, a nasal speculum must be used to investigate the cause.

Finally, examine the cervical glands, and also test the integrity of the second division of the fifth cranial nerve.

Ordinary clinical examination of the upper jaw can be supplemented by transillumination of the maxillary antra (*Figs.* 134, 135).    This readily available method may yield valuable information, but it is less reliable than radiography.    Rhinoscopy is also advisable in most cases.

**Special Signs.—**

*Rockey's sign* detects even very slight depressions of the malar bone.    Two straight edges are placed at the outer edge of the orbit from the prominence of the malar bone.    If depression exists, the difference in the angle is obvious (*Fig.* 136).

## EXAMINATION OF THE ACCESSORY NASAL SINUSES

*Unilateral Purulent Nasal Discharge.*—Especially in a child, the possibility of a foreign body being the cause must first be excluded (*Fig.* 137). A discharge of pus from *one* nostril when the patient bends down—for instance, to do up his boot laces—is said to indicate an open empyema antri (Fränkel).    More frequently it will be found to be the accompaniment of chronic suppurative frontal sinusitis.    At least

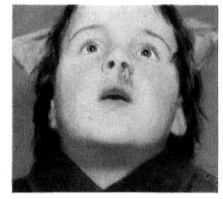

*Fig.* 137.—Unilateral excoriated nostril.

ALPHA EUGENE ROCKEY, 1857–1927, *Surgeon, Samaritan Hospital, Portland, Oregon, U.S.A.*
BERNHARD FRÄNKEL, 1836–1911, *Professor of Oto-rhino-laryngology, University Polyclinic, Berlin.*

it indicates suppuration in one of the accessory sinuses, exact location of which must be confirmed by more refined methods of diagnosis.

*Œdema* over the affected sinus is usually more conspicuous in children than in adults. Swelling of the eyelids often accompanies severe infection of the frontal, and particularly of the ethmoidal (*Fig.* 138) sinuses.

*Tenderness* over the frontal, ethmoidal or maxillary sinuses (*Fig.* 139) may be present, especially if free drainage is obstructed. In the case of the frontal sinus, the finger tip must be insinuated beneath the roof of the orbit towards the medial extremity of the sinus and pressure directed upwards (*Fig.* 140)

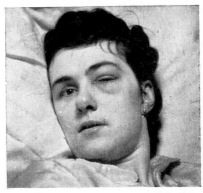

Fig. 138.—Œdema of the eyelids in acute left ethmoiditis.

(Ballenger). In the case of the ethmoidal cell labyrinth, pressure should be directed over the area indicated in *Fig.* 139 (2). In the case of the maxillary antrum, pressure should be applied not only

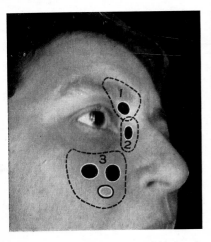

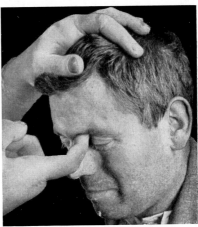

Fig. 139.—Surface markings of (1) frontal, (2) ethmoidal, (3) maxillary sinuses. The black areas show where to palpate for tenderness on the cutaneous surface ; white area, where to palpate from inside the mouth.

Fig. 140.—Eliciting tenderness over the floor of the frontal sinus.

William Lincoln Ballenger, *Contemporary Professor Emeritus, Department of Otology, Rhinology and Laryngology, University of Illinois, Chicago.*

from the cutaneous surface, but also from within the mouth above and just behind the apex of the canine tooth (*Fig.* 139) (3). Tenderness over the frontal sinus is a more reliable sign than a corresponding degree of tenderness over either the ethmoidal or maxillary sinuses.

## EXAMINATION OF THE LOWER JAW

The horizontal ramus is accessible to the palpating fingers both from without and from inside the mouth, where the examination is intimately blended with that of the teeth of the lower jaw. The base of the ascending ramus and the angle of the mandible are

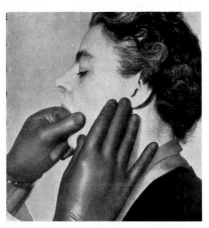

Fig. 141.—Bimanual examination of the ascending ramus of the lower jaw. One finger is within the mouth.

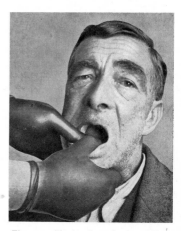

Fig. 142.—Testing for a fracture of the mandible.

also readily examined. On the other hand, the upper portion of the ramus and its condylar and coronoid processes lie deeply. With one finger inside the mouth and the fingers of the free hand applied externally (*Fig.* 141) this comparatively inaccessible portion becomes reasonably accessible. The coronoid process, in particular, can be examined thoroughly in this way.

**Fracture.**—That the patient has fractured his jaw is usually evident. He endeavours to support the fragments with his hands. Speech is impossible, and the saliva is usually blood-stained, for the fracture is nearly always *compound* into the mouth. Ninety-five per cent of fractures of the jaw occur in the horizontal ramus. By inspection within the mouth some deformity in the contour of the alveolus may be seen—frequently a tooth appears out of alinement. On closer inspection with the aid of a torch the gum is sometimes found to be lacerated in this situation. If the jaw is grasped behind and in front of the suspected fracture (*Fig.* 142), mobility and crepitus confirm the diagnosis at once ; this manœuvre should be attempted only if it is not otherwise apparent that the jaw is fractured.

**Median Mental Sinus** is so characteristic as to make diagnosis at first sight almost a certainty. On the point of the chin, exactly in the middle line, there is a discharging sinus (*Fig.* 143). Pain is not a feature of the case. Particularly in males, it is usual for the patient to have a well-developed 'strong' bifid type of chin surmounted by a dimple. In the dimple lies the sinus. A radiograph of the mandible reveals nothing abnormal, but a dental film of the lower incisor teeth, which on clinical examination often appear to be sound, shows

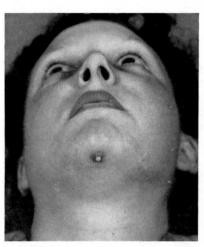

*Fig.* 143.—Median mental sinus.

an area of rarefaction around one or both roots. The case is one of parodontal abscess ; pus has tracked between the two halves of the lower jaw to the point of the chin.

When the clinician is unfamiliar with this condition, almost invariably a diagnosis of infected sebaceous cyst is made.

## THE MANDIBULAR JOINT

**Routine Examination.**—Place the fingers over the joint while the patient opens and closes his mouth ; note if there is any crepitus or clicking. Crepitus signifies osteo-arthritis, and clicking suggests a loose meniscus. Auscultation over the joint and comparison with the side not complained of may yield more valuable information than the fingers can provide.

**Trismus** (*Clenching*).—The patient cannot open his mouth because of muscular spasm. Severe trismus may complicate inflammatory processes in the neighbourhood of the mandibular joint. Chief among these is an erupting wisdom tooth or a dental abscess. Insert a spatula gently along the buccal aspect of the cheek, and inspect the alveolus with an electric torch.

Trismus is also seen in tetanus.  The tonic contraction of the musculature about the jaw gives the patient a painful smiling appear-

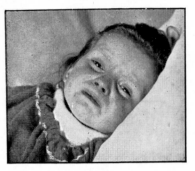

ance—the risus sardonicus (*Fig.* 144)—that is helpful in the diagnosis of early cases of tetanus.

**Ankylosis.**—In old-standing cases of ankylosis of the mandibular joint, incurred during infancy, the lower jaw atrophies (*Fig.* 145).  The receding chin gives a characteristic ' shrewmouse ' profile (Dufourmentel).

Unilateral ankylosis of the jaw

*Fig.* 144.—The risus sardonicus of tetanus.

may be difficult to recognize, and when present is not always demonstrable in a radiograph.  In cases of some standing, when the face at rest is viewed from in front, the facial furrows are more marked on the healthy side (Murphy).  The condition should not be confused with facial paralysis (Kennon).  In old-standing cases the jaw atrophies as in bilateral cases.  In more recent examples the same degree of atrophy is not observed, but attempts to open the mouth are associated with a slight but definite deviation of the lower incisors towards the ankylosed joint.

**Dislocation** of the mandibular joint may be bilateral or unilateral.

*Bilateral Dislocation.*—When the dislocation is bilateral the prognathous★ deformity is so evident as to attract attention immediately.  The mouth is

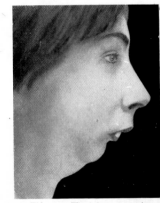

*Fig.* 145.—The ' shrewmouse ' profile.  Case of ankylosis of the jaw following scarlet fever in childhood.

open and fixed, with the lower teeth protruding.  Upon examination of the mandibular joints, a distinct hollow will be seen and felt in front of the tragus.  A prominence is sometimes observed above

---

★ *Prognathous.*  Greek προ in front of, γνάθος jaw = having a projecting jaw.

L. Dufourmentel, *Contemporary Professor of Maxillo-Facial Surgery, University of Paris.*
John Benjamin Murphy, 1857–1916, *Professor of Surgery, Northwestern University, Chicago.*
Robert Kennon, *Contemporary Surgeon, Royal Infirmary, Liverpool.*

the zygoma in cases of dislocated jaw ; this is due to spasm of the temporal muscle.

*Unilateral Dislocation (Fig.* 146).—Here the signs are much less manifest. William Hey stated :

" One would expect that the chin would be turned to the opposite side, but I have repeatedly seen the disease (accident) when I could discern no alteration in the position of the chin. The sign which I have found to be the best guide, is a small hollow which may be felt behind the condyle that is dislocated. This does not subsist on the sound side."

If the little finger is inserted into the auditory meatus, the examiner can feel the movement of the head of the mandible when the patient opens and closes the mouth. This movement is not felt when the jaw is dislocated (Bauer).

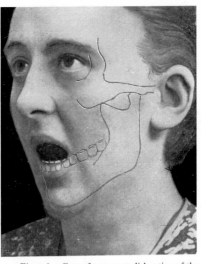

Fig. 146.—Case of recurrent dislocation of the jaw. Every time the patient yawned and sometimes when she ate, dislocation occurred.

## EXAMINATION OF THE FIFTH CRANIAL NERVE

*Motor.*—Palpate the temporal and masseter muscles. Ask the patient to clench his teeth and note whether these muscles contract. Next direct him to open his mouth as widely as possible. If there is weakness of the pterygoid muscles of one side, the jaw will deviate to the paralysed side.

*Sensory (with Particular Reference to Trigeminal Neuralgia).*—Trigeminal neuralgia begins in either the second or third division of the fifth nerve. Ask the patient where the neuralgia began. Patients with this terrible affliction can often map out accurately the distribution of the pain. " Eating will bring it on in some persons ; talking, or the least motion of the face, in others. The gentlest touch of the hand or the handkerchief will bring on the pain, while strong pressure has no effect " (John Fothergill).

*During an attack* the affected area is hyperæsthetic, as can be shown by stroking it with cotton-wool.

6

WILLIAM HEY, 1736–1819, *Surgeon, Leeds Infirmary.*
FRANTISK BAUER, *Contemporary Registrar, Ear, Nose and Throat Department, Hospital for Sick Children, Aberdeen.*
JOHN FOTHERGILL, 1712–1780. *a highly successful London practitioner.*

*Between the attacks.* When the patient is examined carefully one or more *trigger zones of Patrick* will be found. Somewhere in

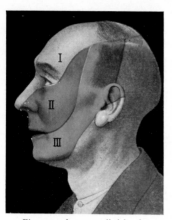

Fig. 147.—Areas supplied by the 5th cranial nerve.

the area supplied by the fifth nerve—on the skin of the face (*Fig.* 147) or the mucous membrane of the cheek or gum—a hyperæsthetic area can be demonstrated, and a light touch on this zone initiates an attack. Curiously, the trigger zone is often in an area supplied by one division of the fifth nerve, and the pain commences in another.

In the earlier stages of the disease the patient believes she has toothache, and one tooth after another, sound or carious, is removed. By the time the patient reaches the surgeon she is usually edentulous.

## EXAMINATION OF THE SEVENTH CRANIAL NERVE

Ask the patient to shut the eyes tightly, and at the same time to show the front teeth. In cases of a complete lesion of the seventh nerve the immobility of one-half of the face becomes obvious. The patient cannot shut the eye on the affected side, and in the attempt to do so, the eyeballs are rolled upwards, giving rise to the well-known unsightly ' blind man ' appearance (*Fig.* 148).

When a patient neither bears the scar of a mastoid operation or of an operation for removal of a parotid tumour, nor gives a history of a severe head injury, Bell's palsy is a probable diagnosis, in which

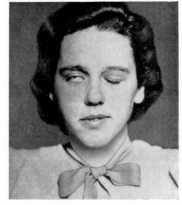

Fig. 148.—Complete facial palsy following a fracture of the base of the skull.

case a history of exposure to cold or to a draught is relevant.

In cases of incomplete palsy, a more painstaking examination is required. It is advisable to divide the examination into two parts :—

Hugh Tabot Patrick, *Contemporary Neurologist, Northwestern University, Chicago.*

Sir Charles Bell, 1774–1842, *Surgeon, Middlesex Hospital, London, later Professor of Surgery, Edinburgh.*

*A. The Examination of the Upper Face.*—On the affected side the eye usually contains " the tear which does not fall " (*Fig.* 149). Ask the patient :—

1. To raise his eyebrows. In facial paralysis the forehead will remain smooth owing to paralysis of the occipito-frontalis.

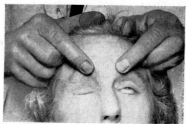

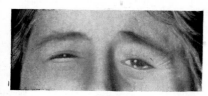

*Fig.* 149.—Showing the " tear that does not fall " and partial paralysis of orbicularis oculi. Case of complete removal of the parotid gland for malignant disease.

*Fig.* 150.—Testing the strength of the orbicularis oculi. (Same patient as *Fig.* 149.)

2. To frown. There will be no furrowing owing to the loss of power in the corrugator supercilii.

3. To shut his eyes. The strength of the orbicularis oculi is tested by attempting to open the eyes against the patient's efforts to keep them shut (*Fig.* 150).

*B. The Examination of the Lower Face.*—The muscles of the lower part of the face are now tested. Ask the patient :—

1. To puff out his cheeks.
2. To whistle.
3. To show the teeth (*Fig.* 151).

The upper facial muscles are represented on both sides of the cortex ; the lower facial muscles have only a unilateral representation. Therefore it follows that in a unilateral supranuclear lesion of the seventh nerve the upper facial muscles tend to escape.

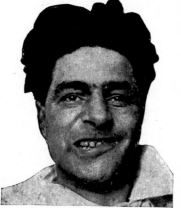

*Fig.* 151.—Left-sided facial paralysis ; the answer to the request, ' Show your teeth '.

## EXAMINATION OF THE NINTH CRANIAL NERVE

Trigeminal neuralgia and glossopharyngeal neuralgia are alike, except for the localization of the paroxysms of agonizing pain

6*

and the areas of the trigger zones. In glossopharyngeal neuralgia the pain is brought on more frequently by swallowing than by any other stimulus. The trigger zones include the pharyngeal wall, the base of the tongue, and especially the tonsillar region. There is no difficulty in differentiating trigeminal neuralgia affecting the first and second divisions of the fifth nerve, from glosso-pharyngeal neuralgia, but when the third division of the fifth nerve is affected, considerable care must be exercised in elucidating the exact area maximally involved.

## EXAMINING A LOCALIZED SWELLING IN THE CHEEK

The following procedure should be carried out :—

1. Observe the outside of the cheek, and make certain whether or not the swelling in question is situated in the skin.

2. Observe the buccal aspect, and satisfy yourself whether or not the swelling originates in the buccal mucosa (*Fig.* 152).

3. Palpate between the finger and thumb.

In the case of a swelling not in the skin and not in the mucosa, remember the sucking pad of the infant, which sometimes persists. There is also an inconstant lymph node along the course of the facial artery (*Fig.* 153).

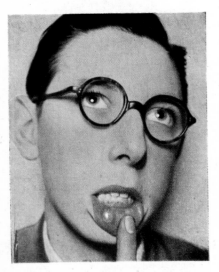

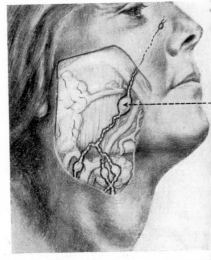

*Fig.* 152.—Retention cyst of a buccal mucous gland.

*Fig.* 153.—The relations and connexions of the bucco-facial lymph node.

# CHAPTER IX

## THE HEAD

### EXAMINATION OF THE CRANIUM

**The Anterior Fontanelle.**—Normally this fontanelle closes between the fifteenth and the eighteenth months (*Fig.* 154).

During the first year of life the anterior fontanelle is a gold-mine of clinical information. Like the eyeball, the anterior fontanelle has a normal tension. This tension can be estimated by pressing the fingers gently over the space. When the child cries, the tension is increased noticeably. In shock the normal tension is diminished, and to some extent the degree of shock present in a case of, say, intussusception or burns, can be estimated by this method. When the child is dehydrated by diarrhœa and vomiting, the anterior fontanelle is depressed, often visibly.

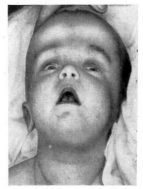

*Fig.* 154.—Eighteen-months-old child with hydrocephalus. The anterior fontanelle is widely open and tense. The somewhat bulging eyes are downcast ; the child appears always to be looking towards the floor (pressure on the orbital plates).

In cases of spinal meningocele, fluctuation should be sought from meningocele to anterior fontanelle (*Fig.* 155). If present, it signifies that a wide-mouthed channel communicates with the cerebrospinal canal and the meningocele.

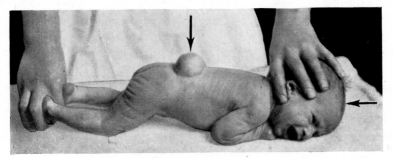

*Fig.* 155.—Fluctuation could be obtained from the anterior fontanelle to the cystic swelling in this case of syringo-myelocele.

Delayed closure of the fontanelle is seen in several metabolic diseases, especially rickets, of which it is good confirmatory evidence.

**The Scalp.**—Scalp wounds never gape unless the aponeurosis has been divided.  Therefore we can tell at a glance if this structure has been involved.  A collection of blood or pus underneath the aponeurosis (dangerous area) tends to involve the whole area between the attachments of the occipito-frontalis.  In these cases fluctuation can be detected over the whole scalp, from frontal to occipital region.  On the other hand, effusion beneath the pericranium is limited by the

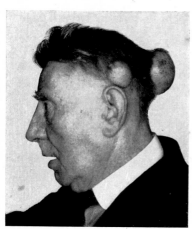

Fig. 156.—Sebaceous cysts of the scalp, sometimes called wens.

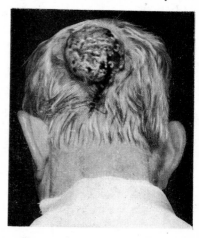

Fig. 157.—Cock's ' peculiar ' tumour looks like squamous-celled carcinoma ; in this case it bled easily too. Cock's ' peculiar ' tumour is a suppurating sebaceous adenoma.

suture lines.  A hæmatoma of this region is often exceedingly deceptive to the palpating fingers : *it feels exactly like a depressed fracture.*  An attempt should be made to indent the edge with the thumb-nail, but often this sign is inconclusive.

A localized swelling in the scalp can be made to move on the skull (*Figs.* 156, 157) : conversely, the scalp can be made to move over a swelling springing from the skull.  An obscure cystic swelling in this region should be watched carefully for pulsation.  The sign of emptying (meningocele and cavernous hæmangioma), translucency (meningocele), the application of a stethoscope (bruit of cirsoid aneurysm), and percussion of the swelling (pneumatocele), may have a place in the elucidation of the diagnosis.

**Cranial Percussion.**—Sir William Macewen found cranial percussion a useful method (*Fig.* 158).  In July, 1922, he said : " The note elicited on percussion of the skull has been used by me since the early seventies, in aiding in the determination of certain pathological conditions which alter the physics of the cranial contents." According to Macewen, it is useful especially in children and those whose skulls are thin. *Percussion is best done over the pterion.* A differential percussion note is found when the ventricles are distended, as may

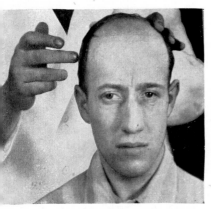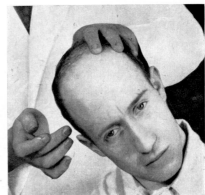

*Fig.* 158.—Differential cranial percussion (Macewen). I. Percussion over pterion in vertical position. II. Percussion over pterion with head tilted.

be occasioned by a cerebellar tumour. Its pitch alters according to the position of the head : the side that is undermost gives the clearer hollow note. This differential percussion note is not found in hydrocephalus where the bones of the skull have not united.

## EXAMINATION OF A CASE OF RECENT HEAD INJURY

**1. The Patient is Unconscious.**—Examine the scalp for a wound or local bruising. Inspect the external auditory meatuses and nostrils for evidence of bleeding. Compare the sizes of the pupils. Make a general survey of the body for other injuries, e.g., fractures.

*Cranial Percussion (Macewen).*—Very occasionally in fractured skull there is a ' cracked-pot ' note. When present it usually signifies an extensive fracture invading the vertex from the base.

Coma is a state of absolute unconsciousness in which the patient does not respond to any stimulus. In semi-coma the patient responds only to painful stimuli. To some extent the depth of unconsciousness can be judged by exerting pressure over the supra-orbital nerves (*Fig.* 159). If unconsciousness is not profound, this

SIR WILLIAM MACEWEN, 1848–1924, *Professor of Surgery, University of Glasgow.*

will cause the patient to contract the facial muscles.  Usually it is unnecessary to make any further examination for the time being.

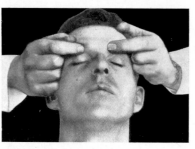

*Fig.* 159.—Exerting pressure over the supra-orbital nerves.  A useful method of determining the depth of unconsciousness, for it causes pain.

Have the pulse and temperature recorded every half-hour, and await developments.  Re-examine later.

**2. The Patient is Conscious or Semi-conscious.**—Should the patient be mentally confused, the degree of confusion at the time of the examination should be recorded.

*Severe Confusion.*—No sensible answers can be obtained, but now and then simple commands forcibly given, such as ' Hold my hand ', will be obeyed.

*Moderate Confusion.*—Although out of touch with his surroundings, relevant answers to obvious questions such as ' How old are you ? ' ' What is your work ? ' will be forthcoming.

*Mild Confusion.*—Some degree of coherent conversation is possible (McConnell).

Proceed to make a clinical test of the cranial nerves.  A rough but efficient examination of the main points takes but a few moments.

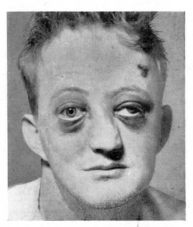

*Fig.* 160.—Injury to the third nerve. Note the ptosis and external strabismus.  The patient fell off his motor-cycle and sustained a fracture of the anterior cranial fossa.

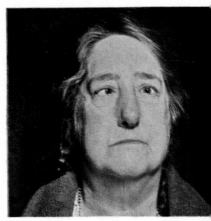

*Fig.* 161.—6th nerve palsy following a head injury.

ADAMS ANDREW MCCONNELL, *Contemporary Professor of Surgery, Royal College of Surgeons, Dublin.*

1st *Nerve.*—Can he smell ?  (Of little practical value.)

2nd  ,,  —Vision.

3rd  ,,  —Movements of lids.  Reaction of pupils.  Is there external strabismus ?  (*Fig.* 160).

4th  ,,  —Deviation of the eye upwards and outwards. Double vision.

5th  ,,  —' Clench your teeth.' Feel the masseter contract (*see* p. 81).

6th  ,,  —Is there internal strab- ismus ?  (*Fig.* 161).

7th  ,,  —' Show the front teeth.' Observe the con- traction of the facial muscles (p. 83).

8th  ,,  —Can he hear ?  Test each side.  Is nys- tagmus present ?

9th  ,,  —Does the palate move when the patient says " Ah " ?

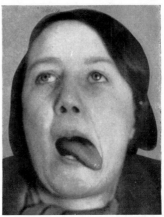

Fig. 162.—The answer to the re- quest ' Put out your tongue ', in a case of paralysis of the left twelfth nerve (hypoglossal).

10th  ,,  —(Cannot be tested con- veniently.*)

11th  ,,  —' Shrug your shoulders.'

12th  ,,  —' Put out your tongue '  (*Fig.* 162).

The integrity of the spinal nerves can be tested quickly by asking the patient to move his legs and his arms.

**Differential Diagnosis between Orbital Hæmorrhage conse- quent upon a Fractured Anterior Cranial Fossa and a ' Black Eye '.—**

1. Examine the eyelids.  In a fracture of the anterior cranial fossa the extravasated blood is limited abruptly to the orbital margin by the palpebral fascia.  It tends, therefore, to be circular.  In ' black eye ' there is no such limitation.

---

* *Vagus.*—The most characteristic sign of a lesion of the vagus is paralysis of its recurrent laryngeal branch.  On the affected side the vocal cord is immobile, fixed in the cadaveric position.  Other tests for the integrity of the vagus are : (1) Direct the patient to swallow ; test the force with which the larynx is drawn up.  (2) Ask the patient to say ' Ah ' with the mouth open, and observe the move- ment of the palate.

The escape of blood, however, is not pathognomonic of a fracture of the middle fossa, for it also occurs when the tympanic membrane is ruptured.

**Fracture of the Posterior Cranial Fossa.**—There is usually respiratory derangement.

*Battle's Sign in Fracture of the Posterior Cranial Fossa.*—Blood accumulates beneath the deep fascia, producing discoloration in the line of the posterior auricular artery. This discoloration first appears near the tip of the mastoid process.

**On Which Side is the Lesion?**

*Hutchinson's Pupils.*—The pupils require observation with scrupulous care. In advanced cases of cerebral compression they are both paralysed and dilated. From the time of the onset of the hæmorrhage, the pupils pass through a series of changes—namely :—

| Stage | Pupil on Opposite Side to the Lesion. | | | Pupil on Side on which Compression Commenced |
|---|---|---|---|---|
| 1 | Normal | ● | ● | Slightly contracted, sluggishly reacts to light. |
| 2 | Normal | ● | ⬤ | Moderately dilated. Reacts to light. |
| 3 | Moderately dilated. Reacts to light. | ⬤ | ⬤ | Widely dilated. Does not react to light. |
| 4 | Widely dilated. Insensitive. | ⬤ | ⬤ | Widely dilated. Insensitive. |

The first stage is rarely seen. It is the second (*Fig.* 165) and third stages that are of signal diagnostic importance.

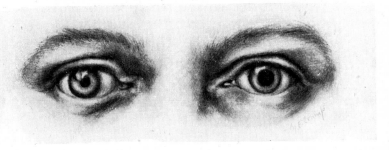

Opposite side to lesion : Normal.   Side of lesion : Dilated ; reacts to light.
*Fig.* 165.—Hutchinson's pupils : second stage.

WILLIAM HENRY BATTLE, 1855–1936, *Surgeon, St. Thomas's Hospital, London*
SIR JONATHAN HUTCHINSON, 1828–1913, *Surgeon, London Hospital.*

*Victor Horsley's Sign.*—Take the temperature first in one axilla and then in the other, using the same thermometer. The temperature in an advanced case of middle meningeal hæmorrhage often registers a degree of difference on the two sides. If a difference exists, it is higher on the paralysed side.

**Acute Cerebral Compression.**—*The half-hourly pulse-rate which we have been observing, gradually becomes slower.* In advanced cases the respirations are stertorous, and the cheeks are puffing in and out.

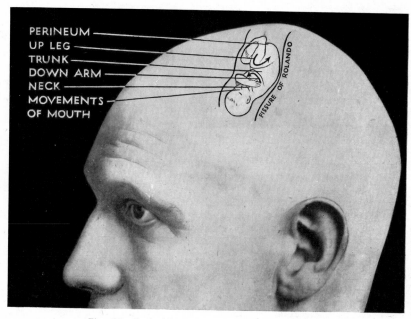

PERINEUM
UP LEG
TRUNK
DOWN ARM
NECK
MOVEMENTS
OF MOUTH

FISSURE OF ROLANDO

*Fig.* 166.—Cerebral localization in the pre-Rolandic cortex.

*Meningeal Hæmorrhage.*—A classical sign of middle meningeal hæmorrhage is a lucid interval. By this is meant that the patient rouses from his unconsciousness and shortly afterwards lapses once more into unconsciousness ; this can be a period of one to 24 hours.

Again examine the head, and with a pocket torch look for a hæmatoma or bruise. If the signs point to a lesion on one side, and the hæmatoma or bruise is on the other side, remember the possibility of a *contre-coup* injury.

One may be fortunate enough to observe a ' fit ', but we are rarely so favoured : usually we have to trust to a description by

SIR VICTOR HORSLEY, 1857–1916, *Surgeon, University College Hospital, London.*

the nurse. Try to find out where the fit *began*. In conjunction with this, it is useful to recall the localization of the various centres in the pre-Rolandic area. In this connexion *Fig.* 166 is a valuable aid to memory.

In middle meningeal hæmorrhage the fit is of the Jacksonian type and unilateral. In hæmorrhage from the superior longitudinal sinus the fits may be bilateral. I had the opportunity of observing a case of the latter in which repeated fits passed up both legs and down both arms.

Search for paralysis. Pick up the arms and allow them to fall. Pick up the legs and do the same. One side may be more flaccid. If this is the case, it is likely that the cerebral lesion is on the opposite side. Rub or pinch the soles of the feet. As a result one leg may be drawn up, whilst the other is not. This is a good test in determining which side is paralysed in an unconscious patient. Vigorously rub both cheeks and then observe the face, particularly the corners of the mouth. Even in deep unconsciousness, the corner of the mouth on the non-paralysed side tends to be drawn upwards after a ' facial massage '.

The examination should be completed by testing the knee-jerks and plantar reflexes. In an unconscious patient, reflexes, as a rule, are not so helpful in determining the side of the lesion as the signs that have been described above.

## CEREBRAL IRRITATION

Cerebral irritation is a clinical concept without exact underlying pathology. Usually it asserts itself about thirty or forty hours after the injury. The patient lies curled up in bed (*Fig.* 167), his face turned

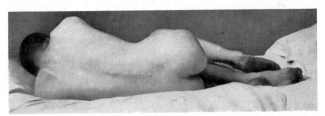

*Fig.* 167.—Cerebral irritation. The patient has turned away from the light.

from the light, because he hates the light (photophobia). The eyelids are closed. The temperature is raised, and may be different on the two sides of the body. The patient resents being aroused. He is abusive and irritable. No further examination is necessary, or, indeed, possible.

Luigi Rolando, 1773–1831, *Professor of Anatomy, Turin.*
John Hughlings Jackson, 1835–1911, *Physician, London Hospital.*

# CHAPTER X

## THE EAR

**The Pinna.**—Those who indulge in detective literature are wont to believe that, by scrutinizing the conformation of the pinna, hereditary tendencies, criminal and otherwise, are revealed to gifted observers. Admittedly, the conformation of the pinna is interestingly variegated, but after years of close observation I have got no further than the detection of the cauliflower ear of the boxer ; that tophi occur in this situation in gouty subjects ; that protuberant ears,

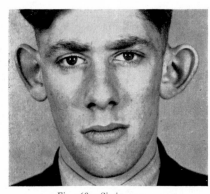

*Fig.* 168.—Simian ears.

*Fig.* 168, are due to nursing babies on their backs with a soft pillow behind the head ; and that Darwin's tubercle is fairly common.

What *is* of general surgical importance, and is but little known, is the clinical entity *pre-auricular ulcer. Fig.* 169 is a typical example. The patient had been treated in a sanatorium for three years as cutaneous tuberculosis associated with an infected pre-auricular lymphatic gland. By focusing attention on the root of the helix a pre-auricular sinus can be seen. A pre-auricular sinus is a congenital abnormality due to imperfect fusion of the tubercles that form the pinna. The ulcer refuses to heal, for infection is maintained from the sinus (Stammers). In this case, after the sinus was excised, the ulcer healed within three weeks. If we bear in mind the embryological derivation of the pinna from five tubercles, it is not difficult to appreciate that it is possible for a *dermoid cyst* (*Fig.* 170) to occur in this situation. If diagnosed early, *squamous-celled carcinoma of the pinna* (*Fig.* 171) responds favourably to surgical treatment.

CHARLES ROBERT DARWIN, 1809–1882, formulated the theory of evolution by natural selection.
FRANCIS ALAN ROLAND STAMMERS, *Contemporary Professor of Surgery, University of Birmingham.*

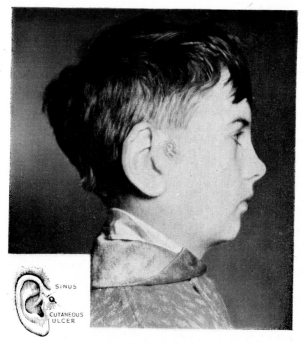

Fig. 169.—Pre-auricular sinus with ulcer. The orifice of the sinus can be seen on the root of the helix ; sometimes it is situated on the tragus.

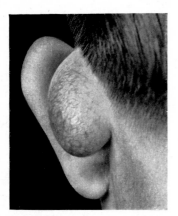

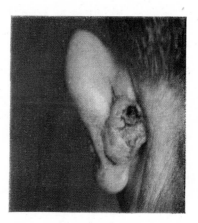

Fig 170.—Dermoid cyst of the pinna.

Fig. 171.—Advanced carcinoma of the pinna. A secondary growth was present in the pre-auricular lymphatic gland.

## EXAMINATION OF A CASE OF ACUTE MASTOIDITIS

In acute mastoiditis a patient will often say that an aural discharge has ceased recently. Look at the external auditory meatus.

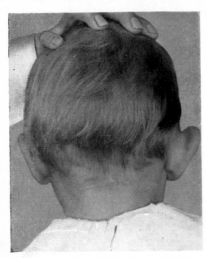

Fig. 172.—Examination from the back in mastoiditis. Note that the ear on the affected side is pushed forward.

In acute mastoiditis the meatus is often narrowed from behind forwards—so it is in furuncle of the auditory canal.

Observe the patient from behind, and particularly note the angle of inclination the two pinnæ make to the side of the head (*Fig.* 172).

In acute mastoiditis the pinna is pushed forward—so it is in suppurating posterior auricular glands.

If, however, the pinna is pushed forward *and* the meatus is narrowed, it is highly suggestive of acute mastoiditis. Auditory furuncle (narrows the external auditory meatus) and posterior auricular adenitis (pushes the pinna forward) claim one point each, but neither of these conditions gives the dual phenomenon. Therefore an almost pathognomonic sign of acute mastoiditis is an ear that is pushed forward and at the same time has a meatus narrowed from behind forward.

### POINTS OF TENDERNESS

*Points of tenderness* are tested next. Before attempting this we must make sure that we know exactly what we are going to do. There are three points at which to apply pressure (*Fig.* 173) :—

1. *Over the Eustachian Tube.*—Perform an experiment upon yourself to prove this. Press a finger on the depression between the tip of the left mastoid process and the angle of the jaw. Now hold your nose and blow. You will hear the right drum (if normal) go

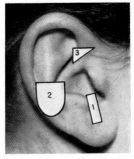

Fig. 173.—Transparent pinna, showing the various structures beneath which need special examination. (1) Eustachian tube ; (2) Mastoid process ; (3) Mastoid antrum.

'bang' before the left. The reason is that you are compressing the left Eustachian tube with your finger.

2. *Over the Mastoid Process.*—The mastoid process is a variable structure : it is absent at birth, and grows slowly until puberty. In the early stage of its development it is full of marrow cells. At this time, should it become seriously infected, pus penetrates the bone into the digastric fossa, forming an abscess in the neck beneath the mastoid process (Bezold's mastoiditis).

3. *Over the Suprameatal Triangle of Macewen.* Pressure can be applied over this by one of two methods. The method most generally used is to draw the pinna forward (*Fig.* 174). This gives access to the posterior part of the triangle. The second method is to place a finger in the fossa triangularis (*Fig.* 175). This brings the finger up directly over the triangle. I have found this latter method of exerting pressure over the antrum most useful.

Possessed of this knowledge, we will now proceed to apply it.

1. Pressure over the Eustachian tube (*Fig.* 176) always gives rise to an unpleasant sensation : but if extreme pain is brought on (which is at once seen by a spasm of the patient's face), it is an indication of middle-ear disease.

2. Pressure over the mastoid process (*Fig.* 177), even in acute mastoiditis, is not necessarily painful. In Bezold's type this is the point of most acute tenderness. It is over the middle of the mastoid process that the maximum tenderness is elicited in suppurating posterior-auricular adenitis.

3. Pressure over the mastoid antrum is tried by both methods detailed above and shown in *Figs.* 174 and 175. Tenderness here is the sign *par excellence* of acute mastoiditis.

In acute mastoiditis tapping over the region of the mastoid antrum in the same manner as detailed in CRANIAL PERCUSSION (p. 86) causes more pain than steady pressure. The reverse is true for cellulitis overlying the region.

*A Confirmatory Test for Mastoiditis.*—The thumb is placed against the mastoid and the patient is ordered to press against it. The thumb is released suddenly and the movement of the patient's head is observed. If the patient is healthy, the head will follow the movement of the releasing thumb : if the mastoid is diseased, the head will remain stationary (Lowndes Yates).

*A Confirmatory Test for Furuncle of the Meatus : Cirumduction of the Auricle.*—The whole breadth of the pinna is grasped between

FRIEDRICH BEZOLD, 1842–1908, *Aurist in Munich.*

ARTHUR LOWNDES YATES, *Contemporary Assistant Surgeon, Ear, Nose and Throat Department, Prince of Wales' Hospital, London.*

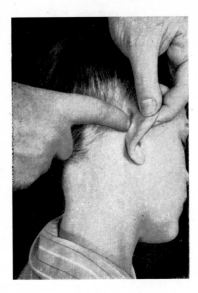

Fig. 174.—Testing for tenderness over the mastoid antrum. Method I.

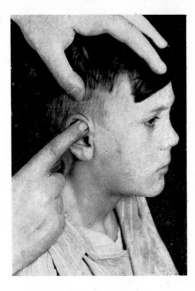

Fig. 175.—Testing for à point of tenderness over the mastoid antrum. Method II, via the fossa triangularis.

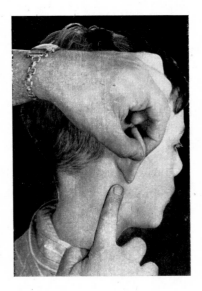

Fig. 176.—Palpating over the Eustachian tube.

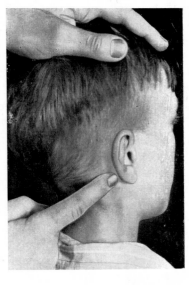

Fig. 177.—Testing for tenderness over the mastoid process.

the finger and thumb. The pinna is rotated gently, the axis being the junction of the cartilaginous with the bony external auditory meatus. In furuncle of the external auditory meatus pain is produced at once, but considerable painless rotation is possible in mastoiditis.

Examination with the auriscope is most desirable, but its description is beyond the limits of this work.

Thrombophlebitis of the lateral sinus is a complication of a neglected acute mastoiditis. Palpate the course of the jugular vein. Very infrequently the jugular vein can be felt like a cord extending down the neck. The most valuable diagnostic sign of lateral sinus

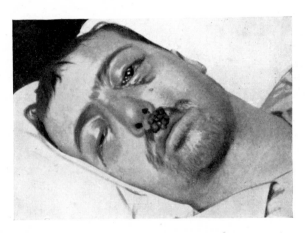

*Fig.* 178.—Thrombosis of the cavernous sinus.
Carbuncle of the upper lip.

involvement is the onset of repeated rigors occurring in a case of acute mastoiditis. Thrombosis of the cavernous sinus may complicate a lateral sinus thrombosis. The cavernous sinus is sometimes infected via the angular (anterior facial) vein from a boil of the upper lip or nose. Infection can also reach this sinus via the pterygoid plexus. *Fig.* 178 shows a thrombosis of the cavernous sinus following a carbuncle of the upper lip. In cases of thrombosis of the cavernous sinus the eye (or eyes) is proptosed, and blood-stained tears may trickle down the cheek.

**Examination of the Eighth Cranial Nerve.**——*It is almost useless to attempt the examination unless we know that the auditory canal is free from wax.*

Stand behind the patient and note the distance at which the ticking of a watch can be heard on each side.  It should be known at what distance the watch can normally be heard.  Each ear is tested separately, one being closed while the other is being examined.

THE DIFFERENTIAL DIAGNOSIS BETWEEN MIDDLE-EAR DEAFNESS AND A LESION OF THE AUDITORY NERVE.—

*Weber's Test.*—Place a vibrating tuning-fork on the centre of the vertex.  Normally the sound is appreciated equally by both ears, and if the patient stops up one ear with his finger the sound is louder on that side.  When the deafness is of the internal ear or of the eighth nerve (nerve deafness), the fork is not heard on the affected side.

*Rinne's Test.*—Place the vibrating fork on the mastoid process, with the limbs of the fork sloping backwards.  The patient is instructed beforehand to signal when he no longer hears the sound.  The tuning-fork is then held close to the external auditory meatus. Normally it is still audible—that is to say, air conduction is better than bone conduction.  In middle-ear deafness, bone conduction is better than air conduction.  In nerve deafness, both are lost.

Giddiness, nystagmus and nausea are signs of involvement of the labyrinth or the vestibular nerve.

ERNST HEINRICH WEBER, 1795–1878, *Professor of Anatomy and Physiology, Leipzig.*
HEINRICH ADOLF RINNE, 1819–1868 *Aural Surgeon, Göttingen.*

*CHAPTER XI*

## THE NECK (EXCLUDING THE THYROID GLAND)

WHEN the neck is to be examined, it should be needless to emphasize that the collar must be removed, and the shirt or blouse unfastened. A better examination can be made when all clothing is removed as far as the axillæ, and this practice is to be recommended : it allows the whole neck to be seen in relationship to the thorax, and permits inspection and palpation of the supraclavicular fossæ.

### EXAMINATION OF THE LATERAL REGIONS OF THE NECK

The key to the lateral region of the neck is the sternomastoid. Bearings are taken from this structure, first with the eye and then with the fingers.

If there is a swelling obviously *in* the sternomastoid muscle, and the patient is an infant, it is an example of the so-called sterno-mastoid 'tumour' (*Fig.* 179).

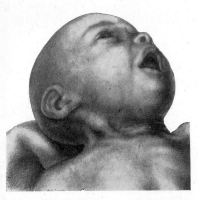

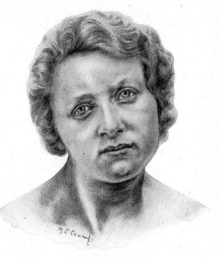

*Fig.* 179.—Sternomastoid ' tumour '.

*Fig.* 180 —Torticollis, often the sequel of a neglected sternomastoid ' tumour ' of infancy.

When one sternomastoid is tense and the patient holds his head even slightly on one side, ask him to try to straighten his neck : he

7

cannot do so, but with the attempt the sternomastoid, especially its sternal head, stands out.  Observe the face critically.  If the case is one of long-standing torticollis (*Fig.* 180), some degree of asymmetry will be present—the features on the affected side will be seen to be, perhaps ever so slightly smaller.  If in doubt, measurements can be taken.

**Determining the Relationship of a Cervical Swelling to the Sternomastoid.**—Frequently it is necessary to determine the relationship of a cervical swelling to the sternomastoid.  Commonly this muscle is thin and flattened out when it flanks a lateral cervical swelling.  Consequently it is sometimes impossible to make out the relationship of the swelling to the sterno- mastoid by mere palpation, un- less the muscle is rendered taut

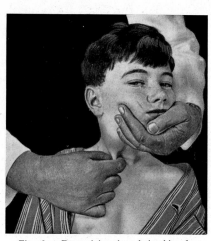

Stand behind the patient Ask him to push his chin as hard as possible against the palm of your hand (*Fig.* 181) This makes the sternomastoid very tense.  With the other hand palpate the sternomastoid

*Fig.* 181.—Determining the relationship of a cervical swelling to the sternomastoid.

from below (where it is normal) upwards, paying special attention to the anterior border.

## PALPATION OF THE CERVICAL LYMPHATIC NODES

Stand behind the patient.  Almost every patient, on learning that his neck is about to be examined, throws back his head, in the belief that he is facilitating the examination.  This extension of the head effectually prevents the examination of the cervical glands, for it renders the sternomastoid and platysma tense, and underlying struc- tures are masked thereby.  Therefore, first adjust the patient's head to a suitable angle, i.e., have it well flexed and inclined slightly towards the side that is being examined.

In order that no lymph-nodes shall be overlooked, it is well to have a routine that scrutinizes every lymphatic group (*Fig.* 182). A useful order with a march of sequence is : (1) Submental ; (2) Submaxillary (*Fig.* 183) ; (3) Jugular chain ; (4) Supraclavicular

*(Fig.* 184) ;   (5) Posterior triangle, which is divided into glandulæ con-
catinatæ and suboccipital ; (6) Posterior auricular ; (7) Pre-auricular.

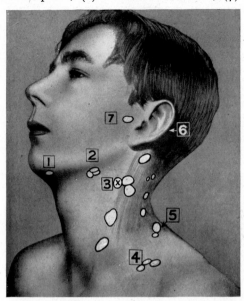

*Fig.* 182.—Order in which the various groups of cervical lymphatic nodes should be
palpated ;  (1) Submental ;  (2) Submaxillary ;  (3) Jugular chain ;  (4) Supraclavicular ;
(5) Posterior triangle ; (6) Posterior auricular ; (7) Pre-auricular.  The gland marked **X**
is the tonsillar lymph-node.

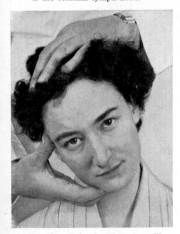

*Fig.* 183.—Palpating the submaxillary
group of cervical lymph-nodes.  The hand
on the head enables the clinician to adjust
the degree of flexion.

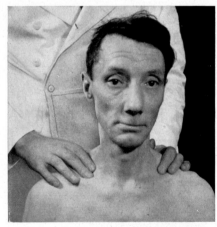

*Fig.* 184.—Palpating the supraclavicular group of lymphatic nodes.   *See* sign of Troisier p. 208.

If the glands are found to be enlarged, the possible sources of infection or primary growth are examined next—scalp, tongue, mouth, tonsil, ear, etc., and particular attention is paid to the area that is drained by the lymph-nodes found to be diseased (e.g., if the posterior triangle and/or posterior auricular region contain enlarged nodes, the scalp must be examined with scrupulous care).

To record the clinical findings graphically is an excellent practice. As I deal with a large number of these cases I make use of a rubber stamp (*Fig.* 185), but a simple diagram of the outline of the neck, which includes the sternomastoid muscle, serves equally well.

When enlarged cervical lymph-nodes are found, but no primary focus is discoverable, there is a tendency to assume hastily that the nodes are tuberculous. Certainly tuberculosis is the commonest cause of chronic inflammation of the lymph-nodes of the neck : any group may be affected, but the upper jugular chain, particularly the tonsillar gland (*Fig.* 186), is attacked most frequently.

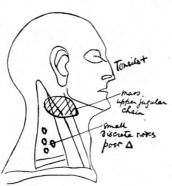

Fig. 185.—Record of a case of tuberculous cervical adenitis.

When the lymph-nodes are large (*Fig.* 187) and feel somewhat discrete and elastic, the question of Hodgkin's disease (*syn.* lymphadenoma) must receive consideration. In such circumstances a wise clinician will palpate the axillæ and the groins : the finding of a similar mass in one or both of these situations tends to support a hypothesis that will be strengthened if an abdominal examination reveals an enlargement of the spleen.

The leading characteristic of malignant lymph-nodes of the neck (*Fig.* 188), especially of secondary malignant nodes, is the stony-hard impression they impart to the palpating fingers.

On many occasions I have seen the great cornu of the hyoid bone mistaken for a hard fixed lymph-node. In elderly subjects the great cornu of the hyoid bone tends to become ossified, when it certainly does simulate a hard node : however, it lies farther forward than the lymph-nodes of the jugular chain, and its true nature can be revealed by asking the patient to swallow.

THOMAS HODGKIN, 1798–1866, *Curator of the Museum, Guy's Hospital, London.*

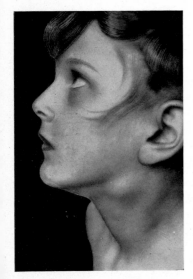

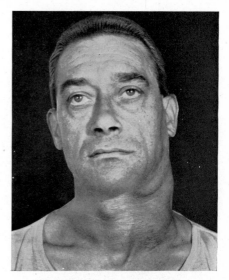

Fig. 186.—The commonest cause of chronic enlargement of the lymph-nodes of the neck is tuberculous lymphadenitis, and the most common lymphatic node to be affected is the tonsillar, which lies in the upper jugular chain.

Fig. 187.—This massive lymphatic enlargement is composed of rather discrete lumps which feel firm, like solid rubber. A case of Hodgkin's disease.

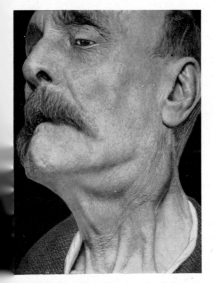

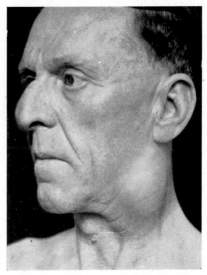

Fig. 188.—These lymph-nodes feel stony hard. The mass behind the sternomastoid is fixed to deeper structures. The primary growth was found on laryngoscopic examination. Case of extrinsic laryngeal carcinoma.

Fig. 189.—This swelling pulsates.* It has been growing slowly for several years. The lump is hard and rather smooth, and the pulsation manifestly transmitted. Case of carotid body tumour.

* Since this patient was under my care I have had four cases of carotid body tumours. Not one of them pulsated.

*If the physical characteristics of the enlarged glands leave little doubt that they are malignant, but no primary growth can be discovered,* remember that the diagnosis of branchiogenic carcinoma (carcinoma developing in a branchial cyst) is a last refuge, and can be entertained only after a fruitless search of the mouth, nasopharynx, extra-laryngeal recesses, and external auditory canal for the primary growth.

## DIFFERENTIAL DIAGNOSIS OF LATERAL CYSTIC SWELLINGS OF THE NECK

The diagnosis of a *cystic hygroma* (*Fig.* 190) is simple : it is the only brilliantly translucent swelling of the neck (*see* p. 11).

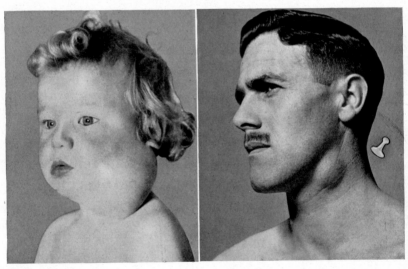

Fig. 190.—Cystic hygroma.        Fig. 191.—Tuberculous ' collar-stud ' abscess.

In addition, by steady pressure, these lymph cysts can be reduced in size, if not emptied entirely. Usually the condition occurs in early childhood.

By far the commonest cystic swelling in the neck is a ' collar-stud ' abscess connected with tuberculous lymphadenitis : the diseased gland, or glands, beneath the cervical fascia are connected by a small opening in the fascia to a more superficially placed ' cold ' abscess (*Fig.* 191).

In about 10 per cent of cases the stem of the ' collar-stud ' is long (*Fig.* 192) : that is to say, the tuberculous glands that feed the abscess are situated some distance away, perhaps in another triangle of the the neck (*Fig.* 193). I note repeatedly that senior students and even graduates usually declare that long-stemmed ' collar-stud ' abscesses are a novelty to them. This is after they have overlooked the causative lesion or failed to associate it with the abscess.

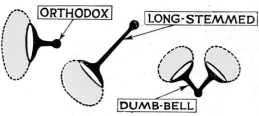

Fig. 192.—' Collar-stud ' abscess ; orthodox and variations.

When, as is not rarely the case, the tuberculous process is entirely limited to a small group of glands, and the abscess is situated directly over them, the diagnosis is far from simple, for the enlarged glands are masked by the abscess. In such a case, provided the overlying abscess is of moderate size, try to palpate deeply behind the swelling with the finger and thumb (*Fig.* 194).

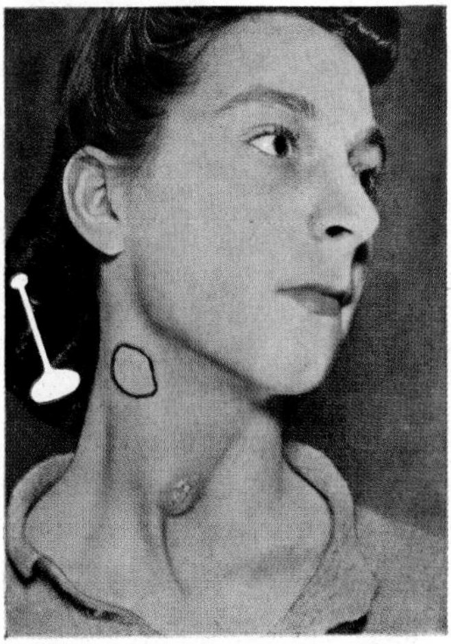

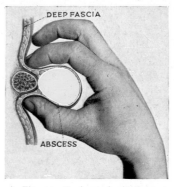

Fig. 194.—By deep palpation between the finger and thumb an enlarged gland can sometimes be felt beneath the cervical fascia.

Fig. 193.—Long-stemmed ' collar-stud ' abscess.

The physical signs of a branchial cyst and tuberculous ' collar-stud ' abscess may be practically identical. The patient presents himself with a cystic swelling in the upper third of the neck deep to the upper third of the sternomastoid, coming round its anterior border.

This is the commonest site for a tuberculous cervical abscess (*see Fig.* 191) and also the constant situation of a branchial cyst (*Fig.* 195). When a branchial cyst is uncomplicated by inflammation—to attacks of which it is prone—it imparts to the palpating fingers what has been described admirably as the sensation given by a half-filled rubber hot-water bottle.

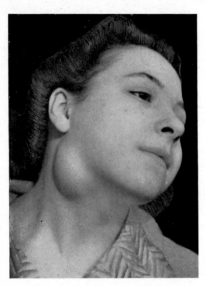

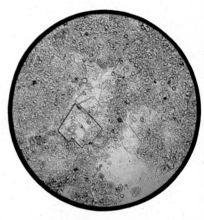

Fig. 195.—A typical branchial cyst. Note its relationship to the upper third of the sternomastoid.

Fig. 196.—Microphotograph of branchial fluid, showing cholesterol crystals and epithelial cells.

If some of the fluid from the cyst is aspirated with a hypodermic syringe, pus-like material will be drawn off in both instances. In the case of a branchial cyst, when this fluid is put in a dish and rocked to and fro, the shimmer of the lipoid content will probably be noted, and a drop placed under the microscope will show an abundance of cholesterol crystals (*Fig.* 196). The finding on microscopical examination of an abundance of cholesterol crystals makes the diagnosis of branchial cyst certain. (*See also* pharyngeal pouch, p. 152.)

## BRANCHIAL FISTULA

A branchial fistula is nearly always congenital, and starts discharging soon after birth. The orifice of the sinus is commonly in the position shown in *Fig.* 197. The amount of excretion varies, and it is inclined to be sticky.

Branchial fistulæ are prone to attacks of inflammation.

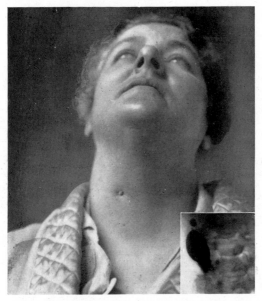

*Fig.* 197.—Congenital branchial fistula, present for thirty years. Inset shows a radiograph after the sinus had been injected with lipiodol.

## SOME RARER CERVICAL CLINICAL ENTITIES

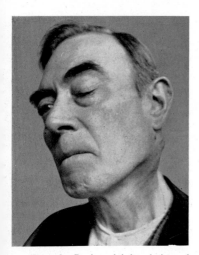

*Fig.* 198.—Ptosis, ophthalmoplegia, and a mass of secondary malignant glands of the neck signify that the primary growth lies in the nasopharynx.

When a patient presents himself with a hard lump in his neck, and a wad of cotton-wool in his ear, it suggests that he is suffering

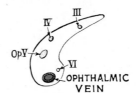

*Fig.* 199.—The sphenoidal fissure. Showing the structures that pass through it.

from *carcinoma of the deep pharynx* (Mollison).

When a *carcinoma of the nasopharynx* has progressed sufficiently to give rise to a secondary mass of glands in the neck, the primary

WILLIAM MAYHEW MOLLISON, *Contemporary Consulting Surgeon, Guy's Hospital, London.*

growth has almost certainly invaded the sphenoidal fissure. Through the sphenoidal fissure pass the third, fourth, ophthalmic divisions of the fifth, and sixth nerves (*Fig.* 199) ; these become implicated. Armed with this knowledge a precise diagnosis of this seemingly obscure and depressing condition becomes a matter of simplicity (*Fig.* 198).

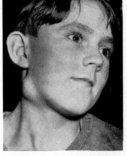

Fig. 200.—A cavernous hæmangioma. At the time of the examination the swelling did not subside on compression ( ? thrombosis). The skin over the swelling has a faint bluish hue.

Largely on account of the rarity of the condition, the diagnosis of *carotid body tumour* (*see Fig.* 189) is seldom made correctly in the first instance. Confined in its comparatively early stages to the fork of the carotid artery, it often gives the sign of transmitted pulsation. A localized, partly calcified mass of tuberculous glands in this area can also give rise to similar signs. As they get larger carotid body tumours extend in an upward direction, they cease to pulsate and tend to involve the twelfth, ninth, eleventh and tenth (recurrent laryngeal) nerves, usually in that order.

*Cavernous hæmangioma of the neck.* Like cavernous hæmangiomata in other situations, the sign of emptying, together with the absence of translucency, should make the diagnosis clear. More often the swelling does not empty indisputably, and is in evidence only for days or weeks at a time *Fig.* 200. By scrutinizing the skin over the swelling a faint bluish hue with, perhaps, an enlarged superficial vein, may be the key to the diagnosis. Aspiration after the insertion of a hollow needle produces pure venous blood.

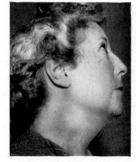

Fig. 201.—Laryngocele.

*A laryngocele* should be suspected if a swelling of the neck appears when the patient blows his nose. This rare condition is due to a narrow-necked pouch connected with some part of the larynx, and is analogous to the air sac of the orang-outang. The patient shown in *Fig.* 201, in addition to exhibiting the classical sign, about once a year had a swelling the size of a tangerine orange in the position shown. On each occasion (eleven to be exact) after ten to twelve days there was a discharge of mucus into the back of the throat, and the swelling subsided with great relief. During the attacks she almost lost her voice.

*CHAPTER XII*

## THE THYROID GLAND

**Inspection.**—Inspection should never be hurried, for it is a highly important method of obtaining information regarding swellings of the thyroid gland. Sometimes it is obvious that the whole thyroid gland is enlarged (*Fig.* 202). When there is a swelling that *may* be

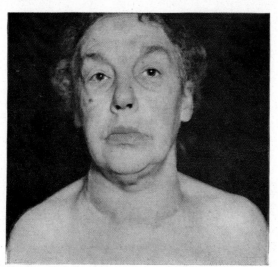

Fig. 202.—Adenoparenchymatous goitre. Enlargement of both lateral lobes and of the isthmus can be seen on inspection.

within the thyroid capsule, ask the patient to swallow. A thyroid swelling moves upwards on deglutition (*Fig.* 203).

In obese and bull-necked individuals, inspection of the thyroid is rendered easier by the patient throwing her head backwards, and pressing her occiput against her clasped hands (Pizillo) (*Fig.* 204).

**Palpation.**—Routine palpation should be performed from behind. In order to relax the musculature, instruct the patient to lower the chin. Using both hands, place the thumbs upon the nape of the neck. In this way, a considerable portion of the fingers comes

GIUSEPPE PIZILLO, *Contemporary Assistant to the Professor of Medicine, University of Palermo.*

to overlie the lateral lobes of the gland (*Fig.* 205). Begin by determining the limits of the lower edges of the lateral lobes, if necessary requesting the patient to swallow. When doubt exists as

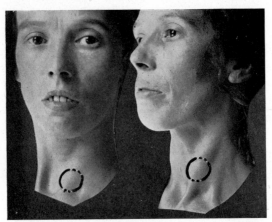

Fig. 203.—Showing how a thyroid swelling moves upwards as the patient swallows.

to whether the thyroid gland is enlarged, palpate the lateral lobes *with the index* fingers directed towards the flat thyroid cartilages (*Fig.* 206). In this way, even a normal thyroid gland can be felt.

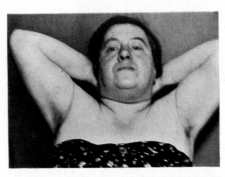

Fig. 204.—Pizillo's method of making the thyroid gland more prominent in cases where a short neck or a thick layer of subcutaneous fat renders inspection of the thyroid by the usual method unsatisfactory.

Having definitely determined the shape and position of the lower limits of an enlarged thyroid, palpate the anterior surfaces of the lateral lobes. These are examined one at a time, the head being inclined slightly to the side that is being examined in order to relax the sternomastoid. In a small proportion of cases it will be found that the pyramidal lobe can be defined.

**A Good Supplementary Method of Palpating the Lateral Lobes of the Thyroid Gland.**—In contrast with the preceding method this examination is conducted from the front. Place the pulp of the thumb against the side of the upper part of the trachea and the lower border of the thyroid cartilage and gently push these structures laterally. This manœuvre throws the opposite lobe of the thyroid gland into prominence and renders it more accessible. Increase the pressure until the patient shows signs of slight discomfort. The fingers of the unoccupied hand are insinuated deeply behind the sternomastoid and so reach the posterior aspect of the prominent lobe. At the same time the unoccupied thumb comes into contact with the anterior surface of this lobe. Thus the examiner is enabled to grasp the lobe (Lahey's method) (*Fig. 207*). At this juncture ask the patient to depress the chin in

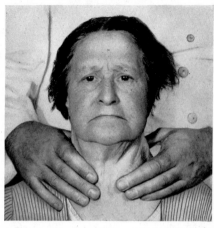

Fig. 205.—Routine palpation of the thyroid gland.

order to relax muscle and fasciæ. It is now possible to make out the size, shape, and consistency of the lobe under consideration. If doubt exists as to whether it is the thyroid gland that is being grasped, tell the patient to swallow, and the matter is settled.

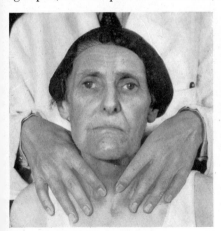

Fig. 206.—Method to be employed in doubtful enlargement of the thyroid gland. It is usually possible to palpate the normal gland by employing this technique.

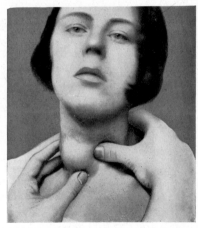

Fig. 207.—Dislocating the trachea, in order that the contralateral lobe of the thyroid may be palpated thoroughly.

FRANK HOWARD LAHEY, *Contemporary Director of Surgery, Lahey Clinic, Boston, Mass.*

**The Whole Thyroid Substance is Enlarged.**—Determine if its surface is smooth, as is found in exophthalmic and colloid goitres, or nodular, which is characteristic of adenoparenchymatous goitres. In large goitres where pressure on the trachea may reasonably be expected, Kocher's test should be applied.

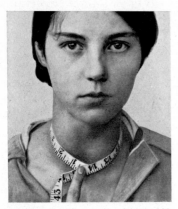

Fig. 208.—Mensuration of the thyroid. A useful method of determining the result of medical treatment of colloid goitres.

*Kocher's Test.*—Slight compression on the lateral lobes produces stridor. If this test is positive it signifies that the patient has a scabbard trachea.

*Mensuration of the Thyroid (Fig. 208)* at intervals is sometimes of value, particularly in cases of colloid goitre of puberty, so that the result of expectant treatment can be noted. The enlargement may progressively decrease.

**A Localized Swelling (Adenoma) is Present.**—If the swelling is visible it will be seen to move upwards when the patient swallows (*see Fig. 203*). Define the lump and make out its relationship to the rest of the thyroid gland. Next, ascertain its relationship to the trachea (*Fig. 209*): the latter is displaced in extravagant cases. By far the most common situation for a solitary adenoma is at the junction of the isthmus with one lateral lobe. Try fluctuation, but remember that an adenoma of the thyroid is paradoxical as far as fluctuation is concerned; the solid variety feels cystic, and the cystic variety feels solid (*see* p. 11).

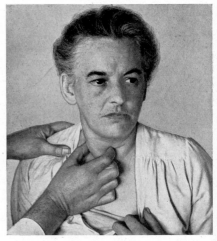

Fig. 209.—Determining the relationship of an adenoma of the thyroid to the trachea.

*When the lower edge of an enlargement of the thyroid cannot be defined*, it is advisable to take the trouble to examine the patient lying down. Arrange her so that the head is slightly extended, but supported. This ensures relaxation of the cervical musculature. Again attempt to reach the lower limit of the thyroid swelling. If one or both lower margins of the lateral lobes still cannot be defined, it is highly probable that the patient has a retrosternal prolongation of the gland.

## RETROSTERNAL (SUBMERGED) GOITRE

Because it is out of sight, a retrosternal goitre is notoriously difficult to diagnose. Dilated veins over the upper part of the

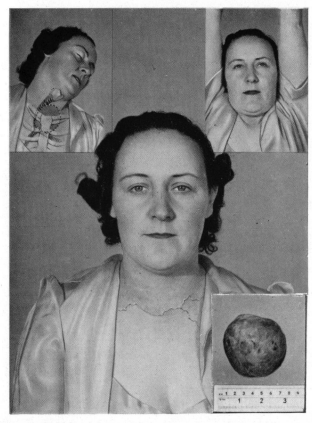

*Fig.* 210.—Retrosterna goitre. Dilated veins over the thoracic inlet were the key to the diagnosis. Inset, the cause of nocturnal dyspnœa when the patient sleeps on her left side.

thoracic wall (*Fig.* 210) due to pressure upon the internal jugular veins sometimes provide a clue to the diagnosis. Occasionally (for reasons obvious on reference to *Fig.* 210 (inset) ), tilting the head strongly to one side produces a sensation of dyspnœa.

Ask the patient to elevate both arms until they touch the sides of the face. After a few moments, congestion of the face, some cyanosis, and lastly distress, become apparent—presumably from narrowing of the thoracic inlet and consequent obstruction to the great veins (Pemberton).

## TOXIC GOITRE

Having determined that some form of thyroid enlargement exists, the clinician's next duty is to decide whether the goitre is toxic or non-toxic.

It should be remembered that toxicity can, and often does, accompany thyroid adenomata of long standing. This is secondary Graves' disease. In the case of primary Graves' disease (*syn.* exophthalmic goitre) the manifestations of toxicity are often striking.

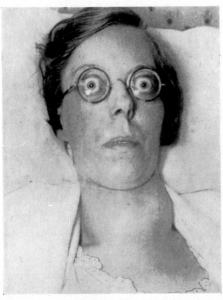

Fig. 211.—Primary Graves' disease (exophthalmic goitre).

**Searching for Toxic Manifestations.—**

*The pulse* should be counted. In hyperthyroidism it is rapid : probably the rate will be exaggerated by nervousness occasioned by examination. In addition to the rate of the pulse, great attention should be paid to the regularity or otherwise of the heart-beat. At this juncture, take the opportunity to feel the hands : in exophthalmic goitre they are inclined to be hot and moist.

*Tremor* may be present. Ask the patient to put her hands straight out in front and spread the fingers. A fine tremor will be observed in hyperthyroidism. Another satisfactory test is to ask the patient to put out her tongue.

*Exophthalmos.* In primary Graves' disease, exophthalmos is often obvious (*Fig.* 211). In secondary Graves' disease it is usually lacking. There are a number of signs connected with exophthalmos : most of them are purely of academic interest.

Forty-three of 100 consecutive cases of chronic Bright's disease showed the nephritic stare with some degree of proptosis.

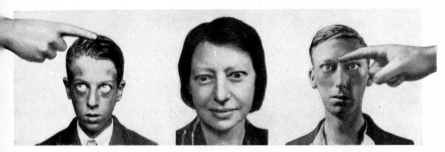

Fig. 212.—Joffroy's sign.  Fig. 213.—Von Graefe's sign.  Fig. 214.—Moebius's sign.

Exophthalmos, therefore, is not synonymous with Graves' disease. A nephritic stare is indistinguishable from that seen in toxic goitre, from which it must be differentiated (Hanes).

*Joffroy's sign* is an absence of wrinkling of the forehead when the head is bent down and the patient looks upwards (*Fig.* 212).

*Von Graefe's sign* is a lagging behind of the upper lid when the patient is requested to look down (*Fig.* 213).

*Moebius's sign* is a difficulty of convergence when the patient is asked to look at a near object (*Fig.* 214).

*Stellwag's sign* is a retraction of the upper lid, often very pronounced, and due to a spasm of the levator palpebræ superioris.

*Naffziger's Method of Examining for Exophthalmos.*—Have the patient seated. Stand behind the patient, and tilt her head

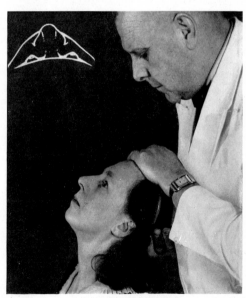

Fig. 215.—Method of looking for minor degrees of exophthalmos.

RICHARD BRIGHT, 1789–1858, *Physician, Guy's Hospital, London.*
FREDERICK MOIR HANES, *Contemporary Professor of Medicine, Duke University, Durham, N. C., U.S.A.*
ALEX JOFFROY, 1844–1908, *Physician to the Hospitals of Paris.*
ALBRECHT VON GRAEFE, 1828–1870, *Professor of Ophthalmology, Berlin.*
PAUL JULIUS MOEBIUS, 1853–1907, *Neurologist, Leipzig.*
CARL STELLWAG VON CARION, 1823–1904, *Ophthalmologist. General Hospital, Vienna.*
HOWARD C. NAFFZIGER, *Contemporary Surgeon-in-Chief, University of California Hospital, San Francisco.*

backwards, holding it in the manner shown in *Fig.* 215, which will keep the hair out of the way.    Observe the eyeballs, your plane of vision

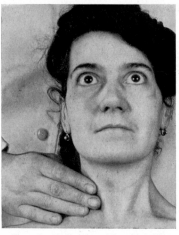

being that of the superciliary ridges.

As opposed to the signs above (small print), this is a really useful, practical test, particularly in doubtful cases and those where unilateral exophthalmos must be confirmed.

**Thyroid Thrill.** — Usually in exophthalmic goitre the thyroid is enlarged evenly.    If the fingers are laid lightly over the gland, a palpable thrill due to vascularity and known as the 'thyroid thrill' can often be felt (*Fig.* 216).    Auscultation will often reveal a systolic bruit in these cases.

*Fig.* 216.—Feeling for a 'thyroid thrill'.

## MALIGNANT GOITRE

When the whole or a portion of the gland feels stony hard, carcinoma of the thyroid should cross the clinician's mind, and particular attention must be paid to fixity to, or freedom from, surrounding structures.    Arising here, it should be remembered that Hashimoto's thyroiditis (*syn.* struma lymphomatosa), which is not malignant, causes a very hard, fixed, somewhat irregular enlargement of the whole gland. In this connexion, Berry's sign may prove useful.

*Berry's Sign.* — When the thyroid gland enlarges it displaces the carotid tree backwards and outwards.    Consequently, in many cases of large goitre the pulsation of the carotid artery

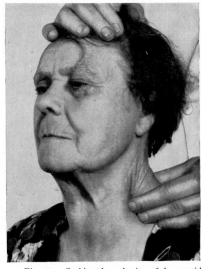

*Fig.* 217.—Seeking the pulsation of the carotid artery.  Berry's sign.  The pulsation could not be detected in this case of carcinoma of the thyroid.

HIROTOSHI HASHIMOTO, *Contemporary Surgeon, Okayama, Japan.*
SIR JAMES BERRY, 1860–1946, *Surgeon, Royal Free Hospital, London.*

can be felt behind the posterior edge of the swelling. The displaced artery is much less in evidence when the thyroid is the seat of malignant disease, for it tends to become surrounded by the tumour (*Fig.* 217).

Remember that carcinoma of the thyroid sometimes gives rise to distant metastases, especially in bones.

## SUSPECTED HYPOTHYROIDISM : CONFIRMATORY SIGNS

The bloated, sallow facies with bagginess of the eyelids—well likened to that of a wax doll that has been in the shop window too long (Marshall)—combined with some degree of mental apathy, awakens in the mind of the clinician the possibility of myxœdema (*Fig.* 218). The subcutaneous tissues everywhere are firm and podgy (pseudo-œdema). The hair is dry and scanty, especially in the outer thirds of the eyebrows. The pulse is slow. The temperature is often subnormal. One examines the supraclavicular regions for pads of fat, but their absence does not disturb the diagnosis. The neck is scrutinized, but owing to pseudo-œdema it is often most difficult to be certain whether any thyroid gland can be made out or not. This is in contrast to the examination of the neck of an infant cretin, where

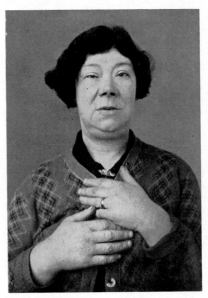

Fig. 218.—Myxœdema.

one can feel the rings of the trachea so plainly that it is possible to be confident of an absent thyroid gland.

## LINGUAL THYROID

While on the subject of ascertaining whether or not a thyroid gland is present in front of the trachea, one should remember that when the thyroid occupies an aberrant position, the aberrant thyroid is often the only thyroid. An aberrant thyroid gland can be situated anywhere in the thyroglossal tract : that is, from the foramen cæcum of the tongue to where the isthmus of the normal thyroid should be situated.   It behoves one, therefore, when confronted with a central swelling at the back of the tongue (*Fig.* 219) or a swelling believed to be a thyroglossal cyst (*see below*) to make it a rule to ascertain by palpation whether a thyroid gland is present in the normal situation.

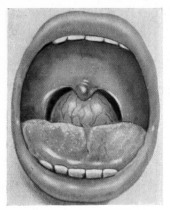

*Fig.* 219.—Lingual thyroid.

## THE  PARATHYROIDS

An enlarged parathyroid is seldom palpable upon clinical examination. It can be found only by exploration when the whole thyroid gland has been displayed at operation.

However, in relevant cases, particularly in examples of recurrent renal calculus and in osteitis fibrosa, an attempt should be made by systematic palpation to discover a possibly enlarged parathyroid.

Tetany can follow removal of the parathyroids at thyroidectomy.

**Trousseau's Sign.**—A sphygmomanometer cuff is placed around the arm and the pressure raised to 200 mm. Hg. If tetany is present, in five minutes typical contractions of the hand are seen— the so-called ' obstetrician's hand ' (*Fig.* 220).

**The Chvostek-Weiss Sign.**—Percuss one side of the face lightly.   A spasm of the facial muscles is brought on.   The sign is seen particularly in tetany, but it is also occasionally seen in cases of tetanus.

*Fig.* 220.—Tetany ; the ' obstetrician's hand '.

## THYROGLOSSAL  CYSTS  AND  FISTULÆ

**A Thyroglossal Cyst** above the thyroid cartilage (*Fig.* 221) is usually in the middle line.   Between the isthmus of the thyroid and the superior border of the thyroid cartilage, it is never exactly median : it lies in the course of the levator glandulæ thyroideæ, which is usually on the left side of the ala of the thyroid cartilage.

A thyroglossal cyst must be distinguished from an enlarged pre-tracheal lymph-node.   A sign that is often helpful in this differential diagnosis is as follows : A thyroglossal cyst moves upwards when the tongue is protruded.   Request the patient to open his mouth.

Grasp the swelling between the finger and thumb (*Fig.* 222). Then instruct him to put out his tongue : to put it in and put it out again. As the tongue is fully protruded (*Fig.* 223) a certain amount of movement of all swellings in this region is to be expected, but in the case of a thyroglossal cyst the upward tug is unmistakable.

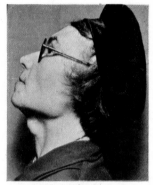

Thyroglossal cysts are prone to attacks of inflammation, and when seen in the acute stage are liable to be mistaken for abscesses. When inflammation is severe the overlying cellulitis spreads around the neck in a necklace-like manner.

**A Thyroglossal Fistula** may result from bursting (or incision) of an inflamed thyroglossal cyst. More often, the fistula is an aftermath of incomplete extirpation

*Fig.* 221.—Subhyoid thyroglossal cyst. This is the most common situation for a thyroglossal cyst.

of the thyroglossal tract, i.e., local removal of a thyroglossal cyst.

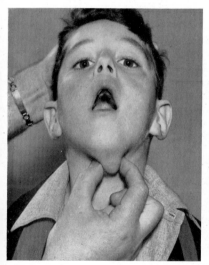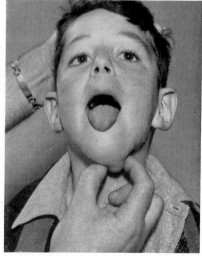

*Figs.* 222 and 223.—If the swelling is a thyroglossal cyst, the upward tug when the patient fully protrudes his tongue is characteristic. Note that the mouth must be open when the swelling is grasped.

Usually the fistula is situated strictly in the middle line (*Fig.* 224) but in cases following incomplete removal of the thyroglossal tract the fistula may present itself at one or other extremity of a tranverse scar. In such cases and when the fistula is situated low in the neck (I have encountered several examples in Burns's space), the condition is liable to be confused with a sinus connected with a tuberculous

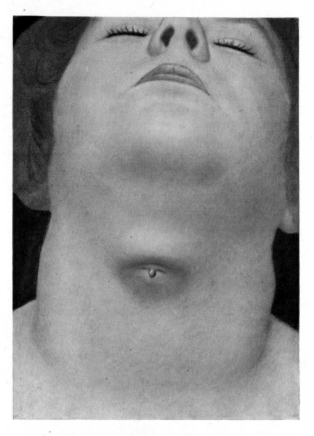

*Fig.* 224.—Thyroglossal fistula. An inflamed cyst was incised in early childhood and the discharge continued. Attacks of inflammation recurred at frequent intervals.

lymph-node. Endeavour to express a bead of the discharge from the fistula ; usually the discharge is purulent and a scab must be removed to give it exit ; less often a glairy yellow or brown fluid runs more or less freely from the fistula.

## CHAPTER XIII

# THE BREAST AND AXILLARY LYMPH–NODES

## EXAMINATION OF THE BREAST

It is customary to meet two classes of patients. The first is the out-patient, in whom the breasts are examined while the patient, undressed as far as the waist, sits with a shawl or blanket over her shoulders. The second is the patient in bed. Unless there is some contra-indication, the examination of the patient in bed should be made comparable with that of the out-patient, and thus, standardizing our technique, findings will tend to become uniformly accurate.

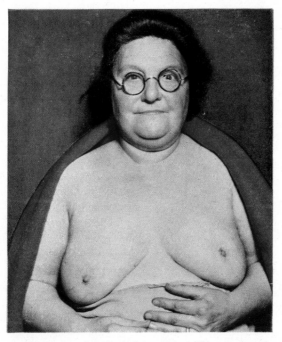

*Fig.* 225.—Comparison of the level of the nipples. This case of neoplasm of the left breast shows the nipple raised on the affected side.

**Preparing for an Examination of the Breasts of a Patient in Bed.**—The patient is required to remove her nightdress to the waist. The nurse then puts a shawl over the patient's shoulders. A pillow is adjusted with its flat surface against the head of the bed, and the patient is instructed to sit bolt upright with her back against the pillow.

## ROUTINE EXAMINATION OF THE BREASTS

**Inspection.**—See that the patient sits 'square'. If the skin over the breast is reddened, inquire if counter-irritants have been applied. Observe the level of the nipples (*Fig.* 225): remember that sometimes the left breast normally hangs lower than the right.

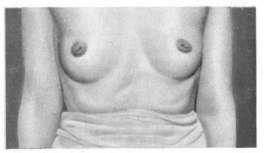

Fig. 226.—Retraction of the nipples.

*The Nipples.*—The normal nipple points slightly downwards and outwards. If retraction of the nipple is observed (*Fig.* 226), immediately ask the patient how long this has been present: retraction is of cardinal importance only if it is recent (*Fig.* 227), when it indicates that neoplastic (or rarely inflammatory) fibrosis is proceeding in the breast.

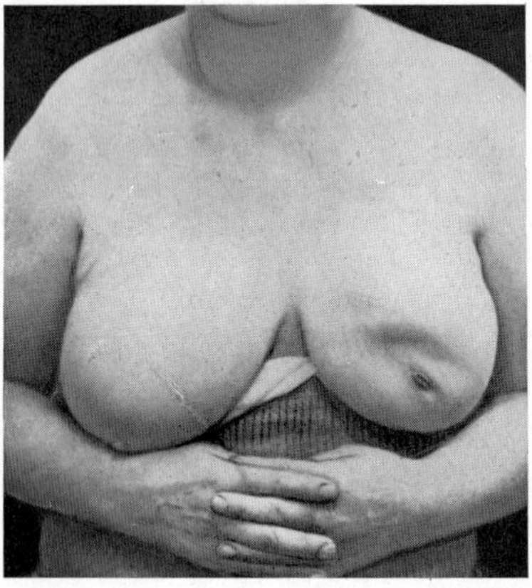

Close inspection of the nipple may reveal a crack, which is sometimes of considerable diagnostic importance in cases where a deep-seated breast abscess is in question. In this connexion one should not always hastily conclude that, because the breast looks inflamed, a more serious condition can be

Fig. 227.—Recent retraction of the nipple. Note also the dimpling of the skin above the nipple.

ruled out. In cases of mastitis carcinomatosis (*Fig.* 228) the proliferation of carcinoma is so rapid that heat and redness are present. A dry eczema of the nipple suggests Paget's disease (*Fig.* 229).

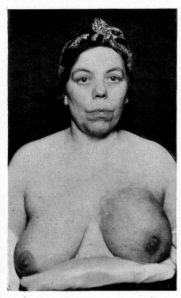

*Fig.* 228.—Mastitis carcinomatosis.

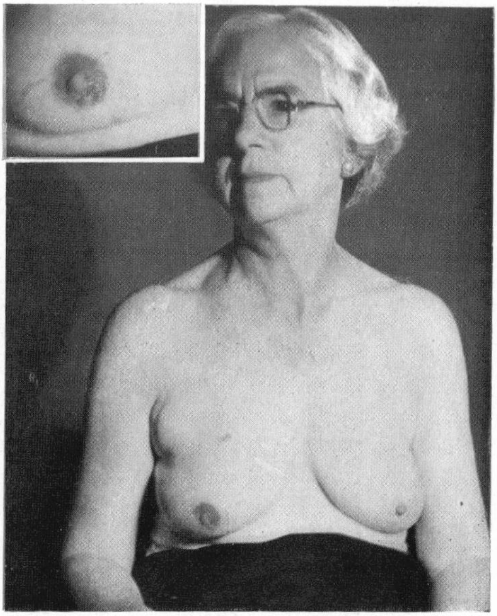

*Fig.* 229.—Early Paget's disease of the nipple.

*The areola* should be inspected and the degree of pigmentation, if any, noted. It is well to remember that the specialized glands of Montgomery are subject to the same affections as other sebaceous glands. *The remainder of the integument of the breast* now receives attention.

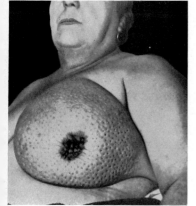

*Fig.* 230.—*Peau d'orange.*

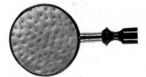

*Fig.* 231.—*Peau d'orange* is conspicuous when viewed through a magnifying glass.

In addition to general observation—e.g., the presence of signs of inflammation or of a lump—look for

Sir James Paget, 1814–1899, *Surgeon, St. Bartholomew's Hospital, London.*
William Montgomery, 1797–1859, *Professor of Midwifery, Dublin.*

alteration in the quality of the skin (*peau d'orange*) (*Fig.* 230). The earliest manifestation of this phenomenon is seen best with the aid of a magnifying glass (*Fig.* 231). *Peau d'orange* is rendered more obvious by squeezing the skin gently (*Fig.* 232).

When the arms are raised fully above the head, visible signs of carcinoma of the breast (e.g., tethering of the skin) frequently become more apparent (Auchincloss).

If the patient has noticed a lump, ask her to find it herself, before you attempt to do so.

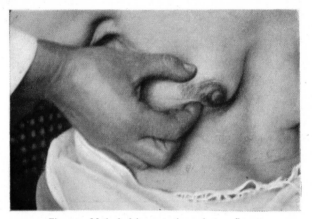

*Fig.* 232.—Method of demonstrating early *peau d'orange*.

**Palpation.**—Commence by examining the opposite breast. Palpate the whole breast with the flat of the hand (*Fig.* 233). Next,

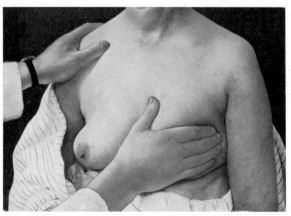

*Fig.* 233.—Palpating the breast with the flat of the hand.

HUGH AUCHINCLOSS, *Contemporary Professor of Clinical Surgery, College of Physicians and Surgeons, Columbia University, New York.*

palpate the four quadrants of the breast (*Fig.* 234) systematically between the finger and thumb. A useful routine is ; (1) Upper and inner quadrant : (2) Upper and outer quadrant, including axillary tail : (3) Lower and inner quadrant : (4) Lower and outer quadrant.

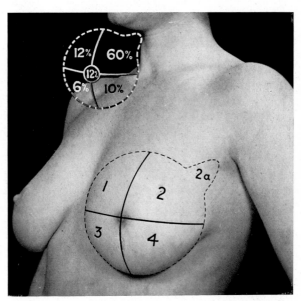

*Fig.* 234.—The quadrants of the breast. It should be noted that the upper and outer quadrant includes the axillary tail (*2a*). Inset shows the relative frequency of carcinoma in the various quadrants.

Finally, palpate directly behind the nipple, during which man-œuvre it should be noted whether any secretion can be expressed from the nipple (*see* p. 130). Afterwards examine the axilla (*see* p. 133).

Proceed in exactly the same manner on the affected side. If there is a lump, note ;—

*Its position*—in which quadrant of the breast.*

*Consistency and shape*—hard or soft, regular or irregular, and so on.

*Fixity to the skin* is tested by gently pinching up the overlying skin : this should be done systematically over the whole surface of the lump (*Fig.* 235). The principal exception to the infallibility of this sign of malignancy is when the lump is situated immediately behind

---

* It is valuable to remember that the breast occupies the interval from the 2nd to the 6th ribs. Swellings of a doubtful nature situated above or below these levels are unlikely to arise from breast tissue.

the nipple.   A swelling in this situation, whatever its nature, is usually superficially adherent, because, if it is not an integral part of the duct mechanism, some or all of the sixteen or so ducts that are about to open upon the surface of the nipple of necessity traverse the substance of the swelling.   *Consequently, the most benign of lumps may be attached to the nipple.*

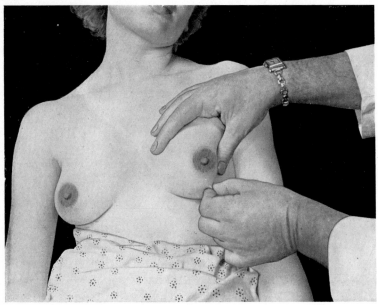

*Fig.* 235.—Testing the mobility of the skin over the lump.   Areas of skin are picked up as in pinching.   By this method early tethering of the skin to the lump can be detected.

*Special Method in Doubtful Cases.*—Valuable information can sometimes be obtained by placing the patient in the knee-elbow position, and inspecting the breasts from the front and the sides.   Displacement of the nipple or indrawing of the skin in the neighbourhood of the lump often becomes apparent in this posture (Basil Rooke).

*Fixity to deep structures (the pectoral fascia).*   By far the best method of putting the pectoralis major into full contraction is by pressing the hand firmly into the side : the truth of this assertion can be confirmed upon oneself.   Ask the patient to place her hand lightly upon her hip with the thumb behind ; feel the pectoralis major : it is quite loose and soft.   Pick up the lump between the fingers and try its mobility, first in a horizontal, then in a vertical direction.   Now ask the patient to press her hand firmly into the side (*Fig.* 236), and feel the pectoralis major ; it is in full contraction.   Try the mobility of the lump once more in two planes.   It should be

A. BASIL ROOKE, *Contemporary Surgeon, Royal Victoria and West Hants Hospital, Milford-on-Sea, England.*

noted that the mobility of the normal breast upon the pectoral muscle is limited to a considerable extent by the full contraction of the muscle, and it requires a certain amount of experience to appreciate minor degrees of pathological fixity.

Swellings towards the periphery of the lower and outer quadrant lie on the serratus magnus, and that muscle should be put into contraction, when testing for mobility of a lump in this situation. Ask the patient to place the hand of the affected side upon your shoulder, and to press. This puts the serratus magnus in full contraction.

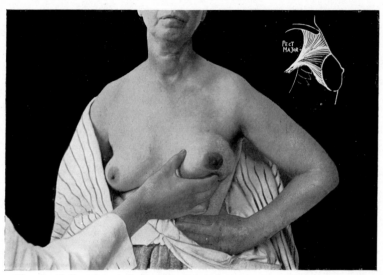

*Fig.* 236.—Testing a lump in the breast for fixity to deeper structures. The patient presses her hand firmly into her side. This puts the pectoralis major into full contraction.

When the breasts are large and pendulous, and the lump is deeply placed, it is well worth taking the trouble to persuade the patient to submit to an examination with the breasts in a hanging position. For this purpose she must kneel on a couch, lean forwards and support herself with her outstretched arms.

At the conclusion of every examination of a tumour of the breast where the signs leave little doubt as to malignancy, the lungs and the liver should be examined for secondary deposits.

*      *      *      *      *

**Chronic Interstitial Mastitis.**—Often the whole breast, indeed both breasts, are inclined to be ' lumpy ' and they may be slightly tender.  At other times the lumpiness is confined to a sector of the breast (*Fig.* 237), this variety usually being associated with a

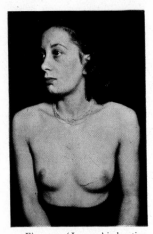

*Fig.* 237.—'Lumpy' induration confined to a sector of the breast. Note the inverted nipple on the affected side.

retracted nipple, which in turn has obstructed a lactiferous duct or ducts. In still other cases there is an ill-defined lump in an otherwise tolerably normal breast.

The differential diagnosis between chronic interstitial mastitis and early carcinoma of the breast is sometimes exceedingly difficult. This is not surprising, for the first is a pre-carcinomatous condition, and tends to merge into the second in patients belonging to the later age groups. If, after a thorough examination, no conclusion can be reached, it is safer to assume a carcinoma and leave the diagnosis to be settled at operation.

**Cyst of the Breast.**—If the physical examination suggests a cyst of the breast, endeavour to elicit fluctuation.  In order that this may be tried, it is necessary for an onlooker to 'fix' the swelling (*see* p. 10). Translucency should be sought (*Fig.* 238) : it often yields valuable information, particularly when carried out in a darkened room.

Large breasts may be trans-illuminated with advantage with the breasts in the pendulous position (Clapham Coates).

**A Discharge from the Nipple.**—When a patient gives a history of a discharge from the nipple, the breast is squeezed gently in an endeavour to express some of the fluid.  The character of this fluid is of great diagnostic significance.  An obviously blood-tinged fluid is pathognomonic

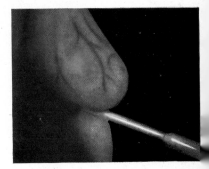

*Fig.* 238.—Appearance of a simple cyst filled with clear fluid as seen on transillumination.

of a duct papilloma or a duct carcinoma : a thin dark-brown discharge suggests the same diagnosis, but also that the blood has been pent up in the duct for some time.  Dark-green mucoid material usually means that a retention cyst associated with chronic interstitial mastitis communicates with a lactiferous duct. Often a discharge can be expressed only when the breast is pressed at a particular place (*Fig.* 239), i.e., behind the obstructed duct.

**Milk engorgement** is a condition which causes much confusion, particularly when one breast or a portion of one breast alone is involved. If the patient is, or recently has been, lactating, and a cystic swelling without obvious signs of acute inflammation is present, try to express a little milk from the *other* breast.

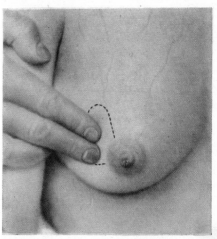

*Fig.* 239.—Duct papilloma of the breast with retention cyst. Pressure over the cyst causes a blood-stained discharge to appear at the nipple.

If milk appears apply a breast pump to the affected breast. If the swelling in question is due to milk engorgement it will subside as the milk is drawn off.

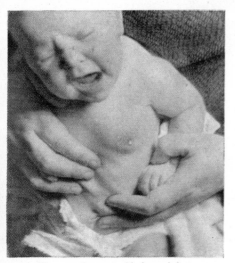

*Fig.* 240.—Acute mastitis in an infant.

**Acute Mastitis.**—The diagnosis of mastitis of infants is obvious by inspection alone (*Fig.* 240). In other examples of acute mastitis the examination of the breast is usually simple ; it does not entail the painstaking care outlined already. Examine the nipple carefully for a crack or abrasion, a finding that is comparatively rare. Most breast abscesses are due to staphylococci entering the lactiferous ducts : such infection is favoured by a retracted or poorly developed nipple. Palpate the inflamed breast with extreme gentleness, the object being to ascertain which portion is most indurated, for there will lie the maximum purulent accumulation. When the breast is not as tender as we might expect, but the induration is greater and the history is somewhat prolonged, it is expedient to try to eliminate the possibility of mastitis carcinomatosis, that galloping cancer of young, pregnant, or lactating women.

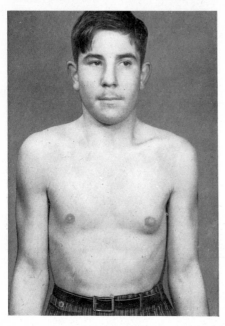

Fig. 241.—Mastitis of puberty.

*Mastitis of puberty* (*Fig.* 241). One breast is tender, slightly swollen, and inflamed. Curiously, the condition is usually seen in boys and is hardly ever bilateral.

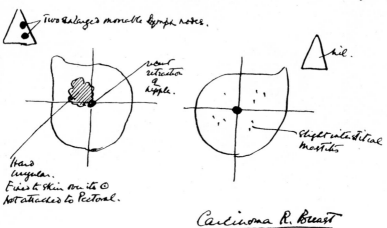

Fig. 242.—Facsimile record of a clinical examination of the breast. (N.B. ☉ = centre.)

**Record of the Clinical Examination of the Breast.**—The record of the examination may be entered conveniently in the graphical manner of which *Fig.* 242 is an actual example. The breast is divided into four quadrants, and a triangle represents the axilla. The clinical findings registered in this way form an accurate record that is more valuable than much description.

## THE MALE BREAST

The examination of the male breast is carried out in the same manner as in the female. There is one sign I have found of value in mastitis in the male. Ask the patient to take off all the clothing above the waist, and then to re-place his braces (*Fig.* 243). The cause of the mastitis is sometimes evident.

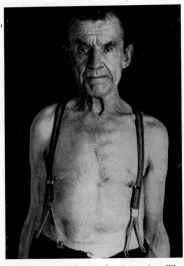

*Fig.* 243.—Mastitis in the male. The patient has been asked to put his braces on without his shirt. This sometimes reveals the cause of the mastitis, as in the accompanying figure. A braces button being lost, the remaining button draws the brace inwards, and the buckle against the nipple.

## EXAMINATION OF THE AXILLARY LYMPH-NODES

The patient should be seated slightly to the right, but facing the surgeon. The right axilla is palpated with the left hand, and vice versa. Let us assume that the left axilla is to be palpated. The various groups of lymph-nodes are indicated in *Fig.* 244.

**The Central Group.**—Raise the patient's arm from her side, and pass the extended fingers of the right hand high up into the apex of the axilla, directing the palm towards the lateral thoracic wall (*Fig.* 245). The patient's arm is now brought to her side once more, and the forearm rests on the examiner's forearm. She is asked to let the arm hang loosely in this position (*Fig.* 246). When this instruction has been carried out, the non-examining hand is free to place upon the patient's right shoulder, and serves to steady and control subsequent manœuvres. The fingers in the axilla are pressed upwards again to be sure that the highest limit is reached. The fingers (the pulps of which are applied to the lateral thoracic wall) pass downwards with a firm, sliding movement.

9

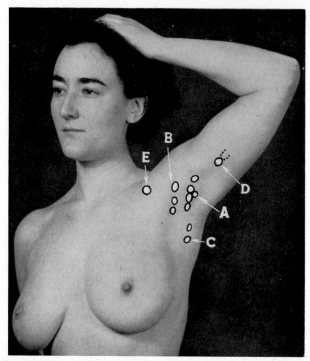

*Fig.* 244.—The axillary lymph-nodes from a clinical standpoint.  **A,** Central group ;  **B,** Pectoral group ;
**C,** Subscapular group ;  **D,** Lymph-nodes around the hiatus semilunaris ;  **E,** Costo-coracoid group.

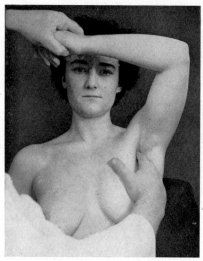

*Fig.* 245.—Examining the axilla (I). The
arm is raised, and the fingers are inserted as
high as is possible.

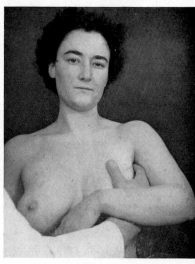

*Fig.* 246.—Examining the axilla (II).
Note that the patient's arm rests comfortably
over the examiner's arm.

If the central axillary lymphatic nodes are enlarged, they will be felt momentarily imprisoned between the thorax and the examining fingers (*Fig.* 247) : their number, size, and consistency are noted.

**The Pectoral Group** of lymph-nodes is next examined. The patient's arm is elevated, and the fingers are insinuated beneath the pectoralis major. This time the pulps of the fingers are directed forwards. The pectoralis minor muscle can frequently be detected, and between the two pectorals are situated the pectoral lymphatic nodes. Finally palpate around the insertion of the pectoralis major and the hiatus semilunaris for

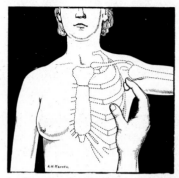

*Fig.* 247.—A node high in the axilla momentarily imprisoned between the thorax and the examining fingers.

enlarged lymph-nodes lying upon the third part of the axillary artery.

**The Subscapular Group.**—The subscapular lymphatic nodes lying in the posterior axillary fold are best examined from the back (*Fig.* 248). Standing behind the patient, the examiner palpates the

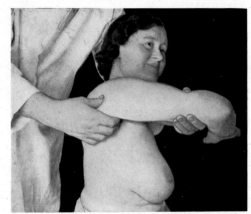

*Fig.* 248.—Examining, from the back, the subscapular lymph-nodes lying in the posterior fold of the axilla.

antero-internal surface of the latissimus dorsi, and if these lymph-nodes are enlarged they will be found at the bottom of the fold. The apex of the axilla may be palpated from this aspect, which gives good access to the more posterior of the central group of lymph-nodes.

**Costocoracoid Group.**—Occasionally the costocoracoid group of lymph-nodes is enlarged when those of the axilla are not. Enlargement of lymph-nodes lying on the costocoracoid membrane may be suspected when there is an obliteration of the infraclavicular hollow. In addition, there may be unilateral prominence of the veins in this region.

\*        \*        \*        \*        \*

Sometimes it is difficult to be sure whether a given lump is situated in the axillary tail of the breast, or whether it is due to a secondary growth in the lowermost of the pectoral group of lymphatic lymph-nodes (*Fig.* 249).

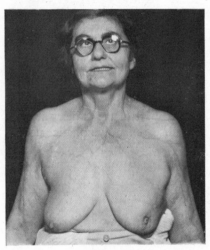

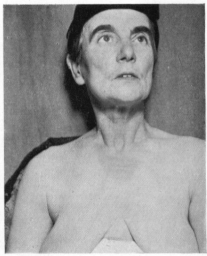

*Fig.* 249.—Massive secondary involvement of the lowermost pectoral group of lymphatic nodes. There is a primary growth the size of a hazel-nut in the breast proper, causing retraction of the nipple.

*Fig.* 250.—A tender swelling under the right pectoralis major is present. Temperature 100·8°F. The patient attributed the condition to lifting a bag of potatoes ten days previously. Subpectoral abscess.

When the axillary lymph-nodes are the seat of bacterial invasion (often due to an infected lesion of the hand or arm) they are wont to break down and form an axillary abscess. Particularly if it is the subpectoral group that is involved (*Fig.* 250), the abscess may escape a cursory examination.

## CHAPTER XIV

# THE THORAX

THE thorax is considered so fully in medical works that no purpose would be served by embarking upon a detailed consideration of physical signs connected with intrathoracic disease. We will, therefore, focus attention on various points of particular surgical significance.

Much information can be obtained from general inspection of the thorax, and an astute surgeon will not fail to notice the thoracic build and respiratory expansion in every relevant case.

*The barrel chest*, the most striking feature of which is an increased antero-posterior diameter of the thorax, suggests chronic emphysema, but kyphosis can cause a similar appearance.

*Pigeon breast (Fig.* 251) is the result of some bygone obstruction to inspiration at a time when the ribs were pliable.

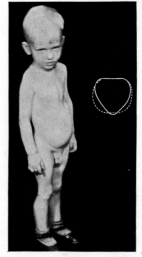

*The flat chest* is, on the whole, a mis-leading guide to chronic pulmonary disease, notably phthisis. Special attention should be given to the conformation of the supra-clavicular fossæ.

*The visceroptotic chest.* The sloping shoulders and great obliquity of the ribs, combined with a narrow subcostal angle

*Fig.* 251.—Pigeon breast.

(*see* p. 206), are a regular accompaniment of the virginal type of visceroptosis. This type of thorax must be distinguished from the flat chest.

*Harrison's sulcus* is a transverse depression, situated at the xiphisternal junction and passing laterally towards the mid-axillary lines (*Fig.* 252). It corresponds to the line of attachment of the diaphragm, and the cause is bygone rickets.

EDWARD HARRISON, 1766–1838, *General Practitioner, Horncastle Lincolnshire.*

*Funnel chest* is due to a depression of the lower part of the sternum, which may extend as high as the third rib. It is usually congenital, and of no clinical importance (*Fig.* 253).

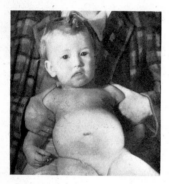

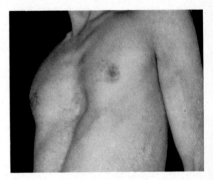

Fig. 252.—Harrison's sulcus.

*Fig.* 253.—Funnel chest.

Elderly shoemakers are apt to have a depression in the lowest part of the sternum from long-continued pressure of the last.

The ' *rickety rosary* ' is the term given to enlargement of the costochondral articulations in children suffering from rickets (*Fig.* 254).

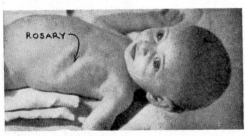

Fig. 254.—The rickety rosary.

*Unilateral contraction of the thorax* suggests chronic pulmonary disease. The retracted side is obviously smaller than its fellow, and the corresponding shoulder droops. The ribs, especially in the mid-axillary line, can be felt crowded together ; they may nearly overlap. The spine is curved with its concavity towards the diseased side. Such changes due to disease of a lung are somewhat similar to those of scoliosis (*see* chapter XXXI) arising from other causes. Without attempting to enter into the diagnosis of chronic pulmonary disease, the surgeon should determine the position of the apex beat and also palpate the trachea.

By applying a thumb in the suprasternal notch (*Fig.* 255) the trachea can easily be felt and deviation of the trachea be readily detected. Deviation of the trachea to one or other side is a most valuable sign of contracted lung, and it is present in most cases of pulmonary tuberculosis, even in the early stages (Webb).

*Unilateral bulging of the thorax* can be due to gas or fluid in the pleural cavity, as well as to intra-thoracic cysts, tumours, or a dia-phragmatic hernia.

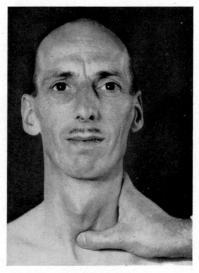

Should the thorax be under-developed or deformed, almost in-stinctively one looks at the hands. Clubbing of the fingers (*Fig.* 256) is a sign of chronic anoxæmia from any cause ; if the cause can be removed, the clubbing often gradually disappears. The nails of such fingers are curved longi-tudinally like a parrot's beak. Hippocrates described them as one of the signs of chronic empyema.

*Fig.* 255.—Palpating the suprasternal notch for tracheal deviation.

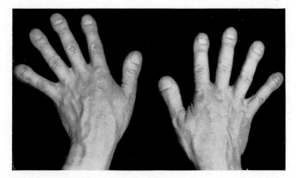

*Fig.* 256.—Clubbing of the fingers.

## OBSERVING RESPIRATORY EXCURSIONS

After noting the way the thorax expands under normal conditions, ask the patient to breathe deeply, and continue the observation. Note the expansion in an upward direction (apices) and downward direction (abdominal movement), as well as the more obvious lateral movement.

GERALD BERTRAM WEBB, *Contemporary Physician, Colorado Springs, U.S.A.*
HIPPOCRATES, *born on the island of Cos about* 460 B.C., *is justly regarded as the Father of Medicine.*

Still continuing the determination of the extent of respiratory excursions, place the hands over each apex and then over each base.

## METHOD OF COUNTING RIBS

Often it is necessary to know which rib is injured or diseased. Running the finger downwards from the suprasternal notch, a transverse ridge can be felt, and often seen—the angle of Louis. The finger, moved to the left or the right along this ridge, will pass directly on to the second rib. Ribs are counted from this point (*Fig.* 257).

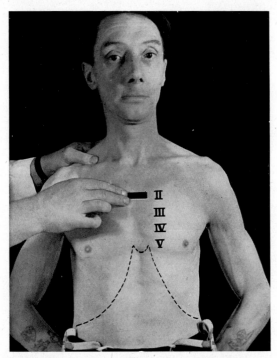

*Fig.* 257.—Method of counting ribs. The angle of Louis is found ; this is opposite the second costal cartilage. Bearings are taken from this point.

Posteriorly, ribs may be counted upwards, starting with the 12th, which can usually be felt, but in obese individuals only with difficulty. When the arm rests by the side, the lower angle of the scapula lies upon the 7th rib. The spine of the scapula lies over the 3rd rib or 3rd intercostal space, but these scapular surface markings are not absolutely reliable guides.

PIERRE CHARLES ALEXANDRE LOUIS, 1787–1872, *Physician in Paris. Some consider that it was* ANTOINE LOUIS (1723–1792), *Surgeon to the Charité Hospital, Paris, and designer of the guillotine, to whom the Angle of Louis should be attributed.*

*The costal margin* is of considerable surgical importance. The subcostal angle is considered on p. 206, and the sign of tender costal cartilage in gall-stones on p. 212.

*Slipping Rib.*—The pain is referred to the exact position of the rib, which is usually the tenth. The tip of the tenth cartilage can be moved upwards freely, and this movement causes pain. Patients with slipping rib are usually women (Davies-Colley).

## CYANOSIS

Particularly if the patient's normal complexion is known to the clinician, and provided the light is good, even a tinge of cyanosis is discernible at once. When cyanosis is perceived, focus your attention on respiratory movement—Are respirations laboured? Do they appear painful? Then proceed to count the respirations. Probably because my memory for numbers is poor, I am not above refreshing it from the following table.

| | | | |
|---|---|---|---|
| 1st year | .. | 35–45 | To be of value the respira- |
| 1–2 years | .. | 20–45 | tory rate of small children |
| 3–4 ,, | .. | 20–40 | must be taken when they |
| 4–5 ,, | .. | 30 | are at rest (Holt). |
| Adults | .. | 16–20 | |

As the count is made over half a minute, attention is riveted on the nostrils for movement of the alæ nasi. The contents of the sputum pot, if available, are scrutinized in the manner taught so thoroughly on the medical side.

**Laryngeal Obstruction.**— Dyspnœa and cyanosis are, of course, cardinal signs of obstruction of the larynx, but I wish to direct attention to another very important sign—

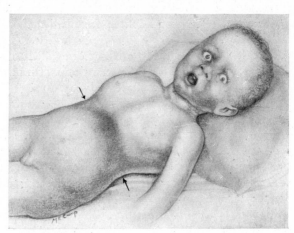

Fig. 258.—Laryngeal diphtheria. At each inspiration the dyspnœic child's lower ribs are sucked in. The sign of recession.

ROBERT DAVIES-COLLEY, *Contemporary Consulting Surgeon, Guy's Hospital, London.*
LUTHER E. HOLT, 1855–1924, *Professor of Diseases of Children, Columbia University, New York.*

*The Sign of Recession.*—The lower end of the sternum, together with the adjacent costal framework, the supraclavicular fossæ and epigastrium, is sucked in during inspiration. This sign is especially noticeable in young children (*Fig.* 258). In older children and adults, owing to the greater rigidity of the chest wall, recession is rarely much in evidence. Considerable and persistent recession is the surest guide that tracheotomy (or intubation) is required urgently.

**Obstruction to a Large Bronchus** (usually due to a foreign body or a plug of mucus).—Collapse of the corresponding lobe may be produced within a short time. The trachea is apt to be pulled towards the affected lobe, therefore examine the trachea in the supra-sternal notch (*see Fig.* 255). A more reliable and constant sign is displacement of the apex beat—a fact that is helpful in differentiating this condition from pneumonia (Brock). In post-operative cases massive collapse of a lung should be suspected in a patient who, within 48 hours of having an inhalation anæsthetic, has a rapid pulse-rate and an abrupt rise of temperature combined with respiratory distress.

A point in the diagnosis of bronchial carcinoma first suggested by Chevalier Jackson is to get the patient to breathe through his open mouth : then, if one listens close to his mouth, an inspiratory and expiratory stridor is audible.

**Pulmonary Embolism.**—The patient (who has usually had an operation ten to fourteen days previously and apparently is progressing favourably) suddenly cries out. There is a feeling of impending death from suffocation, and usually a great desire to defæcate. The condition is frequently, though not necessarily, rapidly fatal.

We will assume that we have been called to a case in which the diagnosis is in doubt, for pulmonary embolism may simulate an intra-abdominal catastrophe, and vice versa.

After examining the pulse, look in the sputum pot, for sometimes blood-stained sputum is coughed up : this, however, appears not to be the rule. The next duty is to *look at the legs and feet*. Here will be found tell-tale evidence in a percentage of cases—not a very large one in my experience. If one leg is œdematous and pits on pressure, it is highly probable that there is thrombosis in the corresponding iliac vein, and this sign, in conjunction with the sudden thoracic symptoms, is often sufficient to establish the diagnosis. Physical signs of infarction of the lung may be present in the thorax, but it is not advisable to disturb the patient in order to elicit them.

RUSSELL CLAUDE BROCK, *Contemporary Surgeon, Guy's and Brompton Hospitals, London.*
CHEVALIER JACKSON, Senior, *Contemporary Emeritus Professor of Laryngology, Jefferson Medical College, Philadelphia.*

## INJURIES TO THE THORAX

**Fractured Rib.**—Ask the patient, who is stripped to the waist, to take a deep breath. If a rib or ribs are fractured, pain is likely to be experienced in the region of the fracture before the zenith of inspiration, and he at once clasps a hand to the injured part in an endeavour to support it. Careful palpation along each rib in this region will often reveal evidence of a breach of bony continuity, especially in a thin subject and when the fracture is of one of the upper ribs. Such evidence is frequently more reliable than a radiograph. In fat or muscular individuals, particularly when the fracture is situated somewhere in the middle of the series, which is quite a common situation, the compression test is valuable.

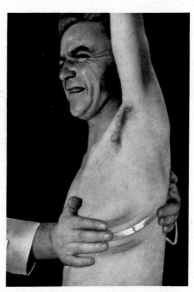

*Fig.* 259.—The compression test for fractured rib.

*The Compression Test.*—The base of one hand is placed over the sternum, and the base of the other over the spine, the thorax is then compressed antero-posteriorly (*Fig.* 259). When a rib has been fractured this manœuvre causes pain at the site of the lesion.

Auscultation for crepitus has some value in obscure incomplete fractures : in doubtful cases this method should be employed.

**Fracture of the Sternum.**—The posture is characteristic : the body is bent forwards with the shoulders rotated inwards, and the head held forwards and downwards. Thanks to the comparative accessibility of the sternum to the palpating fingers, the deformity associated with a fracture of this structure is usually detected without difficulty. The spinal column must be examined for a concomitant injury.

**Traumatic Asphyxia** occasionally complicates compression injuries of the thorax, and forms a striking clinical picture which, once seen, is never forgotten (*Fig.* 260). The face is purple : the cyanosis is confined mainly to the face and neck, although it may be seen to a lesser extent on the thorax. The conjunctivæ are bright red from conjunctival hæmorrhages, and small petechial hæmorrhages are seen in the skin.

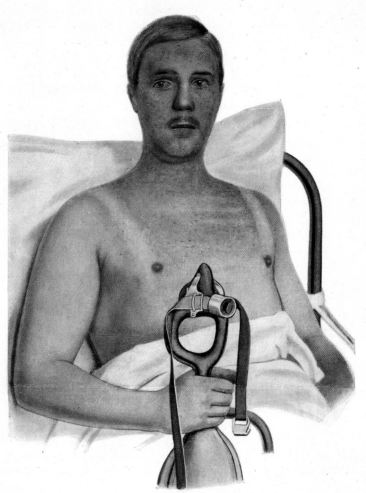

*Fig.* 260.—Traumatic asphyxia.

**Blast Injuries** due to high explosives are borne, to a great extent, by the lungs. In patients who survive, the symptoms and signs are few : consequently, the condition may be overlooked, especially when other lesions are in evidence. Always suspect the presence of lung injury in every patient involved in an explosion. An expanded appearance of the lower chest is a fairly regular accompaniment (*Fig.* 261).

**Surgical Emphysema** has been referred to already (p. 13). A more or less localized emphysema accompanies fracture of the rib with lung penetration by a fragment.

In cases of tension pneumothorax, or a valvular leak in the chest wall, subcutaneous emphysema spreads visibly with each cough, usually in an upward direction. The most extreme examples of surgical emphysema are to be seen when a wound or rupture of the trachea or bronchi allows a communication to exist with the areolar tissue of the mediastinum. In this case the whole of the subcutaneous plane of the neck and face may become distended with air and threaten life by pressure on the great veins.

Every case of thoracic injury with surgical emphysema should be regarded seriously, especially if the answer to the question, " Have you coughed up any blood ? " (an interrogation that must never be omitted) is in the affirmative. The proper procedure in such cases is to look very closely at frequent intervals for signs of hæmo-pneumothorax, having due regard, when the injury is on the left side, for a concomitant rupture of the spleen (*see* p. 306).

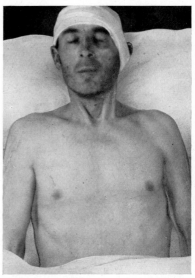

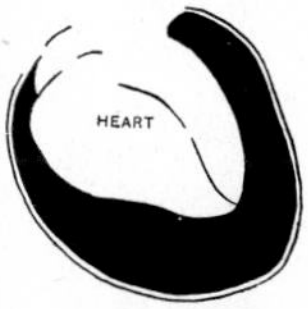

*Fig.* 261.—Blast injury. Appearance of the chest in full inspiration, showing fullness of the lower thorax and over-action of the accessory muscles, notably the sternomastoid.

**Thoracic Wounds.**—'Sucking' wounds indicate that the pleura has been opened. Bloody froth issuing from a wound, coupled with respiratory distress, suggests increased tension.

*Fig.* 262.—
Heart tamponade.

*Heart Tamponade.*—In penetrating wounds of the pericardium the heart may be wounded and bleeding occur into the pericardium. This sometimes gives rise to a precordial bulge. As the hæmopericardium develops, the systemic circulation fails correspondingly, the pulse becoming variable and progressively weaker. The veins of the face and neck become engorged, and the cardiac dullness increases (*Fig.* 262).

## CHRONIC EMPYEMA SINUS

An empyema has been drained, but the sinus continues to discharge indefinitely (*Fig.* 263). Among the common causes of this troublesome complication are ineffectual drainage (*Fig.* 264), a retained drainage tube, necrosis of ribs, thickening of the pleura with fibrosis of the lung, actinomycosis, and tuberculosis. The elucidation of the problem is impossible without the aid of radiography and other diagnostic adjuvants. Nevertheless, at the clinical examination we note the level of the sinus, palpate the bony thorax around it for undue callus formation, percuss and auscultate, and examine the pus for actinomycotic granules (p. 52).

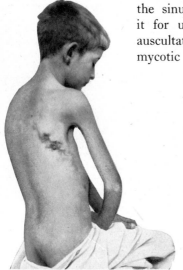

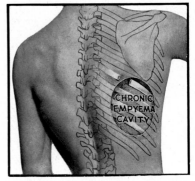

*Fig.* 263.—Chronic empyema sinus of seven years' duration. The opening is at a comparatively high level. This patient's hands are shown in *Fig.* 252 (p. 139).

*Fig.* 264.—An empyema sinus, even when the orifice is pin-point, often communicates with a cavity of considerable size.

## EXAMINATION OF A
## CYSTIC SWELLING OF THE THORACIC WALL

A patient with a cystic swelling connected with the deeper layers of the thoracic wall is presented. After confirming that the swelling fluctuates, apply the following tests : ask the patient to cough, and by inspection and palpation note if there is any impulse.

A favourite location for an *empyema necessitatis*, i.e., one in which the pus has escaped subcutaneously, is the fifth interspace. " I see many empyemata necessitatis, but have yet to meet one with the physical sign of reducibility present. There is nearly always a fluid thrill when the patient coughs, and in such a case occupying the left

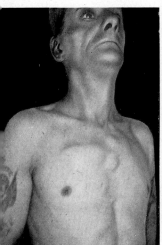

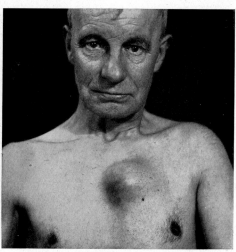

Fig. 265.—Tuberculous abscess connected with the third right costal cartilage. The enlarged costal cartilage can be seen, and the abscess, situated over the gladiolus sterni, is the lower separate swelling.

Fig. 266.—Aortic aneurysm eroding the thoracic wall. The patient had little complaint. His Wassermann reaction was strongly positive.

chest, I have seen it mistaken for an aneurysm because of transmitted pulsation. The thrill on coughing distinguishes it from an aneurysm." (Andreasen.) These signs are absent in the case of *an abscess connected with a tuberculous rib* (*Fig.* 265). Occasionally this cystic swelling is partially reducible into an extrapleural pocket of the abscess cavity.

*A hernia of the lung* is of great rarity : it gives rise to a tympanitic cystic swelling that is completely reducible. It is possible for *an aortic aneurysm* to give rise to a cystic swelling near the sternum (*Fig.* 266), but it is unlikely that such a pulsating swelling will cause diagnostic perplexity.

## SWELLING IN BURNS'S SPACE

By far the commonest cystic non-pulsating swelling situated in Burns's space is a dermoid cyst (*Fig.* 267). This cyst is not connected with the thyroglossal tract nor with the thymus gland.

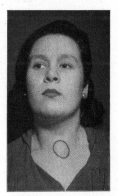

Fig. 267.—Dermoid cyst of Burns's space.

Anthony Turner Andreasen, *Contemporary, formerly Professor of Surgery, Calcutta.*
Allan Burns, 1781–1813, *Extramural Lecturer in Surgery and Anatomy, Glasgow*

## COSTOCHONDRITIS

The patient, always a woman, complains of a varyingly painful swelling of the chest wall.   More often than not she considers that

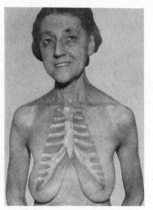

the lump is in the breast, and this is the real cause of the concern, which may be shared by her medical attendant, particularly when the swelling is associated with the fourth or fifth costal cartilages.   The most common costal cartilage to be affected is the third.   On palpation with the pulps of two fingers applied vertically, it becomes quite evident that the swelling in question is caused by an expansion of the costal cartilage as it joins the rib.

In a very small proportion only of these cases which contribute a common clinical entity is the chronic inflammation due to tuberculosis.

*Fig.* 268.—The disposition of the costal cartilages and the over-lying breast.

## RETROMAMMARY  SWELLING

Swellings connected with the bony thorax (*Fig.* 269), when situated immediately behind the breast, are very liable to be confounded with swellings within the breast itself.   *Fig.* 270 shows a case in point. The breast is obviously enlarged.   If the hand be placed over the breast the whole breast will be found to be movable on the swelling

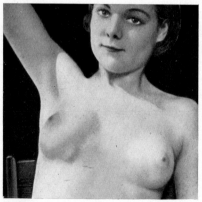

*Fig.* 269.—A retromammary tuberculous swelling connected with a costal cartilage. Mistaken by several observers for a fibro-adenoma of the breast.

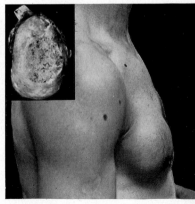

*Fig.* 270 —A tumour of the rib causing enlargement of the breast.   *Inset*—the excised tumour, which proved to be a chondro-sarcoma.

behind it. This is the method by which is settled the important point—"Is the swelling in or behind the breast?"

## RETROCLAVICULAR SWELLINGS

I am referring to swellings situated in the supraclavicular fossa that plunge beneath the clavicle (*Fig.* 271) rather than to enlarged lymphatic nodes in this situation.

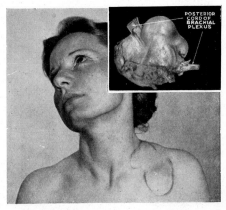

Retroclavicular swellings often present difficulties in diagnosis. A tumour of one of the cords of the brachial plexus appears to be a clinical entity that is liable to be confused with a deep-seated lipoma.

More than once a stony-hard mass in this deep recess beneath the clavicle has proved to be, not malignant lymph-nodes of unknown origin, but an ecchondroma arising from the first rib and containing so little calcium as to make it radio-translucent.

*Fig.* 271.—This retroclavicular swelling was soft and fluctuation could be elicited from the supra-clavicular fossa to below the clavicle. *Inset*—the specimen, which proved to be a neuromyxofibroma of the posterior cord of the brachial plexus.

## SUBDIAPHRAGMATIC ABSCESS

Although not a thoracic lesion, it is more instructive to deal with this condition here for reasons that will be obvious.

Thanks to the adoption of Fowler's position in treatment, sub-diaphragmatic abscess is now comparatively rare.

Nevertheless, subdiaphragmatic abscess remains extremely diffi-cult to diagnose, and clinical methods are still the best guides in arriving at the vital conclusion that, concealed in this inaccessible recess, there is a quantity—often a surprisingly large quantity—of pus. Pain is conspicuous by its absence, but there is always a hectic temperature.* "Signs of pus somewhere, signs of pus no-where else, signs of pus *there*" was Barnard's aphorism regarding subdiaphragmatic abscess, and it is a marvellous compendium of the situation. Having followed his advice regarding the exclusion of pus in other situations, proceed as follows :

---

* This important sign may be masked by penicillin therapy.

10

*Litten's Diaphragmatic Shadow.*—The patient, stripped to the pubes, lies upon his back, with his feet pointing directly towards a window. Cross lights are excluded by darkening all other sources of illumination. The observer stands at the patient's side and watches the respiratory movements (*Fig.* 271). As the ribs *rise* with inspiration a narrow shadow moves *down* the axilla from the seventh to approximately the ninth or tenth rib. By observing this shadow it is possible to tell whether diaphragmatic excursions are taking place normally. The sign can be elicited upon either side.

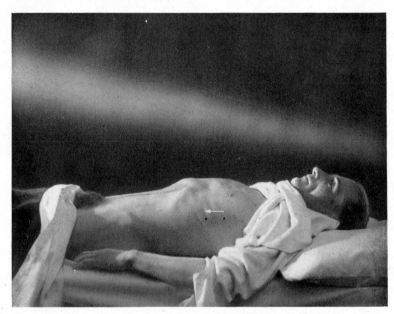

*Fig.* 272.—Observing Litten's diaphragmatic shadow.

**Abdominal Signs.**—Provided the patient is not obese, the information gained by observing Litten's diaphragmatic shadow (*Fig.* 272) is often more reliable than repeated radiographic examinations.

In post-operative cases, where the primary lesion was situated in the right upper quadrant of the abdomen (e.g., perforated duodenal ulcer), there is nearly always a purulent discharge from the wound. In cases of a right posterior abscess (the commonest situation) there is often tenderness over the 11th intercostal space. To elicit this

atisfactorily the patient must be turned on to his face. When the
bscess is left-sided, there is usually tenderness and sometimes a
welling in the position shown in *Fig.* 273.

**Thoracic Signs.**—Just as in acute osteo-
nyelitis there is a sympathetic arthritis of
he near-by joint, so in subdiaphragmatic

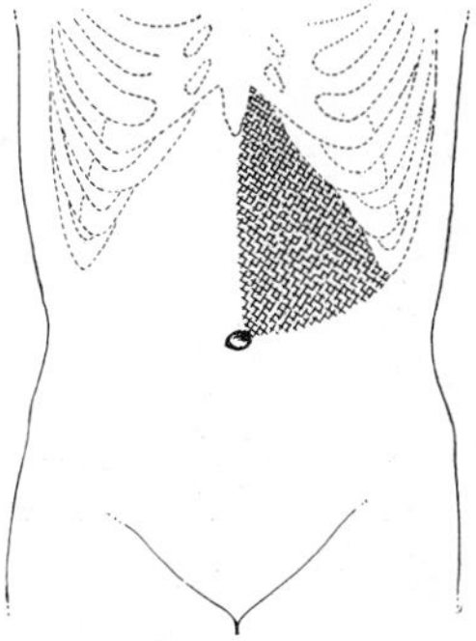

*Fig.* 273.—Left anterior subdiaphragmatic abscess.
Area of tenderness and sometimes fullness.

bscess there is a concomitant basal pleurisy
r pleuro-pneumonia. It must, therefore, be
learly understood that *signs of pneumonia at
he base of the lung favour, rather than hinder,
he diagnosis of subdiaphragmatic abscess.*

*Percussion.*—When gas is present, percussion may yield the
lassical four areas of altered resonance (*Fig.* 274), which are, from

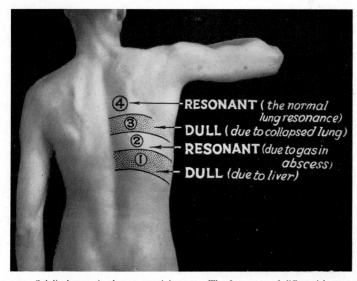

*Fig.* 274.—Subdiaphragmatic abscess containing gas. The four areas of differential percussion.

elow upwards ; (1) Dull—due to liver : (2) Resonant—due to gas
the abscess : (3) Dull—due to collapsed lung : (4) Resonant—the
ormal lung resonance. Unfortunately it is not usual to find this
lassical picture.

*Differential Diagnosis between Subdiaphragmatic Abscess an Primary Empyema.*—The curve of the area of dullness in subdia phragmatic abscess is the curve of the diaphragm, which is dome shaped. The curve of the dullness in empyema is S-shaped. I should be noted also that there is no displacement of the heart laterall in even the largest subdiaphragmatic abscess.

## EXAMINATION OF A CASE OF DYSPHAGIA

Undoubtedly the main points in the examination of a case c increasing dysphagia can be ascertained only by laryngoscopica œsophagoscopical, and radiological methods. Nevertheless there ar certain points to which attention should be directed at the preliminar clinical examination.

Ask the patient where he thinks the food is arrested. If h is intelligent, he can often throw much light upon his own case Examine the mouth. Palpate the neck, particularly for enlarge glands. Eliminate the possibility of aneurysm—for instance, fee both radial pulses simultaneously, and try for a tracheal tug. Examin the abdomen, and at the same time look for signs of wasting as evince by laxity of the subcutaneous tissues.

Another moderately rare cause of dysphagia, which, if we ar alive to its existence, can be diagnosed clinically, is what is know as the Plummer-Vinson syndrome. The patient is nearly always woman. She may complain that she is unable to swallow anythin solid. She is abnormally pale, for she is profoundly anæmic. He tongue is red, for some of its epithelium is lost. At the angles of th mouth cheilosis* is often in evidence. We examine her finger-nails instead of being convex they are spoon-shaped. The dysphagi anæmia, the raw tongue, and spoon-shaped finger nails constitute th syndrome (*Fig.* 275).

Occasionally a pharyngeal pouch is the cause of dysphagia a well-developed pouch can be felt as a soft cystic swelling on th side of the neck (*Fig.* 276, *a* and *b*), usually the left side. B pressure the contents of the pouch—often foul fluid—can be emptie into the pharynx and mouth. Sometimes this is accompanied b audible and palpable gurgling.

Supposing the diagnosis of an inoperable carcinoma of the œs phagus has been proved, and one is undecided whether gastrostomy necessary, have the patient weighed, and examine him in a week

---

* *Cheilosis.* Greek, $\chi\epsilon\hat{\imath}\lambda os$ = a lip. Cracks at the corners of the mouth.

HENRY STANLEY PLUMMER, 1874–1937, *Physician, Mayo Clinic, Rochester, U.S.A.*
PORTER PAISLEY VINSON, *Contemporary Physician, Mayo Clinic.*

me. During the interval he should make out a complete list of the
ourishment he has managed to retain.

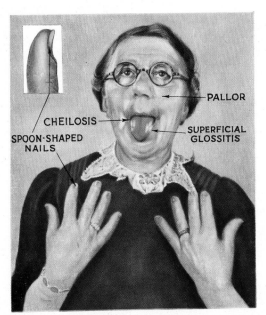

Fig. 275.—Patient exhibiting the signs of the Plummer-Vinson
syndrome. She was able to swallow fluids only.

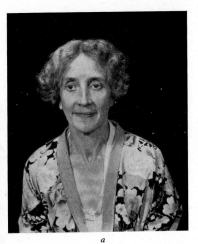

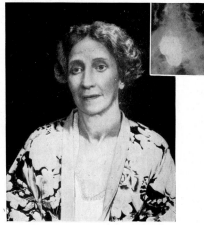

a                                              b

Fig. 276.—(a) Pharyngeal pouch before water has been swallowed ; (b) Pharyngeal pouch after
water has been swallowed.

## CHAPTER XV

## THE SHOULDER, ARM, AND FOREARM

### THE EXAMINATION OF THE SHOULDER GIRDLE WITH SPECIAL REFERENCE TO INJURY

THE patient should sit with both shoulders bare. Inspect the shoulder girdle from in front and also from the side, and compare one side with the other. It is usually convenient to postpone inspection from the back until a later stage of the examination.

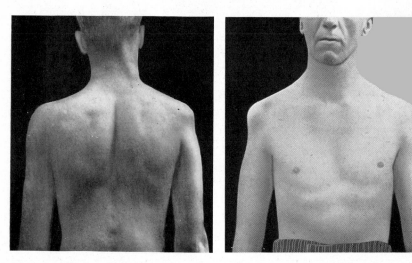

*Fig.* 277.—Right circumflex nerve paralysis. Note the wasting of the deltoid.

**Flattening of the Shoulder** is often seen in dislocation of the joint but it is by no means an infallible sign. *Fig.* 277 shows a case of paralysis of the circumflex nerve which defeated a Fellowship candidate. Unquestionably the shoulder is flattened, but the flattening is due to wasting of the deltoid muscle.

# CONFIRMATORY TESTS FOR DISLOCATION OF THE SHOULDER-JOINT

**The Ruler Test (Hamilton's Test).**—This test is simplicity itself, and is of great practical utility. Normally a straight-edge cannot rest simultaneously upon the acromion and the lateral epicondyle of the humerus, for the great tuberosity of the humerus is in the way. If it can so rest, then the shoulder is dislocated (*Fig.* 278) or the neck of the scapula is broken.

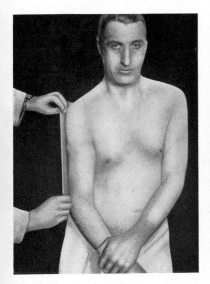 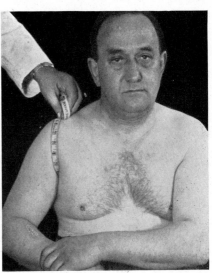

Fig. 278.—Hamilton's ruler test.    Fig. 279.—Callaway's test in dislocated shoulder.

**Callaway's Test** (*Fig.* 279) is of signal value for elucidating obscure dislocation in a fat person. A tape measure is passed over the acromion and through the axilla. The measurement is compared with that of the opposite side. If the shoulder is dislocated there is increased girth on the affected side.

**Dugas's Test.**—The patient places his hand on the opposite shoulder. Normally, when this is done the elbow can readily touch the side of the body ; but if the head of the humerus is dislocated, the action cannot be performed.

FRANK HASTINGS HAMILTON, 1813–1886, *Surgeon, Bellevue Hospital, New York City.*
THOMAS CALLAWAY, JUN., 1822–1869, *English Surgeon ; practised in Algiers.*
LOUIS ALEXANDER DUGAS, 1806–1884, *Professor of Surgery, Medical College, Georgia, U.S.A.*

**Swelling of the Joint.**—Owing to the thick, muscular covering of the capsule, even moderate effusions often are not manifest. A point worth remembering is that, as opposed to an effusion into the shoulder-

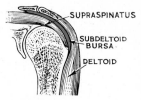

Fig. 280.—Effusion into the subacromial bursa, which must be distinguished from an effusion into the shoulder-joint.

joint proper, an effusion into the sub-acromial (subdeltoid) bursa (*Fig.* 280) is most likely to be recognized if the patient is observed from *behind* and above (Küster).

\*    \*    \*    \*    \*

Continuing with the examination of the shoulder-joint by inspection :

Ask the patient to lift his arms away from his side, at first to a right angle, and then above his head (*Fig.* 281).

1. If the patient can abduct his affected arm to 90° and then raise it perpendicularly above his head, it is proof positive that there cannot be a serious injury to the shoulder-joint or to the shoulder girdle.

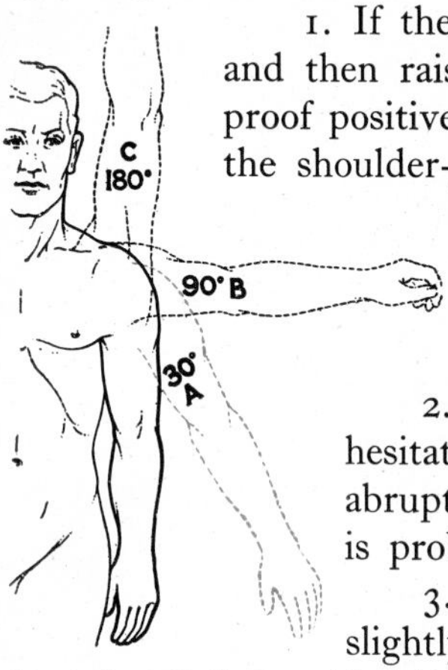

Fig. 281.—Observing the patient's performance of abduction is a mine of information. If he can abduct to 30° only, help him to 60°, and see if he can complete full abduction (*see* text).

2. When the movement B-C is performed hesitatingly, and the endeavour is terminated abruptly by sudden pain, fracture of the clavicle is probable.

3. If the arm can be raised only very slightly, and, above all, if the patient supports the injured limb with his other hand, then a fracture or dislocation is practically certain.

4. **Arthritis.**—Pain begins as soon as abduction is commenced and continues throughout the movement (Codman).

5. **Adhesions.**—The movement A–B is carried out painlessly until nearing B ; pain then commences and tends to increase as further abduction is attempted.

6. **Rupture of the Supraspinatus.**—As the patient attempts to abduct the arm, the deltoid can be seen to be contracting vigorously,

ERNST GEORG FERDINAND VON KÜSTER, 1839–1930, *Professor of Clinical Surgery, Marburg, Germany.*
ERNEST AMORY CODMAN, 1869–1940, *Surgeon, Massachusetts General Hospital, Boston.*

but the arm cannot be abducted by the deltoid alone (Watson-Jones). Consequently, the more the patient struggles to elevate the limb, the more he shrugs his shoulder (*Fig.* 282). In this condition it is the first 30° of A–B that cannot be performed. If the patient is helped over this, he can complete the movement by deltoid action.

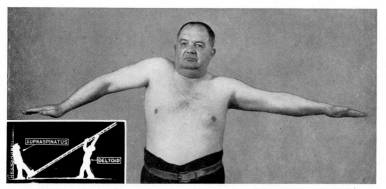

*Fig.* 282.—Rupture of the supraspinatus. The more the patient endeavours to lift his arm, the more he shrugs his shoulder. Inset : Showing the fundamental co-operation of the supraspinatus when the deltoid is at work.

7. **Supraspinatus Tendinitis.**—A–B continues painlessly until nearing B. Pain then starts abruptly, only to pass off after 90° has been surmounted.

### ROUTINE EXAMINATION OF THE MOVEMENTS OF THE SHOULDER-JOINT

The movements of the shoulder-joint cannot be examined properly from in front ; from this aspect it is possible to overlook, and even to pass as normal, a completely ankylosed joint. The clinician must stand *behind* the patient, where he can observe any movement of the scapula, and, if necessary, fix that bone.

*Abduction.*—Commence by testing abduction (*Fig.* 283). It is convenient to grasp the elbow while the various movements of the shoulder are tested, and one should commence by examining the shoulder that is not complained of, so that one can get an idea of the range of movement that is to be expected in that particular patient. The normal degree of maximum abduction is to a right angle. One must be certain that this abduction is taking place entirely at the shoulder-joint ; the scapula must be perfectly still. If the scapula is seen to move before the arm reaches a right angle, then it should be fixed while the arm is at rest by the side, and the movement of abduction carried out again. When the scapula is felt to rotate before 90° is reached, then there is limitation of abduction, and the angle of that limitation is noted and recorded.

## ROUTINE EXAMINATION OF THE SHOULDER-JOINT

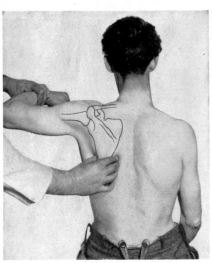

*Fig.* 283.—Abduction.

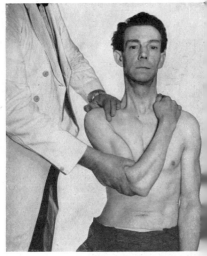

*Fig.* 284.—Adduction.

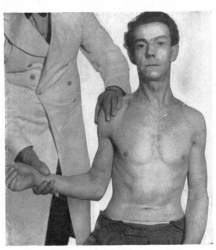

*Fig.* 285.—External Rotation.

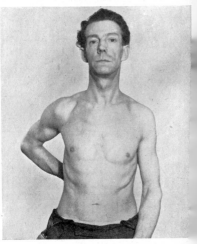

*Fig.* 286.—Internal Rotation.

*Adduction.*—The normal limit of adduction of the shoulder-joint is shown in *Fig.* 284. With the forearm flexed the elbow comes to the umbilicus. The same precaution of watching, and if necessary fixing, the scapula must be observed, as in all tests of movement of the shoulder.

*External rotation* is carried out as shown in *Fig.* 285. "If you have limited movement in every direction, it is due to arthritis. If limited in every direction but one, it is due to adhesions" (Sir Robert Jones).

*Internal Rotation.*—Ask the patient to place the palm of his hand on the lower part of his back (*Fig.* 286).

The routine examination of the shoulder-joint should be completed by passing the fingers, with the pulps directed outwards, well up into the axilla. In spare individuals the head of the humerus can be felt, and the position of the subglenoid synovial pouch can be located.

## THE TRIANGLE TEST

A useful method of investigating the neighbourhood of the shoulder-joint for bony injury is to compare, with that of the opposite side, the triangle formed by three bony points, namely, the tip of the

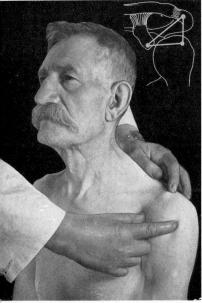

Fig. 287.—Determining the relationship of the ee bony points about the shoulder; (1) The tip the coracoid : (2) The tip of the acromion : (3) e great tuberosity of the humerus.

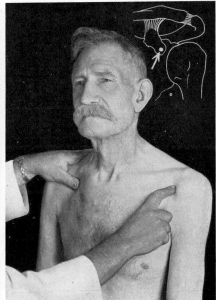

Fig. 288.—Determining the tip of the coracoid process.

Sir Robert Jones, 1858–1923, *Orthopædic Surgeon, Royal Southern Hospital, Liverpool.*

acromion, the tip of the coracoid process, and the most prominent part of the great tuberosity of the humerus (*Fig.* 287). Students are apt to have difficulty in locating the tip of the coracoid process; they are liable to search too medially for this really very obvious structure. *Fig.* 288 shows the finger resting upon the tip of the coracoid process.

### EXAMINATION OF THE CLAVICLE

The clavicle is palpated by running the fingers along its subcutaneous surface. If a breach in continuity is not obvious, stand behind the patient and carry out the manœuvre shown in *Fig.* 289.

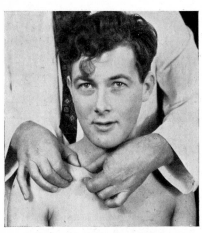

Fig. 289.—Examining the clavicle for an ununited, or obscure recent, fracture.

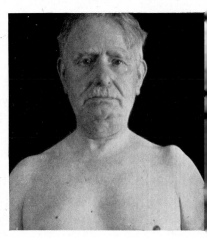

Fig. 290.—Osteo-arthritis of the acromio-clavicular joint with effusion.

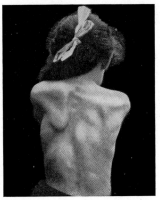

Fig. 291.—Sprengel's shoulder. Note the relatively small, elevated left scapula.

The sterno-clavicular joint and the acromio-clavicular joint (*Fig.* 290) are both readily accessible to the palpating fingers.

### EXAMINATION OF THE SCAPULA

Congenital elevation of the scapula (Sprengel's shoulder) is usually evident on inspection (*Fig.* 291). Winging of the scapula is discussed in Chapter XXXII.

A considerable portion of the scapula is readily accessible to the palpating fingers, and as X-ray examination of this bone is sometimes

---

OTTO GERHARD KARL SPRENGEL, 1852–1915, *Surgical Director, Grossherzogliches Krankenhaus, Brunswick, Germany.*

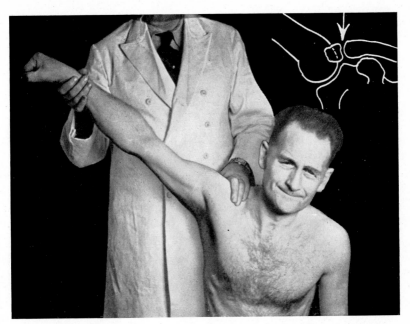

*Fig.* 292.—Testing for fracture of the acromion by hyper-abduction of the arm.

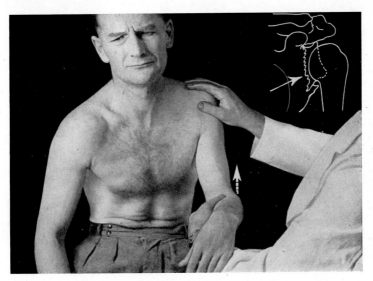

*Fig.* 293.—Testing for a fractured neck of the scapula.

unsatisfactory, clinical methods are all the more important.  The spine and acromion are examined by palpating along this bony ridge while the arm is gently hyper-abducted (*Fig.* 292).  Fractures of the neck of the scapula are particularly liable to be overlooked.  Grasp the patient's arm in such a manner that his forearm rests on the examiner's forearm (*Fig.* 293).  By this means the whole of the upper extremity can be raised and lowered gently.  Provided the clavicle is intact, abnormal mobility and crepitus in the region of the shoulder-joint suggest a fracture of the neck of the scapula.

## EXAMINATION OF THE UPPER ARM

When the arm is viewed from the side a characteristic deformity is often seen in cases of fracture of the anatomical neck of the humerus : the normal rounded curve is replaced by a sharp anterior deformity.

Fractures of the shaft of the humerus are best tested for by gentle abduction of the arm, the forearm being supported during this manœuvre (*Fig.* 294).

Comparative measurement from the tip of the acromion to the lateral epicondyle is sometimes of value (*Fig.* 295), especially when an impacted fracture is suspected.

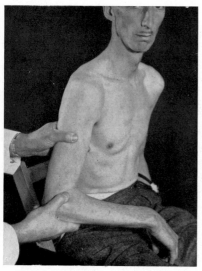

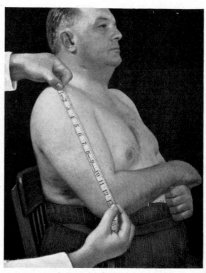

*Fig.* 294.—Testing for fracture of the humerus (upper two-thirds).  The forearm is supported, and the arm is abducted carefully.

*Fig.* 295.—Measuring the length of the arm. The distance between the tip of the acromion and the lateral epicondyle is measured on each side.

Impacted fractures are often overlooked in the first instance through the omission of measurement.

The lower half of the humerus can be palpated readily. The upper half is accessible on the medial side between biceps and triceps.

**Rupture of the Biceps Muscle.**—In rupture of the belly of the muscle there are two lumps separated by a gap. In rupture of the tendon, and also in rupture of the sheath of the muscle, there is but one lump (*Fig.* 296).

When the biceps is ruptured, flexion of the forearm supinated is less powerful than with the forearm pronated.

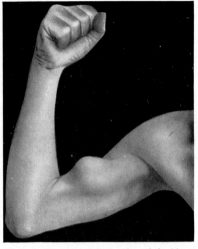

Fig. 296.—Rupture of the tendon of the biceps.

## EXAMINATION OF THE ELBOW-JOINT

Very characteristic is the appearance of a backward dislocation of the elbow-joint (*Fig.* 297). The olecranon protrudes abnormally ; the diagnosis is obvious.

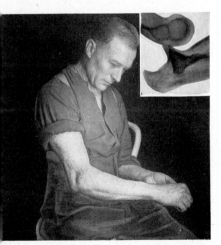

Fig. 297.—Characteristic attitude and deformity in backward dislocation of the elbow-joint.

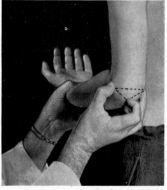

Fig 298.—Examining for a fracture in the region of the elbow-joint. The triangle is formed by the lateral and medial epicondyles and the tip of the olecranon. When the forearm is extended these three points should be in a straight line.

**Testing for more obscure Injuries about the Elbow.**—
A useful method is to determine the relationship of the lateral and

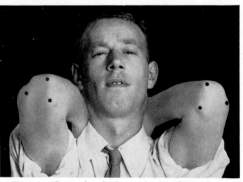

medial epicondyles to the tip of the olecranon. These three bony points form a triangle when the elbow is flexed (*Fig.* 298).

By requesting the patient to clasp hands behind the head, one is enabled to compare the elbow triangle of one side with that of the other (*Fig.* 299).

*Fig.* 299.—Comparing the bony triangles of the elbows.

**Testing the Integrity of the Head of the Radius.**—The head of the radius lies more posteriorly than we are apt to think. To find it, rest the tip of the middle finger on the lateral epicondyle,

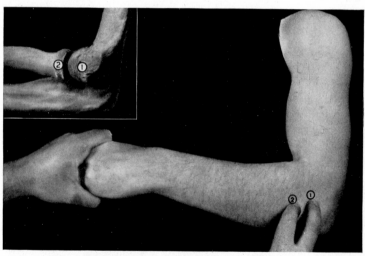

*Fig.* 300.—Testing for the integrity of the head of the radius.

then place the index alongside it, the elbow being at a right angle (*Fig.* 300). The arm is then pronated and supinated, and the head of the radius is felt to rotate beneath the index finger (Alan Todd's method).

ALAN HERAPATH TODD, *Contemporary Consulting Orthopædic Surgeon, General Hospital, Croydon.*

**Tennis Elbow.**—There is tenderness over the lateral epicondyle and in the outer part of the antecubital fossa (*see Fig.* 3, p. 4). Pronation of the forearm accentuates the pain.

When an effusion occurs into the elbow-joint the ulnar nerve, where it abuts against the capsule, is rendered more superficial and is sometimes dislocated from its groove. By palpating both sides simultaneously the phenomenon may be apparent and assist in the diagnosis of arthritis of the elbow-joint (Orbach).

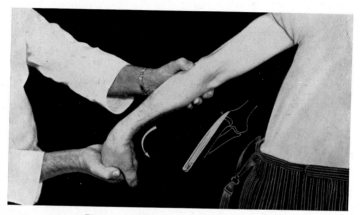

*Fig.* 301.—Confirmatory test for tennis elbow.

*Mills' Manœuvre.*—With the elbow quite straight and the wrist flexed, pronate the forearm (*Fig.* 301). This brings on the characteristic pain, and does so only in cases of tennis elbow.

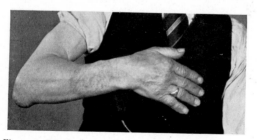

*Fig.* 302.—Effusion into the olecranon bursa. Miner's elbow.

**Miner's** (syn. **Student's**) **Elbow.**—The effusion into the bursa over the subcutaneous surface of the olecranon process can hardly be mistaken (*Fig.* 302).

11

EGMONT J. ORBACH, *Contemporary Surgeon, New Britain, Conn., U.S.A.*
GEORGE PERCIVAL MILLS, *Contemporary Surgeon, Royal Cripples' Hospital, Birmingham.*

## EXAMINATION OF THE SUPRATROCHLEAR LYMPH-NODE

Quite significant enlargements of this lymphatic node are missed, even after a search has been made. It is futile to seek minor enlargements of this node with the arm in the extended position. First of all flex the arm to a right angle, in order to relax surrounding structures. *Fig.* 303 shows the node being palpated ; when enlarged, it will be found slipping beneath the finger and thumb on the anterior surface of the medial intermuscular septum half an inch above the base of the medial epicondyle.

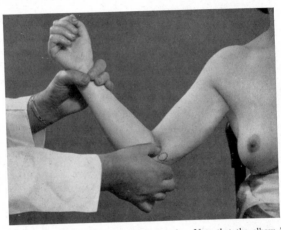

*Fig.* 303.—Palpating the supratrochlear lymph-node.  Note that the elbow is flexed.

Bilateral enlargement of the supratrochlear lymph-nodes suggests syphilis. Of 100 consecutive patients with bilateral enlargement of the supratrochlear lymph-nodes, 50 proved to have a positive Wassermann reaction (Griffith Evans).

## EXAMINATION OF THE FOREARM AND WRIST

The ulna can be palpated along its subcutaneous border throughout its length. The lower two-thirds of the radius is accessible also. The most common fracture in this region is Colles's, which gives rise to the typical ' dinner-fork ' deformity (*Fig.* 304).

In the more obscure injuries of this region the styloid processes of the radius and ulna should be palpated, and their position in relation to each other noted and compared with the opposite side. The styloid process of the radius is $\frac{1}{2}$ in. lower than that of the ulna.

August von Wassermann, 1866–1925, *Director of the Institute for Experimental Therapy, Berlin.*
Griffith Ivor Evans, *Contemporary Surgeon, Caernarvon, Wales.*
Abraham Colles, 1773–1843, *Professor of Anatomy and Surgery, Dublin.*

If there is no obvious deformity, but a fracture of the lower end of the radius is suspected, try to elicit abnormal movement or crepitus by grasping the radius with one hand above and the other hand below the probable site of fracture.

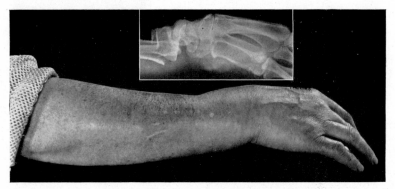

*Fig.* 304.—Colles's fracture. The dinner-fork deformity.

**Ganglion of the Wrist.**—The commonest place for a ganglion to occur is in connexion with one of the numerous tendon-sheaths around the wrist. The swelling is usually so densely filled with gelatinous material that it feels solid. Occasionally fluctuation can be elicited,

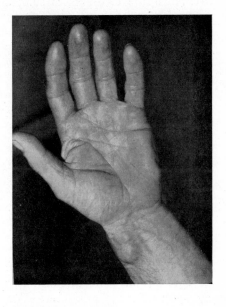

*Fig.* 305.—Ganglion associated with the tendon-sheath of the brachioradialis.

especially on the flexor aspect of the wrist (*Fig.* 305). It is insufficient to make the diagnosis of ganglion ; it is more accurate and a good anatomical exercise to state with which tendon-sheath the ganglion is associated.

*CHAPTER XVI*

## THE HAND

## EXAMINATION OF THE CARPAL BONES
## FOR INJURY

INJURY to the carpal bones is apt to be regarded by students and practitioners as a subject quite beyond their ken. As a consequence, fractured carpal scaphoid, the commonest of these injuries, is frequently overlooked. So it comes about that permanent disability following this accident is rife.

To remedy this it is essential to visualize the location and surface anatomy of two bones—the scaphoid and the semilunar (*Fig.* 306). Once one has grasped the relative positions of these bones in the wrist, half the complexities surrounding the subject disappear like dew before the sun.

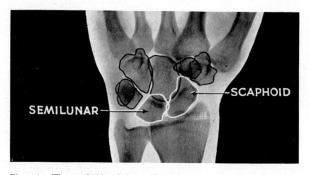

Fig. 306.—The scaphoid and the semilunar bones are the only carpal bones to be frequently injured, and if the clinician orientates them, the subject becomes much easier.

Never begin the examination of the carpal bones as a first step, but rather be assured that the radius and ulna are intact, and particularly that there is not an impacted fracture of the lower end of the radius.

## FRACTURED CARPAL SCAPHOID

*Inspection.*—After fracture of the carpal scaphoid, swelling appears almost at once (*Fig.* 307). It is most marked in the anatomical snuff-box. The swelling is neither great nor widespread (Alan Todd).

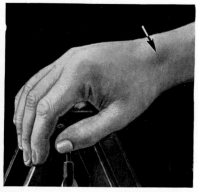

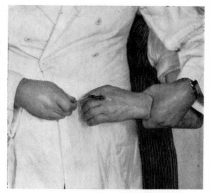

*Fig.* 307.—Typical localized œdema associated with (recent) fracture of the carpal scaphoid.

*Fig.* 308.—Maximum tenderness over the knuckle of the middle finger suggests a fractured scaphoid bone. The hand must be deviated to the radial side while the knuckles are being percussed.

*Indirect Percussion.*—With the hand deviated towards the *radial* side, percussion over the heads of the metacarpals shows maximal tenderness over the middle metacarpal (*Fig.* 308). There may

DIAGNOSIS OF FRACTURED CARPAL SCAPHOID

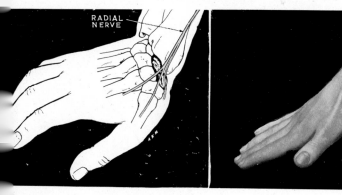

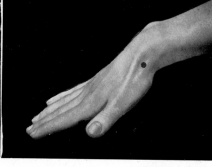

*Fig.* 309.—Bearing in mind that normally firm finger-tip pressure in the anatomical snuff-box causes pain due to compression of the radial nerve . . . .

*Fig.* 310.— . . . . firm finger-tip pressure is applied in the anatomical snuff-box and the findings compared with those of the opposite side.

ALAN HERAPATH TODD, *Contemporary Consulting Orthopædic Surgeon, General Hospital. Croydon.*

be tenderness when the index and thumb knuckles are percussed, but none over the ring and little finger knuckles.

*Palpation.*—Grasp the patient's hand in your left hand, and place the tip of your right index finger in the anatomical snuff-box ; the carpal scaphoid bone is directly beneath the palpating finger. Now deviate the patient's hand to the ulnar side. This makes the scaphoid more accessible ; palpate again firmly. Normally, firm pressure in the box causes pain, due to compression of the radial nerve (*Fig.* 309) ; therefore do not jump to a conclusion until the same amount of pressure has been applied in the contralateral anatomical snuff-box. Firm finger-tip pressure in the anatomical snuff-box (*Fig.* 310) causing pain sufficient to make the patient wince and of a degree that does not appertain on the contralateral side, is indicative of fracture (McCarty).

## FRACTURED CARPAL SEMILUNAR

*Inspection.*—Ask the patient to clench his hands, presenting the backs of them towards you. *Fig.* 311 shows the characteristic shortening of the middle metacarpal due to a fracture-dislocation of the semilunar compared with the opposite side.

*Indirect percussion* is the only method of examination of real value in this instance. Grasp the lower part of the forearm as shown in *Fig.* 312, so that the patient cannot see what is being done. Keeping the injured hand deviated towards the ulnar side, percuss knuckles

DIAGNOSIS OF FRACTURED CARPAL SEMILUNAR

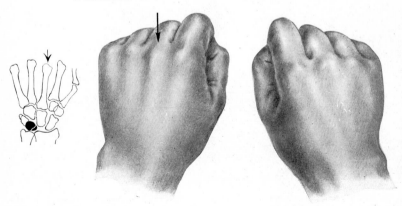

Fig. 311.—Fracture-dislocation of the carpal semilunar. Note the characteristic shortening of the middle metacarpal when the patient makes a fist.

FRANKLIN BENNETT McCARTY, *Contemporary Surgeon, St. Joseph's Hospital, Chicago.*

2, 3, 4, and 5.  Localized tenderness over the fourth knuckle suggests a fracture of the semilunar bone for the reason shown in *Fig.* 312, inset.

*Palpation.*—While visualizing the position of the carpal semilunar bone in relation to the wrist-joint (*see Fig.* 306), move the wrist to and fro.  At the same time palpate the base of the dorsum. When the carpal semilunar bone is fractured this manœuvre will elicit tenderness.  When it is judged that the palpating finger lies over the semilunar bone, extend the wrist and press deeply.

### DIAGNOSIS OF FRACTURED CARPAL SEMILUNAR

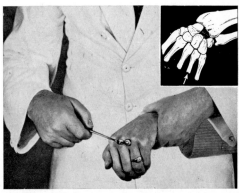

*Fig.* 312.—Indirect percussion.  Maximum tenderness of the ring knuckle suggests a fractured semilunar bone (inset). The hand must be deviated to the ulnar side while the knuckles are being percussed.

## EXAMINATION OF AN INFECTED HAND

Paronychia is a comparatively minor infective lesion of the hand. Almost always the diagnosis can be made on inspection alone.  Inflammation is seen around the nail (*Fig.* 313), and in about 60 per cent of cases under the base of the nail also.

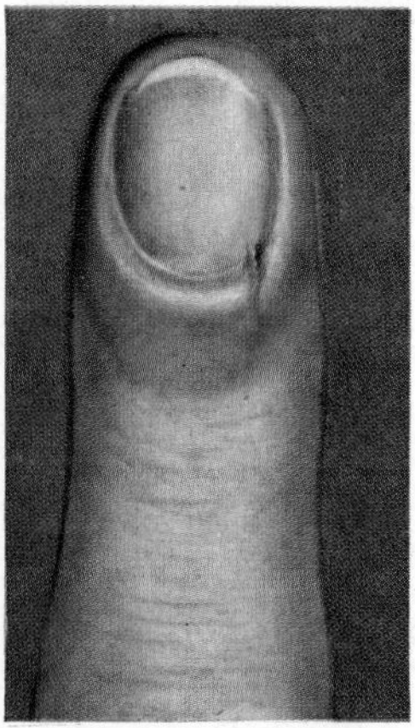

Nearly as common as paronychia is infection of a *terminal pulp compartment.* The pulps of the fingers and thumb are subjected to more pricks, and therefore infections, than any other part of the body. Nature has provided in this situation a closed fascial com-

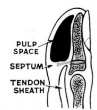

PULP SPACE
SEPTUM
TENDON SHEATH

*Fig.* 314.—The terminal pulp compartment.  It is separated from the rest of the finger by a fascial septum, at the level of the epiphysial line of the terminal phalanx.

*Fig.* 313. — Paronychia. Often organisms enter through a 'hang nail'.

partment which extends from the tip of the digit to the level of the epiphysial line of the terminal phalanx (*Fig.* 314).  When a terminal pulp compartment is infected there is tenderness limited to the pulp, and later local swelling. The diagnosis presents no difficulty, and, unless the condition is improperly treated, it is seldom serious.

## SERIOUS INFECTIONS OF THE HAND

When the hand is to any extent seriously inflamed it takes up the position of rest (*Fig.* 315). Grave infections of the hand fall into three categories :—

*a.* Lymphangitis.

*b.* Suppurative tenosynovitis.

*c.* A fascial space infection. This is often a sequel of (*b*).

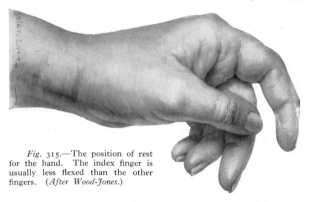

Fig. 315.—The position of rest for the hand. The index finger is usually less flexed than the other fingers. (*After Wood-Jones.*)

It is of cardinal importance to distinguish lymphangitis from suppurative tenosynovitis and fascial space infections. The two latter conditions require urgent operation, while in lymphangitis, at any rate in its early stages, incision is highly mischievous.

Usually the all-important diagnosis can be made if we proceed as follows :—

1. Take the patient's temperature.

2. Observe the hand. This is a convenient place to enunciate a principle so fundamental that it should be shouted from the house-tops : *the greatest swelling does not indicate the position of the pus.* Frequently there is œdema (swelling) of the dorsum (*Fig.* 316), whereas in 90 per cent of cases the pus lies on the palmar aspect. Œdema gives rise to pitting on pressure (*see* p. 6). If pus is present, induration of tissues can be felt.

3. Scrutinize the arm for lymphangitis ; if present, red lines will be seen passing up the limb (*see* p. 43).

4. Palpate the supratrochlear lymph-node (*see* p. 166).

5. Examine the axillary lymphatic lymph-nodes (*see* p. 133).

**Suppurative Tenosynovitis.**—If a tendon-sheath is infected, that finger is likely to be more flexed than the others. The forefinger when inflamed is not so much flexed as the remainder (John Hilton).

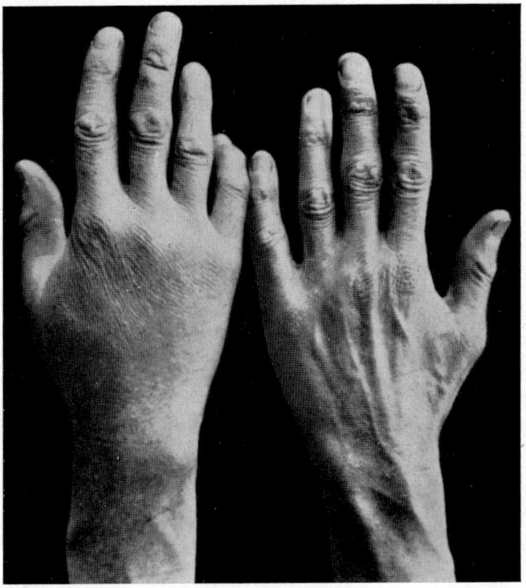

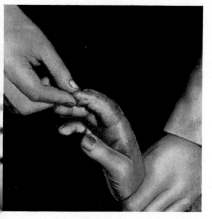

*Fig.* 316.—Œdema of the back of the hand is very common in infections of the palmar aspect.

The essential signs of an infected digital tendon-sheath are :—

1. Swelling and loss of function.

2. Flexion of the finger (*signe de crochet*).

3. Tenderness, maximal over the infected sheath. Bearing these in mind, let us proceed to examine the hand. Ask the patient to move the fingers ; one would think that he would hold the infected digit rigidly. Too often this assumption has beguiled the clinician. Gently—exceedingly gently—extend a finger not suspected. Similarly, test the other digits. Often exquisite pain is produced by the slightest attempt at extension (*Fig.* 317), not only of the infected, but of an uninfected, digit or digits immediately adjacent. So it comes about that although we are now

*Fig.* 317.—Testing for suppurative tenosynovitis. The flexed index finger is being gently extended. When the tendon-sheath is involved, this causes acute pain, most marked over the metacarpo-phalangeal joint.

JOHN HILTON, 1805–1878, *Surgeon, Guy's Hospital, London.*

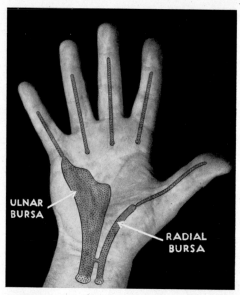

Fig. 318.—Showing the relationship of the flexor tendon-sheaths to the creases of the fingers and palm.

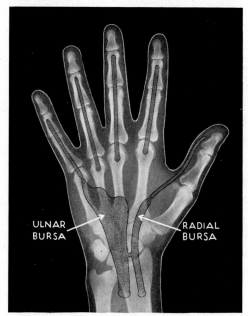

Fig. 319.—Showing the relationship of the flexor tendon-sheaths to the bones of the hand.

almost certain that a tendon-sheath is involved, we are as yet, usually, unable to be certain which. The point of maximum tenderness must be found, and while the search is in progress it is of fundamental importance to be able to visualize the surface anatomy of the tendon-sheaths and their connexions (*Figs.* 318, 319).

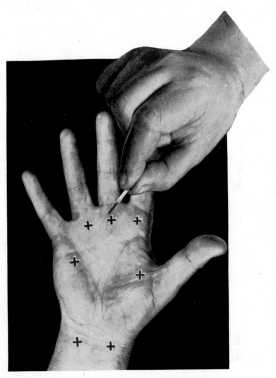

*Fig.* 320.—Seeking the point of maximum tenderness. In suppurative tenosynovitis this point is over the cul-de-sac at the base of the sheath in the case of the index, middle, and ring fingers. The maximum point of tenderness in the case of infection of the sheaths of the thumb and little finger are shown also. (Points of tenderness *after R. Kennon.*)

Ask the patient to lay the hand in the most comfortable position possible, palm upwards, and to take his time in doing so. The point of maximum tenderness is found by palpating systematically with some blunt-pointed instrument ; a burnt match stalk, with the loose charcoal removed, answers the purpose admirably (*Fig.* 320).

Serious as it is at all times, when the tendon-sheaths of the thumb or the little finger are involved, suppurative tenosynovitis becomes a lesion of the first magnitude. In the case of the little finger, almost certainly, the *ulnar bursa* (the palmar bursa of British anatomy) will be implicated quickly. If the infection is primarily in the flexor tendon-sheath of the thumb, simultaneously the *radial bursa* (syn. sheath of the flexor pollicis longus) must be involved totally, that is, right up under the anterior annular ligament to above the wrist (*see Fig.* 318).

Nor is this the whole gloomy story. If the tendon-sheath of either the thumb or the little finger becomes infected, there is an 80 per cent chance that within 48 hours there will be infection of both the ulnar and radial bursæ, for usually, as shown in *Fig.* 318, there is an intercommunicating channel between these bursæ.

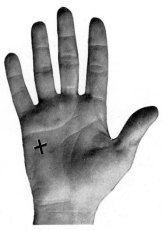

Fig. 321.—Kanavel's sign for ulnar bursitis. Maximum site of tenderness marked with a cross. The sign passes off in a few days.

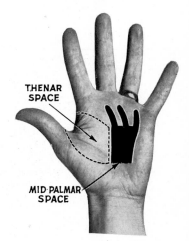

Fig. 322.—The relative positions of the thenar and middle palmar spaces. The three diverticula from the middle palmar space are the lumbrical canals.

*Signs of Involvement of Ulnar Bursa.*—The following signs are indicative of involvement of the ulnar bursa : (1) Œdema of the hand, especially of the dorsum ; (2) Fullness of the palm, but the concavity is still present ; (3) Fullness immediately above the anterior annular ligament ; (4) Kanavel's sign—the most valuable of all—a point of maximum tenderness in the position shown in *Fig.* 321.

*Signs of Involvement of the Radial Bursa.*—These are as follows : (1) There is flexion of the distal phalanx of the thumb, *with rigidity* ; (2) There is swelling just above the anterior annular ligament ; (3) There is tenderness over the flexor pollicis longus sheath. It should be emphasized thoroughly that the radial and ulnar bursæ communicate in over 80 per cent of cases. Reference to *Fig.* 318 is again advised.

**Fascial Space Infections.**—There are many fascial spaces in the hand where pus may accumulate. I wish to draw attention to the two most important (*Fig.* 322): (1) The middle palmar space ; (2) The thenar space.

*Signs of Involvement of the Middle Palmar Space.*—Obliteration of the concavity of the palm with slight bulging thereof is almost pathognomonic of the condition. The middle palmar space infections produce those enormous hands that have been likened to a whale's flipper.

*Signs of Involvement of the Thenar Space.*—This gives rise to the typical ' ballooning ' of the thenar eminence, which is quite characteristic (*Fig.* 323). Flexion of the distal phalanx may be marked in this condition, but it lacks the resistance to extension that is present in tenosynovitis of the flexor pollicis longus.

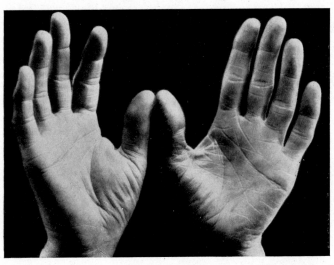

*Fig.* 323.—' Ballooning ' of the thenar eminence : the sign of an infected thenar fascial space.

## DUPUYTREN'S CONTRACTURE

The diagnosis of Dupuytren's contracture is usually very easy because the palmar fascia is obviously thickened and contracted. While typically the condition affects the ring finger (*Fig.* 324) and years

BARON GUILLAUME DUPUYTREN, 1777–1835, *Surgeon, Hôtel Dieu, Paris.*

## Dupuytren's and Volkmann's Contractures and their Differential Diagnosis

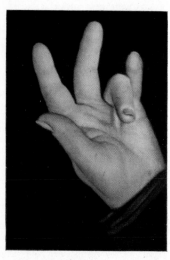

*Fig.* 324.—Dupuytren's contracture.

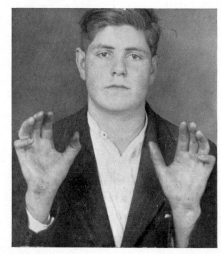

*Fig.* 325.—Congenital contracture of the little fingers.

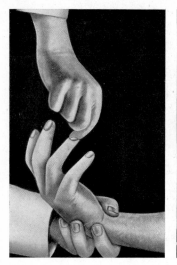

*Fig.* 326.—Differential diagnosis between a Dupuytren's contracture and a contraction of the flexor tendon.

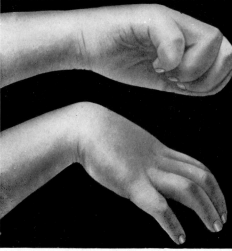

*Fig.* 327.—Showing ; A, Volkmann's contracture : B, That the fingers can be partially extended by flexing the wrist.

ater the little finger becomes implicated, in perhaps 15 per cent of cases t is the little finger that is primarily affected. The only conditions with which it is confused are a contracture of the corresponding flexor tendon and congenital contracture of the little finger (*Fig.* 325). The possibility of the former can be eliminated at once by flexing the wrist and trying to extend the finger (*Fig.* 326). If the contraction is in the flexor tendon, the affected finger can now be straightened.

On the other hand, if the deformity is a Dupuytren's contracture (palmar fascia), the finger still resists extension.

## VOLKMANN'S ISCHÆMIC CONTRACTURE

Ischæmic contracture is liable to follow an injury of the extremity when the arterial blood-supply to the part is impaired by œdema. Such œdema is not necessarily, but too often, the result of a tight plaster cast. In the case of the forearm the fingers are flexed, but can be at least partially extended when the wrist is flexed (*Fig.* 327). This demonstrates that the contracture is in the flexor group of muscles. In extreme cases a complete 'claw hand' may result (*see* Chapter XXXI).

## DACTYLITIS

The spindle-shaped appearance of the finger or fingers (*Fig.* 328) makes the diagnosis extremely simple. The patient is often a very young child. Most of these cases are tuberculous (the so-called spina ventosa\* of the older clinicians); a

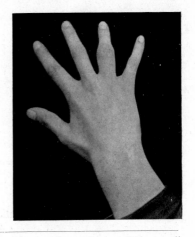

*Fig.* 328.—Tuberculous dactylitis.

minority (very few nowadays) are syphilitic. It is said that hereditary syphilis attacks the metacarpals more often than the phalanges. Dactylitis must be distinguished from multiple central enchondromata.

---

\* " Spina "—an ache, such as that produced by a spike or thorn. " Ventosa " denotes a fusiform outline. This terminology is unsatisfactory and should be discarded.

## SYNDACTYLISM  (WEBBED  FINGERS)

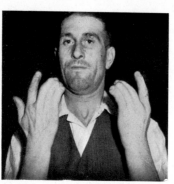

Although occasionally the result of badly treated burns, nearly always webbed fingers are a congenital and a hereditary condition. Two or more fingers may be webbed (*Fig* 329). Ascertain whether the webbing involves skin only, or whether, in addition, there is fibrous or even bony union.

*Fig.* 329.—Bilateral syndactylism.

## COMPOUND
## PALMAR  GANGLION

Compound palmar ganglion is an old term to signify tuberculous tenosynovitis of the ulnar bursa. In cases of some standing the fingers are partially flexed and there is an hour-glass-shaped swelling which bulges above and below the anterior annular ligament. Fluctuation can be elicited from

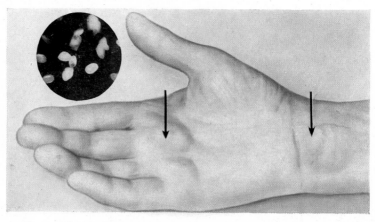

*Fig.* 330.—Compound palmar ganglion. Fluctuation accompanied by a peculiar crepitant sensation (due to the movement of melon-seed bodies) could be obtained between the positions marked by the arrows. *Inset*—Some of the melon-seed bodies removed at operation on this case.

one compartment of the swelling to the other (*Fig.* 330), and very characteristic is the soft crepitant sensation derived from the movements of the melon-seed bodies which abound within the infected bursa.

## IMPLANTATION DERMOID

Because the fingers and thumb are frequently pricked—especially the pulps of the fingers—implantation dermoid cysts are more often encountered in this region than else-where. Under the skin there is a painless, soft cyst (*Fig.* 331), which is neither attached to the skin nor the deeper structures. The over-lying integument is normal. The inference is that at some previous time a fragment of epidermis was driven beneath the dermis and there continued to proliferate.

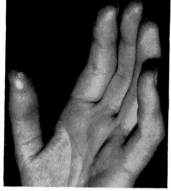

*Fig.* 331.—Implantation dermoid.

## MALLET FINGER*
## AND TRIGGER FINGER

Each of the above clinical entities is so characteristic that once seen their diagnosis never presents the slightest difficulty. (*Figs.* 332, 333.)

When the symptoms so characteristic of 'trigger' finger affect the thumb, the condition is known as 'snapping' thumb.

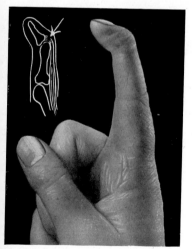

*Fig.* 332.—Mallet finger. The terminal phalanx cannot be extended because the inser-tion of the extensor tendon has been torn.

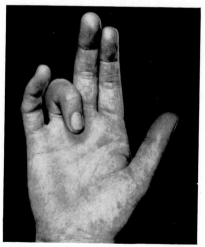

*Fig.* 333.—Trigger finger. After closing her hand the patient was asked to open it, with this result; only when the ring finger was assisted could it be extended: a mere touch towards unflexing and the finger snapped into line with the others.

12

* Mallet finger is known in the U.S.A. as baseball finger.

## CHAPTER XVII

# HERNIA.  LYMPHATICS OF GROIN

## HERNIA

**Preparation of the Patient for Examination of Inguinal and Femoral Herniæ when there is no question of Strangulation.—** The male patient stands while the examiner sits.  The patient lets down his trousers completely, and pulls up his shirt above the umbilicus.

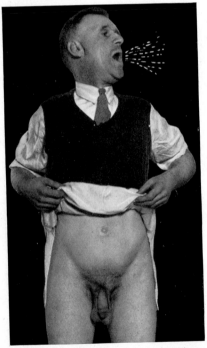

For the examination of this region in the female a good method is practised at the London Hospital.  The patient (under the sister's instructions) removes the garments below the waist, and puts on a pair of ' bathing triangles '.  She then stands with a blanket wrapped around her.

When asked to examine a patient for a hernia, 75 per cent of students commence palpation at once, and disregard the well-known fact that an impulse is much better seen than felt. First adjust the patient.   He will almost certainly be doubled up with his neck craning down to see what is about to be done. Tell him to hold his shirt well up and keep his head erect, then

*Fig.* 334.—Watching for a visible impulse on coughing.  Note that the patient's head is turned to one side.

(in order that you may avoid the salivary shower when he coughs) to turn his head to one side (*Fig.* 334).   Carefully observe his abdominal musculature, and ask the patient to cough. Malgaigne's bulgings (*Fig.* 335) are more than suggestive of weak abdominal musculature which predisposes to hernia, particularly direct inguinal hernia. With the eyes glued on the external abdominal ring, request the patient to cough again. Observe whether there is an impulse. Ask him to cough once more, and compare with the ring of the opposite side. When neither a swelling nor an impulse can be seen, ask the patient to point to the place where he experienced pain or noticed a swelling.

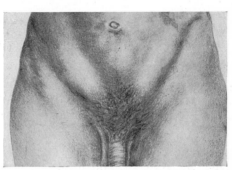

*Fig.* 335.—Malgaigne's bulgings.

**Notes on the Anatomy of the Inguinal Canal.**—Before the inguinal canal is examined a few anatomical points must be recalled. The external abdominal ring lies $\frac{1}{2}$ in. above and external to the spine of the pubis. Define this point by palpating the upper limit of the symphysis and then tracing the crest of the pubis laterally. When the spine of the pubis cannot be felt (a rare event, but not unknown in obese females), ask the patient to lie down. Flex and abduct the thigh, define the adductor longus, and follow up the tendon to its origin.

The internal abdominal ring lies $\frac{1}{2}$ in. above the mid-point of Poupart's ligament.

### INGUINAL HERNIA

**Palpation of the Abdominal Ring, and, in Certain Cases, of the Inguinal Canal Itself.**

1. *If there is no Obvious Lump.*—*In the male*, invaginate the scrotum upon the little finger (*Fig.* 336); then rotate the finger so that the nail lies against the cord, and follow the cord upwards— this will lead the pulp of the finger, with its tactile sensibility, to the external abdominal ring (*Fig.* 337). If the finger is not introduced in this way, it is more than likely that the nail will abut against the ring, and the point of the examination will be missed. A normal ring feels like a triangular slit ; it just admits the tip of the little finger. If more than this is possible, it is not normal. Again ask the patient to cough, and note if there is a *palpable* impulse.

*In the female,* unless the patient is very thin, it is impossible to explore the inguinal canal digitally by invaginating the skin. In the average case the best method of procedure is to lay two fingers over, and just below and to the inner side of, the external abdominal ring, and to test for an impulse when the patient coughs. Valuable as the visible (as opposed to the palpable) impulse is at all times, its necessity becomes apparent in the female, in whom a digital exploration of this ring cannot be performed.

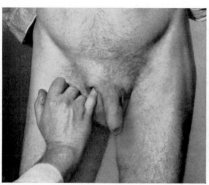 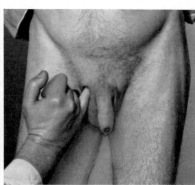

<table>
<tr><td>

*Fig.* 336.—Preparing to palpate the external abdominal ring. The skin of the scrotum is invaginated.

</td><td>

*Fig.* 337.—The finger is then rotated so as to bring the finger-nail against the spermatic cord. The pulp will then be available to feel the external abdominal ring.

</td></tr>
</table>

2. *If there is an Obvious Lump* (*in Both Sexes*).—See whether you can get above the lump ; if you can, it is manifestly not issuing from the inguinal canal and therefore cannot be a hernia. If you cannot get above it, ascertain the relationship of the neck of the sac and its continuity with the inguinal canal. Grasp the neck of the sac between finger and thumb. Ask the patient to cough, and again note whether or not there is an impulse.

The absence of an impulse signifies that the hernia is in all probability irreducible. If it is irreducible, you must decide (on data other than the purely local) whether or not the hernia is strangulated.

**Method of Testing for the Reducibility of an Inguinal Hernia.—** Flex and internally rotate the thigh, and gently manipulate the fundus of the sac between finger and thumb, exerting even pressure. At the same time, with the other hand grasp the neck of the sac and pull it lightly inwards. This is *taxis.* Forcible taxis is fraught with dangers.

**If Reducible, Method of Ascertaining the Contents of Sac.—**
*If the Hernia Contains Omentum.*—In the first place it will give a doughy impression to the palpating fingers. But this is not so valuable as the second sign : the first part of the hernial contents will reduce easily, the last with difficulty (because of adhesions).

*If the Hernia Contains Intestine.*—The first part is difficult to reduce ; the last part is reduced with ease, and returns to the general peritoneal cavity with a characteristic gurgle.

After a diagnosis of inguinal hernia has been made, before advising early operation, examine the abdominal musculature, by getting the patient to contract these muscles (*see* Chapter XIX) ; note the development and tone of the recti, and especially of the obliqui.

**Differential Diagnosis between Direct and Indirect Inguinal Hernia.—**A direct hernia is comparatively uncommon. It is often acquired and usually occurs in patients over 40 years of age. It does not come down the inguinal canal, but passes forward through Hesselbach's triangle (*Fig.* 338).

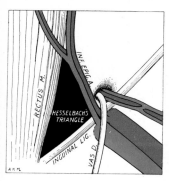
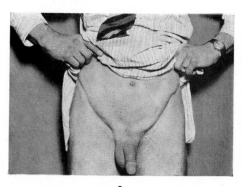

A             B

*Fig.* 338.—A, Hesselbach's triangle, through which a direct inguinal hernia passes. Boundaries ; deep epigastric vessels, Poupart's ligament, and outer border of rectus sheath. (Viewed from within.) B, Bilateral direct inguinal hernia (diagnosis confirmed at operation).

If the finger passes directly backwards into the abdomen instead of obliquely upwards and outwards, it is very suggestive, but not diagnostic, of a direct inguinal hernia. The only sign that can make the diagnosis absolute is feeling the pulsations of the deep epigastric artery to the outer side of the hernial sac. This, as may be imagined, can be done with certainty only about once in a surgical lifetime.

FRANZ KASPAR HESSELBACH, 1759–1816 *Professor of Surgery, Würzburg, Germany.*

## The Signs in the Differential Diagnosis between Inguinal Hernia and Vaginal Hydrocele.—The first thing to determine is : " Is it

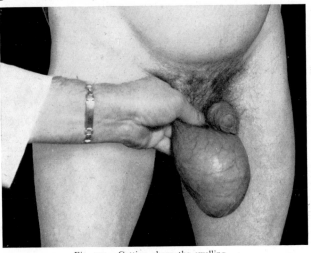

*Fig.* 339.—Getting above the swelling.

possible to get above the swelling ? " If, with the finger and thumb one is able to get above the lump, then obviously it cannot be a hernia (*Fig.* 339). This seems such an elementary point that it is almost an insult to the intelligence to record it ; and yet, if all the men walking about with inguinal trusses when all they are suffering from is a vaginal hydrocele were assembled, their number would be astounding. If one *can* get above it, the swelling is not a hernia. If one *cannot* get above the swelling, and the neck of the swelling is continuous with the inguinal canal, the patient should be made to lie down, and it should be seen if the lump is a *reducible* hernia (*Fig.* 340).

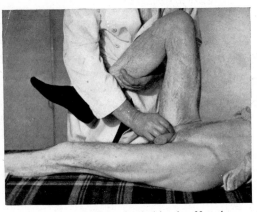

*Fig.* 340.—Reducing an inguinal hernia. Note the thigh is flexed and internally rotated.

Translucency is not an absolute test between hernia and hydrocele. A hernia containing gut, especially in a small child, may be translucent.

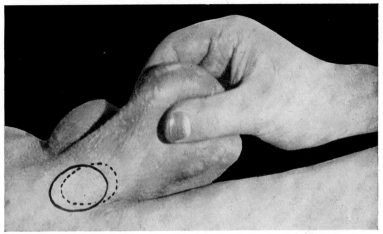

Fig. 341.—When gentle traction is exerted on the testis a hydrocele of the cord moves with the testis.

**Confirmatory Test for Encysted Hydrocele of the Cord** (when such a cyst is situated at the external abdominal ring).—Grasp the testis between finger and thumb and pull gently. When traction is made on the testis, if the swelling is a hydrocele of the cord it will move downwards with the cord (*Fig.* 341). For obvious reasons this test must be carried out with extreme care.

*The Differential Diagnosis between an Inguinal Hernia and Vasitis.*—When the vas deferens is inflamed, the only symptom may be pain and tenderness located at the external abdominal ring (*Fig.* 342). In such cases, an examination of the epididymis, which is at least slightly swollen and usually

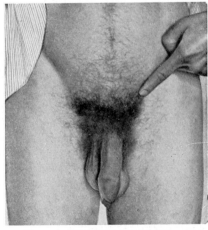

Fig. 342.—The patient stated that he experienced sudden pain in the groin while straining at work. Note that he points accurately to the external abdominal ring as the site of pain and tenderness. Case of subacute epididymo-vaso-vesiculitis.

tender, will quickly eliminate an obscure hernia as the cause of the symptoms.

## FEMORAL HERNIA

**There is no Lump.**—As in the diagnosis of inguinal hernia, so in femoral, look and look again for the presence of a visible impulse.

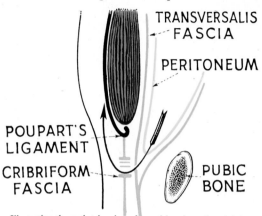

TRANSVERSALIS FASCIA

PERITONEUM

POUPART'S LIGAMENT

CRIBRIFORM FASCIA

PUBIC BONE

Fig. 343.—Illustrating the path taken by a femoral hernia, and explaining the appearance of the fundus above Poupart's ligament, which sometimes occurs when a femoral hernia becomes irreducible.

The bulge of a femoral hernia is below Poupart's ligament, and after a little practice it becomes evident that it is more laterally placed than that of an inguinal hernia. Confirm the presence of an impulse by palpation, and note the relationship of the swelling to the pubic spine.

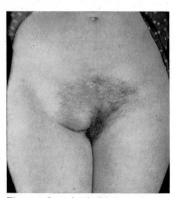

Fig. 344.—Large irreducible femoral hernia.

**There is a Lump.**—Three typical types of swelling are encountered ; to a large extent each is a stage in progressive protrusion along the path of the arrow depicted in *Fig.* 343.

*a.* There is a rounded reducible swelling lying below the inner end of Poupart's ligament (*see Fig.* 345B).

*b.* The hernia, after passing the confines of the femoral canal, bulges into Scarpa's triangle. This variety is usually irreducible (*Fig.* 344).

*c.* Fundamentally the opposite of the foregoing, for the fundus mounts upward in front of Poupart's ligament and overlies the inguinal canal. By the time the contents have pursued so tortuous a course they are usually strangulated.

**Differential Diagnosis between Inguinal and Femoral Hernia.—**

1. *There is no Lump Present.*—Observe once more the visible impulse. *If inguinal*, the bulge is seen at, and below, and to the inner side of, the external abdominal ring (*Fig.* 345A). *If femoral*, the bulge is seen under Poupart's ligament, at the upper and inner extremity of Scarpa's triangle (*Fig.* 345B).

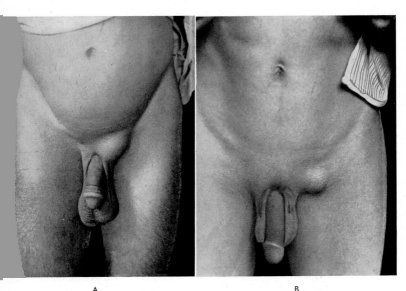

A                                                         B

*Fig.* 345.—A, inguinal and B, femoral herniæ, compared. Note that the femoral hernia is placed more laterally.

Confirm by palpating over the inguinal and femoral rings. If the visible and palpable impulse is indefinite, but the patient gives a history of a lump coming down, ask her (it is usually in the female that difficulty arises in the differential diagnosis) to point to the spot where the lump appeared. Then say, " In which direction does the lump come down ? " If she points over the lateral aspect of the mons veneris towards the labius majus, it is almost certainly an inguinal hernia. I have found this sign (*Fig.* 346, A) both useful and exceptionally reliable. In a femoral hernia, on the other hand, the patient rarely maps out the course (*Fig.* 346, B) accurately.

In other words, if the finger is pointed in the direction of the labium, it is greatly in favour of an inguinal hernia ; if the finger is not so pointed, the sign is without value. The only course is to defer the examination until the lump reappears.

2. *There is a Lump Present.*—*Cardinal rule* : If by the invagination test it is possible to demonstrate that the inguinal canal is empty, then obviously the swelling cannot be an inguinal hernia (*Fig.* 347). Inspection of the lump may prove a veritable trap, for the swelling caused by the hernia sometimes lies above Poupart's ligament ; but even in these cases the knowing eye can often detect that the swelling is placed more laterally than it is in an inguinal hernia.

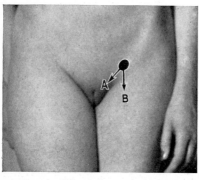

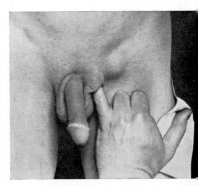

Fig. 346.—The pointing test in the differential diagnosis between inguinal and femoral herniæ. A, Inguinal direction : B, Femoral direction.

Fig. 347.—Differential diagnosis of inguinal and femoral herniæ. The little finger is in the inguinal canal, which is empty. The swelling therefore, obviously cannot be an inguinal hernia.

Palpate the swelling. Endeavour to define the neck of the sac. If the neck can be defined, then it must be contiguous to either the femoral or the inguinal ring, and the diagnosis is clear.

The real case of difficulty arises when there is a strangulated hernia situated above Poupart's ligament in which the invagination test cannot be performed, and the neck of the sac is not palpable. It is in such a case that we have to hark back to inspection, and with a certain amount of experience we can say the lump is too far lateral to be an inguinal hernia. Sometimes this point can be confirmed by determining the relationship of the lump to the pubic spine. A femoral hernia, even when it overlaps Poupart's ligament, must always lie to the outer side of the pubic spine. In fat individuals the landmark can be located by following up the tendon of the adductor longus.

### Differential Diagnosis between a Small Reducible Femoral Hernia and a Saphena Varix* (*Fig.* 348).

This, again, proves a difficult problem, and it has been known to entrap the very elect. Both swellings give an impulse when the patient coughs, and both visibly disappear when the patient lies down. It is, however, improbable that the differential diagnosis of these two conditions will remain in a nebulous state after the following factors have received due consideration.

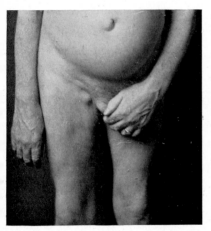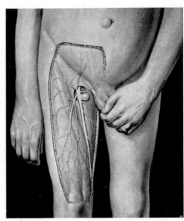

*Fig.* 348.—A saphena varix. The patient has also a para-umbilical hernia.

1. In thin subjects a faint blue coloration of the varix may be apparent.

2. Usually a saphena varix feels softer than a femoral hernia (Milnes Walker).

3. In many cases of reducible femoral hernia, when the patient lies down and the swelling visibly disappears, by skilful palpation and comparison with the opposite side, the pad of fat overlying the sac can be detected.

4. *Cruveilhier's Sign of Saphena Varix.*—In the erect position, when the patient coughs, there is a tremor imparted to the palpating fingers as if " a jet of water is entering and filling the pouch " (Cruveilhier).

---

* These swellings should be handled with great care. I had a patient with a thrombosed saphena varix who died from a pulmonary embolus that became dislodged during a clinical examination.

ROBERT MILNES WALKER, *Contemporary Professor of Surgery, University of Bristol.*
JEAN CRUVEILHIER, 1791–1874, *Professor of Pathological Anatomy, Faculty of Medicine, Paris*

**Differential Diagnosis between an Irreducible Femoral Omentocele and an Enlarged Lymph-Node in the Position of the Femoral Ring.**—This often proves a most perplexing problem, for when the lymph-node in the femoral canal known as the gland of Cloquet (*Fig.* 349) becomes enlarged, it simulates exactly an irreducible femoral omentocele. Indeed, the riddle " strangulated femoral omentocele or inflamed gland of Cloquet ? " is an ever-recurring responsible surgical diagnosis that elevates the gland of Cloquet to the notorious position of the most important lymph-node in the body.

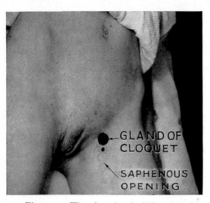

Fig. 349.—The *deep* inguinal lymph-nodes, usually only two in number, are situated within the femoral canal. The gland of Cloquet is unrivalled among lymph-nodes for surgical importance.

GLAND OF CLOQUET

SAPHENOUS OPENING

Search for a possible focus of infection. Examine the feet, the legs, buttocks, perineum, anus, and the genitals for a boil, blister, or an abrasion. If this does not elucidate the problem, there are no physical signs that will. The nature of the lump remains a matter of opinion that is best settled in the operating theatre.

**Differential Diagnosis between a Reducible Hernia and a Psoas Abscess pointing beneath Poupart's Ligament.**—

Fig. 350.—A psoas abscess usually points in Scarpa's triangle *lateral* to the femoral artery. If this relationship is verified, the question of the swelling being a femoral hernia should not arise.

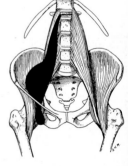

A cold abscess arising from tuberculous disease of the body of one of the lumbar vertebræ tracking along the psoas sheath to the insertion of the psoas magnus (*Fig.* 350) gives rise to a reducible, painless swelling that has, on many occasions, been mistaken for a femoral hernia. Re-examination, which includes inspection of the back and (when the patient lies down) palpation of the corresponding iliac fossa, clarifies the diagnosis and

JULES GERMAIN CLOQUET, 1790–1883, *Professor of Anatomy, Paris.*

serves to remind the clinician that purely localized regional clinical examination of his patients will sooner or later cause him to stumble, perhaps seriously.

**Differential Diagnosis between an Irreducible Femoral Hernia and a Hydrocele of a Femoral Hernial Sac.**—A hydrocele of a femoral hernial sac (*Fig.* 351) is always brilliantly translucent.

Although in the case illustrated the swelling appeared spontaneously, most examples of a hydrocele of a femoral hernial sac occur in conjunction with ascites. Therefore in this condition the abdomen should be examined for the presence of free fluid.

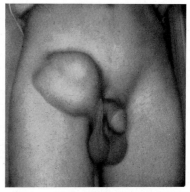

Fig. 351.—Hydrocele of a femoral hernial sac. It is brilliantly translucent.

## THE LYMPH-NODES OF THE GROIN

For clinical purposes there is no better division of the superficial inguinal lymph-nodes than into an oblique set beneath and parallel to Poupart's ligament, and a longitudinal set overlying the femoral vessels (*Fig.* 352). These two groups should be palpated (*Fig.* 353) on each side. If any are found enlarged, seek the primary focus.

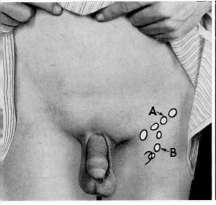

Fig. 352.—The inguinal lymph-nodes from a clinical standpoint. A, Those along Poupart's ligament : B, Those along the femoral vessels.

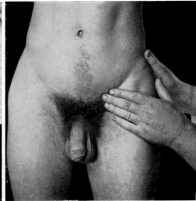

Fig. 353.—Palpating the inguinal lymph-nodes.

The leg, from the toes upwards, is inspected.  Should this prove negative, the abdominal wall, buttocks, anus, and the genitalia must be scrutinized for an infective lesion, because all these areas have

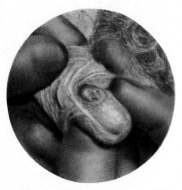

afferent lymphatic vessels draining into the groin.  When the patient has a prepuce, it should be retracted fully, so as to display the sulcus behind the corona.  The region of the frænum requires more than a haphazard glance ; it should be so displayed that no part of it is hidden from view (*Fig.* 354).  Many times has this manœuvre brought to light a primary focus hitherto undiscovered.  This is an excellent opportunity to bring to the notice of those on the threshold of their life-study of human nature how often a patient suffering

*Fig.* 354.—This primary chancre hidden beneath the prepuce was the cause of enlargement of the left inguinal lymph-nodes.

from venereal disease seemingly seeks to beguile his trusting clinician. For instance, the silvery-haired, benevolent-looking possessor of the

lesion displayed in *Fig.* 354 insisted that the lump in the groin (enlarged inguinal lymph-node) appeared as the result of his participation in a parochial cricket match !

Confronted with massive, painless adenitis of one or both groins that cannot be accounted for after carrying out a careful clinical investigation, one should reflect that millions while in the armed forces visited tropical and sub-tropical climes.  Lympho-

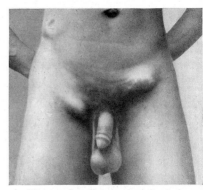

*Fig.* 355.—Lympho-granuloma inguinale (tropical bubo).

granuloma inguinale (tropical bubo★) is a venereal disease (*see* Chapter XXII) that in white people often causes considerable constitutional disturbance, and, unlike the usual manifestations in natives, the lymph-nodes along the iliac vessels share in the inflammation.  The primary

---

★ *Bubo.*  Greek, βουβών = groin.

ELUCIDATING THE CAUSE OF ENLARGED INGUINAL LYMPH-NODES

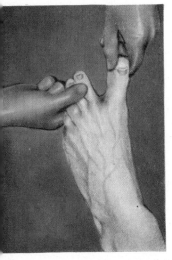

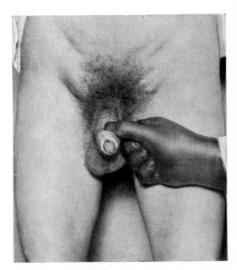

*Fig.* 356.—**Case I.** A patient with enlarged inal lymph-nodes is presented. Scrutiny of corresponding leg and foot reveals the focus ifection.

*Fig.* 357.—**Case II.** Beneath the prepuce, which cannot be retracted, a hard irregular swelling is rolled between the finger and thumb. A spot of blood appears. Carcinoma of the glans penis is the primary source of the stony hard inguinal lymph-nodes.

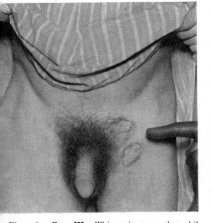

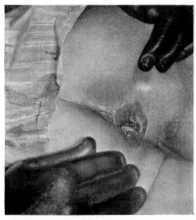

*Fig.* 358.—**Case III.** This patient says that while ng at work he felt pain in the groin. We suspect ernia : instead, two enlarged, slightly tender inguinal ph-nodes are found.

*Fig.* 359.—**Case III,** *continued.* Nothing is discovered to account for these enlarged lymph-nodes until the nates are separated. The patient denies that he has had even discomfort from these grossly inflamed prolapsed hæmorrhoids.

lesion is rather like herpes and is of fleeting duration (Stammers).
When lymphogranuloma inguinale enters the diagnostic arena,
arrangements should be made for a Frei intradermal test.

Attention has been directed already (*see* p. 192) to the importance
of an enlargement of the gland of Cloquet, especially when this enlargement is not shared by the other inguinal lymph-nodes—a state
which, for some unexplained reason, is far from uncommon.

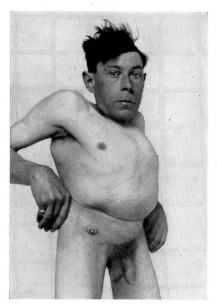

*Fig.* 360.—An ' abscess in the groin ' from Pott's disease via the psoas sheath.
A psoas abscess opening into the groin.

An abscess in the groin, particularly a chronic abscess, sometimes
originates elsewhere ; e.g., a psoas abscess is apt to point here (*Fig.*
360), and is often misdiagnosed.

Francis Alan Rowland Stammers, *Comtemporary Professor of Surgery, University of Birmingham.*
Wilhelm Frei. *Contemporary. Formerly Professor of Dermatology, Berlin. Now a refugee in New York.*

## CHAPTER XVIII

# NON-ACUTE ABDOMINAL CONDITIONS

## GENERAL PRINCIPLES IN THE CONSIDERATION OF THE ABDOMEN

THE patient should lie on his back with one pillow only beneath his head. In passing it may be remarked that it is almost unbelievable how often a presumably intelligent person, when requested to lie on his back, will promptly roll on to his abdomen. Have the patient uncovered from the nipples to the pubes. When a patient, particularly a young man, realizes that he is about to be examined, it is not exceptional for him to arch his back and blow out his chest— no doubt to demonstrate his manly proportions. Tell the patient to deflate his lungs, and by trying

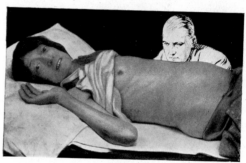

Fig. 361.—Tangential inspection of the abdomen.

to insinuate your hand between the couch and the patient, make certain that his back is resting comfortably upon the couch.

**Inspection.**—A great deal of information can be gathered from inspection (*Figs.* 362, 363). In the demonstrations of abdominal cases that follow, an endeavour will be made to bring out particular points that are revealed thereby. A common error is to scamp this important part of abdominal examination. In addition to observing every quadrant of the abdomen, it is often necessary to sit or kneel in order to get your eye at the level shown in *Fig.* 361. In this way abdominal respiratory movement is seen to advantage.

**Palpation.**—Attention has been directed already to the necessity of not hurrying over inspection. Continue in this calm, methodical frame of mind, and instead of placing the hand upon the abdomen

## THE VALUE OF INSPECTION

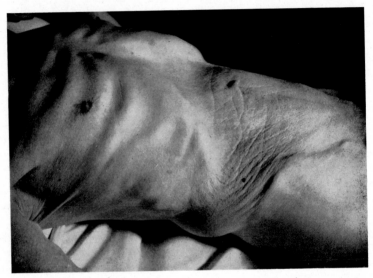

Fig. 362.—By patiently watching the abdomen for about a minute,

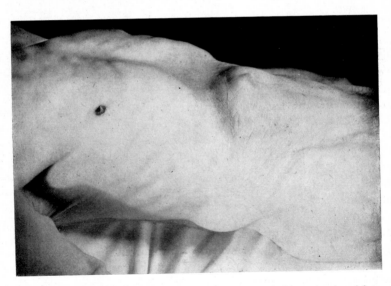

Fig. 363.—This swelling appeared, accompanied by visible peristalsis passing from left to right. Case of carcinoma of the pylorus.

unceremoniously, pay very careful attention to several preliminary details.

1. Routine palpation of the abdomen should be carried out with the flat of the hand. It is the flexor surfaces of the fingers, used collectively, that form the active palpating agent; the tips of the fingers take no part in the manœuvre. In order that the hand may impinge upon the abdomen at the correct angle, it is essential for the forearm to be maintained in a strictly horizontal plane (*Fig.* 364).

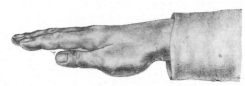

Fig. 364.—Routine palpation of the abdomen. The forearm must be kept in the same horizontal plane as the abdomen.

As beds and couches vary so much in height, the examiner, if need be, must sit on a suitable chair or even kneel upon the floor, no matter how undignified the latter position may appear (Emerson).

2. The great enemy of efficient palpation is muscular rigidity. The hands must be warm, at least as warm as the patient's skin, otherwise he will certainly contract his abdominal muscles. To wash your hands in hot water before the examination is an excellent expedient. Especially in cold weather, I commence palpating with a blanket or the patient's shirt intervening between the abdomen and my hand. By doing this the patient's confidence is obtained, and, realizing that he is not going to be hurt, he tends to relax his muscles. Some clinicians, believing that better relaxation is obtained thereby, make it a rule to have the knees flexed. Personally, I think that any advantage this may have in bringing about initial relaxation is counter-balanced by the effort of maintaining the position. A small pillow beneath the knees has much to recommend it.

3. Ask the patient to breathe quietly through the mouth and keep his hands loosely by his sides. Request him to ' drop his jaw '—this ensures that his mouth is open and it seems to help in obtaining general muscular relaxation. Tell him he is not going to be hurt. Some patients relax better when they are engaged in conversation. Experience, and to some extent native wit, will reveal what manner of man the clinician is palpating.

*Overcoming Rigidity in Refractory Cases.*—In spite of ingenuity and subterfuge, the abdominal wall sometimes continues to remain unrelaxed. In such cases Nicholson's method is of considerable value. The base of the palm of the left hand is placed upon the lower

CHARLES PHILLIPS EMERSON, *Contemporary Research Professor of Medicine, Indiana University, U.S.A.*
NEVILLE JENNINGS NICHOLSON, *Contemporary Medical Superintendent, County Hospital, Louth, Lincoln-shire, England.*

part of the sternum and increasing pressure is exerted. Eventually the examiner is leaning quite heavily upon the chest, with the result that the patient breathes abdominally, while his thorax, held as in a vice, is comparatively still. When he draws in his breath his abdominal muscles necessarily relinquish their tonicity, whereupon the right hand seizes its awaited opportunity (*Fig.* 365). I have achieved success by this method when other expedients to effect efficient abdominal palpation have failed, but I nearly always try the small pillow beneath the knees and plead with the patient to co-operate before resorting to it.

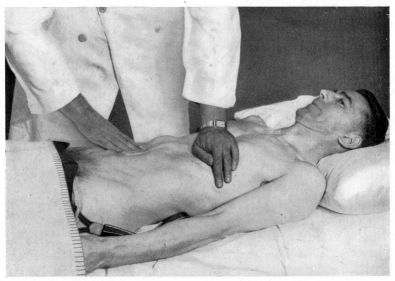

*Fig.* 365.—With the base of the left hand pressing upon the lower part of the sternum, thoracic respiration is impeded and the abdominal muscles relax.

To continue with the examination of an average case. If pain is experienced in any particular part of the abdomen, begin by palpating the region diagonally opposite. For example, if the pain is in the right iliac fossa, commence in the left hypochondrium (*Fig.* 366) and work round, palpating each quadrant in turn, ending with the region of which the patient complains. During this manœuvre there should be intelligent co-operation between the hand and the mind. While the hand is over a particular region the mind should visualize the anatomical structures beneath the hand ; at the same time the examiner's eyes should be directed to the patient's face, for if he winces when a particular area is palpated it may be of ominous diagnostic significance.

*Deep Palpation.*—During the routine palpation of the abdomen just described no attempt is made to palpate deeply ; this is reserved as a confirmatory measure in particular instances. The first essential

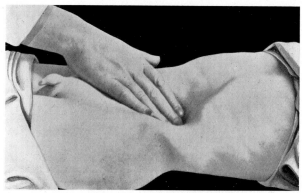

Fig. 366.—If pain is complained of in the right iliac fossa, commence palpating in the region diagonally opposite, viz., the left hypochondrium.

is to overcome the resistance of the abdominal wall. Even a tense abdominal wall tends to relax during expiration or the pause between expiration and inspiration. Continuing palpation, advantage is taken

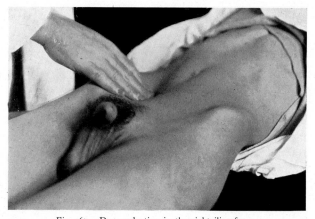

Fig. 367.—Deep palpation in the right iliac fossa.

of the periods of relaxation in order to feel progressively deeper and deeper. The position of the hand and fingers during deep palpation depends on what we wish to feel and how deeply we palpate. Deep palpation is not conducted with the flat of the hand, but rather with the flexor surfaces of the fingers with the hand tilted at a slight angle (*Fig.* 367).  By gentle, even pressure, which becomes progressively deeper and deeper, valuable information, unobtainable by any other method, is sometimes forthcoming.  When an indefinite lump is present the technique shown in *Fig.* 368 sometimes proves useful.

*Gliding palpation* is a manœuvre whereby the pulps of the fingers pass across a hollow viscus ;  in so doing they may perceive its contour.  This is possible only in loops of intestine that are fixed at each end.  So it comes about that the method is of service only in the case of the large intestine and, even in this situation, in comparatively few cases.

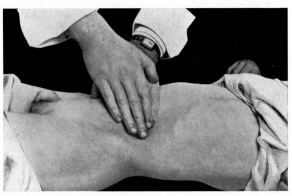

*Fig.* 368.—Using both hands, one superimposed upon the other, pressure is distributed evenly and the method is effective, particularly in deep palpation.

## EXAMINATION OF AN INTRA-ABDOMINAL SWELLING

**Inspection.**—If there is a visible lump, note particularly if it moves on respiration.  In the endeavour to elucidate the nature of a lump in the abdomen, the first step is to exclude a swelling in the abdominal wall.

It is often taught that the abdomen should be palpated before and during the raising of the head from the pillow.  Raising of the head certainly renders the recti abdominis tense, but it fails, sometimes miserably, as a differential sign in the lateral regions of the abdomen.  A good example is afforded by the following case :—

A boy had a painless lump in the right side of the abdomen, the nature of which was obscure.  He was submitted to the individual examination of eight clinicians, including four candidates for the Fellowship.  Each observer tested the lump before and whilst the patient's head was raised from the pillow.  Each came to the conclusion that the tumour was intra-abdominal, and most probably a cyst

of the kidney.   When the patient was asked to shut his mouth, hold
his nose, and then blow, it at once became evident that the lump was
in the abdominal wall.   It can be seen even in the photographs that
the lump, which is barely visible in *Fig.* 369, stands out in *Fig.* 370.

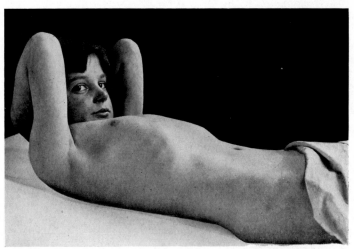

*Fig.* 369.—Is the lump in the abdominal wall ?   Putting the abdominal musculature
into action by asking the patient to raise his head.   (N.B.—The arms should rest by
the side.)

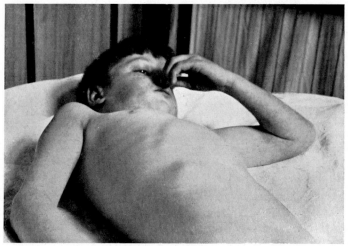

*Fig.* 370.—Putting the abdominal musculature into action.
Patient holding his nose and blowing.

Whilst the intra-abdominal pressure was thus raised, and the abdominal musculature tense, it was quite easy to elicit fluctuation. A diagnosis of tuberculous abscess of the abdominal wall in connexion with a costal cartilage was made, a diagnosis which was confirmed later. The ' blowing test ' is of value whenever it is desired to make the abdominal musculature tense—e.g., when examining for the integrity of a laparotomy scar.

There are two other good methods of rendering the abdominal wall tense, each having its particular sphere of usefulness.

1. *Carnett's Method.*—The patient is asked to extend both legs, and while keeping his knees stiff, to raise his feet from the bed. This procedure renders the abdominal muscles very tense, but the patient must be of a somewhat athletic disposition to carry out the exercise.

2. *Kamath's Test.*—Ask the patient to strain as if at stool.

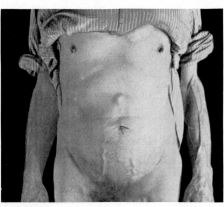

*Fig.* 371.—Fatty hernia of the linea alba that became visible only when the patient was examined standing up. He complained of symptoms that suggested the presence of a peptic ulcer.

Perhaps the most frequent call for this type of test is when a possibility of a small incisional or other hernia through the anterior abdominal musculature enters the diagnostic arena. In such circumstances, I have noticed repeatedly that even candidates for higher qualifications omit to examine the patient standing up. Time and again, standing erect, without other aids, has brought into sight a protrusion through the abdominal musculature that was indiscernible in the prone position (*Fig.* 371).

**Palpation.**—Note the consistency and shape of the lump ; whether it is regular or irregular ; mobile or fixed to the posterior abdominal wall. Further, note whether it moves on respiration. Percuss the lump, and record whether it is dull or resonant. An examination in the knee-elbow position (*Fig.* 372) should always be resorted to in obscure cases, and occasionally this is very helpful, particularly in deciding whether pulsations are transmitted from the abdominal aorta to an overlying swelling, or whether the swelling

John Berton Carnett, 1876–1934, *Professor of Surgery, University of Pennsylvania, U.S.A.*
Manjeshwar Vamanrao Kamath, *Contemporary Assistant Surgeon, Stanley Hospital, Madras, India.*

tself is pulsatile. If the swelling arises from the pelvis, a bimanual ectal or vaginal examination is essential (*see* Chapter XX). It

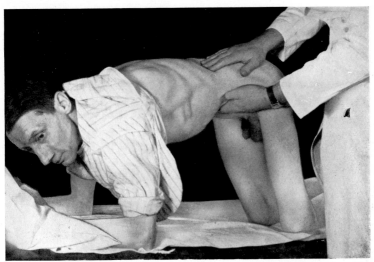

Fig. 372.—Examining the abdomen in the knee-elbow position.

here behoves us to remember a simple but important rule: *Never express an opinion upon a tumour arising out of the pelvis until the bladder has been emptied by a catheter.*

There is one physical sign that occasionally proves helpful in obscure intra-abdominal swellings, and that is the *sign of a mesenteric* cyst. The lump moves in a plane from the right hypochondrium to the left iliac fossa, but not in the plane at right angles to this (*Fig.* 373).

In the demonstrations that follow, the physical signs of swellings connected with particular organs will be considered.

So far as tumours are concerned, the abdomen is indeed a temple of surprise, and it is by our diagnostic humiliations when the abdomen is opened that we learn.

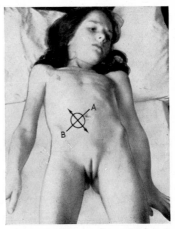

Fig. 373.—The sign of a mesenteric cyst. A–B represents the line of attachment to the mesentery. A mesenteric cyst moves much more freely in the direction of the arrows than in the plane at right angles to this.

## CHAPTER XIX

## NON-ACUTE ABDOMINAL CONDITIONS — SPECIAL DEMONSTRATIONS

### EXAMINATION OF A GASTRIC CASE

WHILE the history is all-important in the diagnosis of a lesion of the stomach or duodenum, physical examination may yield information.

**Examine the Teeth**—particularly for evidence of pyorrhœa. Record the number of teeth present. If the patient has a dental plate, get him to remove it, and examine the jaws again.

**Inspect the Abdomen.**—For examination, the body should be uncovered from the pubes to the nipples. Pay considerable attention to the subcostal angle. A narrow subcostal angle is indicative of *visceroptosis* (*Figs.* 374, 375). If there is a narrow subcostal angle, look

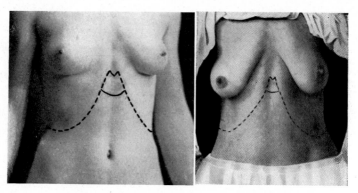

Fig. 374.—Normal subcostal angle.  Fig. 375.—Narrow subcostal angle associated with visceroptosis.

for visible pulsation above the umbilicus. Thorkild Rovsing, speaking of gastroptosis, said : " One perceives a distinct pulsation in the epigastric region. When I place my hand on the epigastrium, I feel the aorta pulsating quite close to my fingers ; you can see, in fact, how my fingers rise and fall simultaneously with the pulse-wave.

THORKILD ROVSING, 1862–1927, *Professor of Surgery, Copenhagen.*

You will never find this with individuals whose stomachs occupy their normal position. It is merely due to the fact that the stomach which usually covers the vertebral column like an air or water cushion, has glided down from its position into the abdomen. It is therefore, a pathognomonic sign of gastroptosis." That the patient has visceroptosis is often demonstrable by viewing her from the side in the erect position (*Fig.* 376).

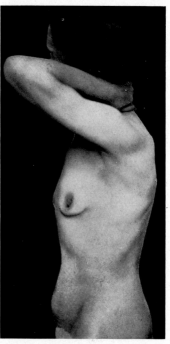

If, from the history, there is any reason to believe that there is pyloric stenosis, particular attention should be directed to watching for visible peristalsis passing from left to right in the epigastrium (*see Fig.* 378).

**Epicritic Hyperæsthesia.**—No importance should be attached to superficial or, for that matter, deep tenderness in the diagnosis of chronic gastric ulcer.

**Palpation.**—Make a routine examination of the abdomen by palpation. In very thin individuals the normal pylorus can sometimes be felt. When thickened by infantile hypertrophy, inflammation, or neoplasm, the impression imparted by a palpable pylorus can be likened to a bobbin lying transversely. A neoplasm of the stomach often possesses very evident transmitted pulsation from the abdominal aorta, and it usually moves with respiration.

*Fig.* 376.—Viewing the abdomen from the side for evidence of visceroptosis.

Neoplasms of the stomach that cannot be felt can sometimes be seen in the epigastric notch, descending at each inspiration, and disappearing during expiration.

**The Sign of Splashing.**—Splashing is of value only when the stomach should normally be empty—that is, three hours after a meal. The hand is laid over the stomach, and short, sudden, dipping movements are made. When the sign is positive it suggests dilatation of the stomach, probably due to pyloric obstruction.

*Scraping Auscultation.*—In order to differentiate between splashing of the stomach and that of the transverse colon scraping auscultation should be used. Place a stethoscope just below and to the left of the xiphoid process, and keep it there.

Make scraping movements with the finger in lines radiating from this point. Wher the confines of the stomach have been passed, the characteristic noise ceases. The size of the organ can be determined by this method.

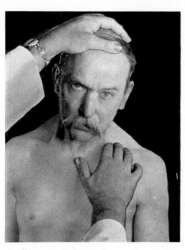

Fig. 377.—Palpating for an enlarged gland in the left supraclavicular fossa. The sign of Troisier. The head should be flexed and the chin inclined to the left shoulder during deep palpation of the fossa.

**The Sign of Troisier.**—In the late stages of carcinoma of the stomach, especially when the primary growth is high up on the lesser curvature, the left supraclavicular glands may be enlarged. Therefore, always palpate this supraclavicular fossa as a routine when examining a gastric case (*Fig.* 377).

Supposing that the probable diagnosis of carcinoma of the stomach has been arrived at, make it a practice not only to try the sign of Troisier, but to perform a rectal examination to exclude the possibility of transcœlomic implantation of secondary growth into the recto-vesical pouch. Also examine the liver with great care for signs of secondary deposits.

## EXAMINATION OF A CASE OF SUSPECTED INFANTILE PYLORIC STENOSIS

It is best to have the infant upon a table. The clinician's chair should be of such a height as to allow his arms to rest upon the table

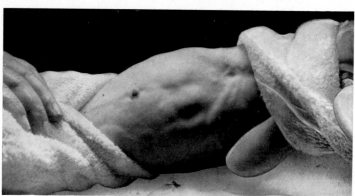

Fig. 378.—Visible peristalsis. A wave could be seen passing from left to right. A case of hypertrophic pyloric stenosis in an infant.

CHARLES EMILE TROISIER, 1844–1919, *Professor of Pathology, Paris.*

n a comfortable position. If the child is crying, rigidity makes it useless to proceed. It is given a feeding-bottle of warm water to suck (Seeger). This often affords an op-portunity to observe a wave of peristalsis (*Fig.* 378), which is sufficient evidence to make a concrete diagnosis. The child usually vomits the water that has been imbibed. During the temporary relax-ation that follows, by bimanual palpation (*Fig.* 379) it is frequently possible to feel the lump, if such be present. A useful procedure is to rest the infant face down-wards on one's hand, so that the pulps

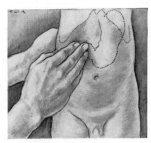

Fig. 379.—Method of palpating an infant's abdomen for a hypertro-phied pylorus (*after Seeger*).

of the fingers lie under the right hypo-chondrium. Sometimes the hypertrophied pylorus can be felt in this way when it has not been palpable with the child lying on its back (Milnes Walker).

## EXAMINATION OF A CASE OF SUSPECTED RECURRENT OR CHRONIC APPENDICITIS

The methods to be employed differ very little from those dealt with fully in Chapter *XXIII*. It is well to bear in mind that an examination of a case of suspected gastric or duodenal ulcer is not complete without thorough palpation of the right iliac fossa, for so often many, if not all, of the symptoms of chronic appendicitis are referred to the stomach or more frequently the duodenum.

In highly strung women it should be noted that deep tenderness in the right iliac fossa does not necessarily signify that the appendix is diseased—indeed, other things being equal, a tender gurgling cæcum negatives this diagnosis in such individuals.

When confronted with a patient who has resided in the tropics and has signs of recurrent inflammation in the right iliac fossa, consider the possibility of chronic amœbic colitis. At the clinical examination seek a tender, palpable segment of the colon other than in the right iliac fossa.

## EXAMINATION OF A COLONIC CASE

The history strongly suggests that the seat of the trouble is in the large intestine.

STANLEY JOSEPH SEEGER, *Contemporary Surgeon, Columbia Hospital, Milwaukee, Wisconsin.*
ROBERT MILNES WALKER, *Contemporary Professor of Surgery, University of Bristol.*

**Examination of a Case of Chronic Constipation ; Suspected Chronic Intestinal Obstruction.**—Time spent in inspecting the abdomen is seldom wasted ; in this instance it frequently brings a

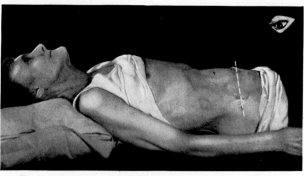

*Fig.* 380.—Inspection of the abdomen in general, and for a fullness in the right iliac fossa in particular, is best undertaken in the manner shown above. It is important to see that the patient is lying quite ' square '. The imaginary line drawn through the iliac spines should be at right angles to the edge of the examining couch.

rich reward. In most cases of carcinoma of the colon with early (chronic) obstruction, there is a slight fullness in the right iliac

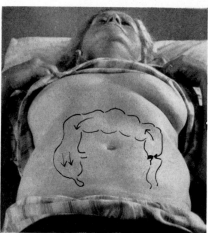

*Fig.* 381.—The cæcum is distended in *all* cases of obstruction to the large intestine, including the rectum.

fossa that is only apparent when looked for especially.

Arrange the patient on the examination couch carefully, so that one anterior superior iliac spine is not higher than the other, and an imaginary line through them is precisely at right angles to the long axis of the examining couch (*Fig.* 380). Ensure that the patient is comfortable and relaxed.

Observe the abdomen intently. Compare the left with the right iliac fossa. A fullness of the right iliac fossa due to a distended cæcum is better seen than felt. The cæcum is distended in *all* cases of obstruction to the large bowel, including the rectum, irrespective of the site of obstruction (*Fig.* 381). When here is even the slightest fullness in the right iliac fossa percuss the area. If a resonant note is obtained, the suspicion of a distended cæcum is strengthened. Commence palpation in the right iliac fossa. If on deep palpation gurgling is heard, the suspicion is confirmed.

Palpate each quadrant of the abdomen systematically.

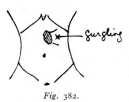

Fig. 382.

On several occasions when a lump (carcinoma) in the line of the transverse colon inclining to the left of the middle line has been presented, the question has arisen "Is this a growth of the stomach, or is it a carcinoma of the colon ?" If gurgling can be elicited on the left side of the lump (*Fig.* 382) assuredly the pyloric end of the stomach is obstructed.

When a lump is detected in the line of the large intestine, it is frequently necessary to eliminate the possibility of a fæcal mass. A fæcal mass can be indented by digital pressure, and many times I have seen students (and graduates) beguiled by omitting this test. At times the mass is not accessible enough for this test to be carried out. If even a lingering doubt exists, reserve your judgement. Arrange for a re-examination on another day after an enema has been administered by a competent nurse. I consider that this somewhat troublesome method yields more reliable information than the usual course of referring the patient to the radiological department.

It is hardly necessary to point out how important is a rectal examination (*see* Chapter XX) in the type of case now under consideration.

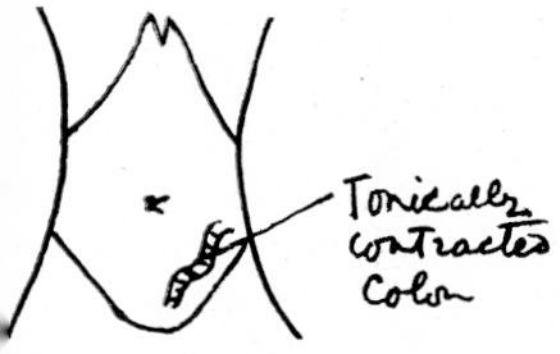

Especially in thin females, the pelvic colon can often be rolled beneath the fingers. In some cases where there is a history suggesting colitis, or one of obstinate constipation, the pelvic colon can be felt tonically contracted (*Fig.* 383)—a state that gives a characteristic sensation to the examining fingers.

Fig. 383.

## EXAMINATION OF THE GALL-BLADDER

**Examination of a Case of Cholecystitis.**—The subjects of this disease are often fat, middle-aged, multiparous women, and this is so well known that it has been remarked that if a bed in a female surgical ward is occupied by a person answering to this description, it is ten to one that she has either gall-stones or a para-umbilical hernia ! This sweeping assumption needs a corrective ; gall-stones are not uncommon even in thin men.

The first thing to look for is the presence of jaundice.* The conjunctiva is the best place to look for minor degrees of this pigmentation, but here let it be emphasized that it is by no means necessary for the patient to have jaundice in order to make the diagnosis of gallstones. The presence of deep, unmistakable jaundice associated with this condition means that a gall-stone is, or has been, obstructing the *common* bile-duct. On the other hand, slight transient jaundice can be accounted for by infection—for instance by cholangitis, which can reasonably be expected to be associated with inflammation of the gall-bladder.

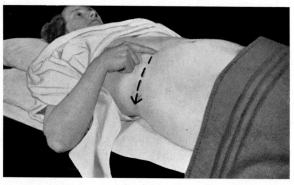

Fig. 384.—The pointing test in cholecystitis. The pain commences in the right hypochondrium and passes round to the back or between the shoulders.

Observe the abdomen. A brownish stain is not infrequently seen in the epigastrium and right hypochondrium. This is due to the application of heat, in the form of hot plates or hot-water bottles, to relieve the pain. Ask the patient to show you where she gets the pain. She will point to the right hypochondrium (*Fig.* 384). Now ask where the pain goes to, and she will run her finger round the right side, saying that it passes to the back or between the shoulders. Palpate the abdomen, beginning in the left iliac fossa and ending in the right hypochondrium.

*Murphy's Sign* (*Moynihan's Method*).—Place the left hand on the costal margin in such a manner that the thumb lies over the fundus of the gall-bladder (*Fig.* 385). The thumb exerts moderate pressure. Ask the patient to take a deep breath. The sign is positive if the

---

* The yellow tinge cannot be perceived by ordinary artificial light.

John Benjamin Murphy, 1857–1916, *Professor of Surgery, Northwestern University, Chicago.*
Berkeley George Andrew, Lord Moynihan of Leeds, 1865–1936, *Professor of Surgery, Leeds.*

patient ' catches her breath ' when the descending diaphragm causes
the inflamed gall-bladder to impinge against the pressure of the
thumb. Murphy's sign may be described technically as a temporary
inhibition of respiration when inspiration is nearing its zenith.

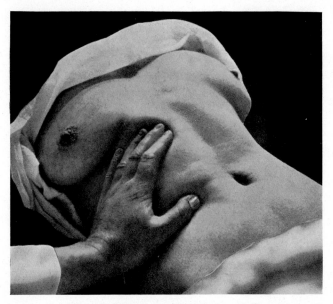

*Fig. 385.*—Murphy's sign (Moynihan's method).

*Tender Rib Cartilage as a Sign of Cholecystitis.*—This sign is
sought for with the hand flat upon the abdomen. Beginning on the
left side, the pulp of a finger is brought into firm contact with the
costal margin. Inch by inch the costal margin is examined in this
way, the examiner saying nothing, but watching the patient's face.
On the right, in cases of cholecysitis, a single tender spot, indicated
by the patient's expression, is often found. Generally this is upon
the 8th rib edge, but is sometimes a little higher or lower.
Professor Carmalt-Jones speaks highly of this sign in the diagnosis
of cholecystitis.

*Boas's Sign.*—In cholecystitis there may be an area of epicritic
hyperæsthesia posteriorly. The tenderness extends from about one
inch lateral to the spines of the vertebræ to the posterior axillary
line, and vertically from the level of the 11th dorsal to the 1st lumbar

14

DUDLEY WILLIAM CARMALT-JONES, *Contemporary Emeritus Professor of Medicine, University of Otago New Zealand.*

ISMAR ISIDOR BOAS, 1858–1938, *Gastro-enterologist, Berlin.*

spine (*Fig.* 386). I have noted in a case of recurrent cholecystitis, with gall-stones, itching in this area, which was not completely relieved by scratching.

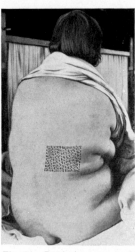

Fig. 386.—Boas's sign—an area of epicritic hyperæsthesia posteriorly.

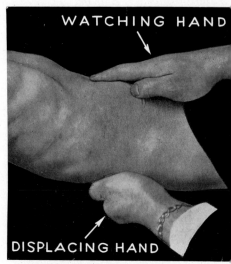

Fig. 387.—Differential diagnosis of a large gall-bladder and a hydronephrosis.

**Differential Diagnosis between a Large Hydrops of the Gall-bladder and a Hydronephrosis.**—Place the hands as shown in *Fig.* 387. With the displacing hand exert *gentle* upward movements with the pulps of the fingers acting in harmony. If the swelling in question is a hydronephrosis, the watching hand will appreciate the upward lift imparted to the swelling. On the other hand a large gall-bladder will be unaffected by these movements. The sign is entirely without value unless the movements are gentle.

## EXAMINATION OF A CASE OF OBSTRUCTION TO THE COMMON BILE-DUCT

The patient is deeply jaundiced (*Fig.* 388), and there is no doubt that the common bile-duct is obstructed. The differential diagnosis we are usually required to make is between a carcinoma of the head of the pancreas and a stone impacted in the common bile-duct. If a stone is a cause of the biliary obstruction, the jaundice will almost always be preceded by an attack of biliary colic, *and, what is more important, the jaundice tends to vary in intensity from day to day.* In carcinoma

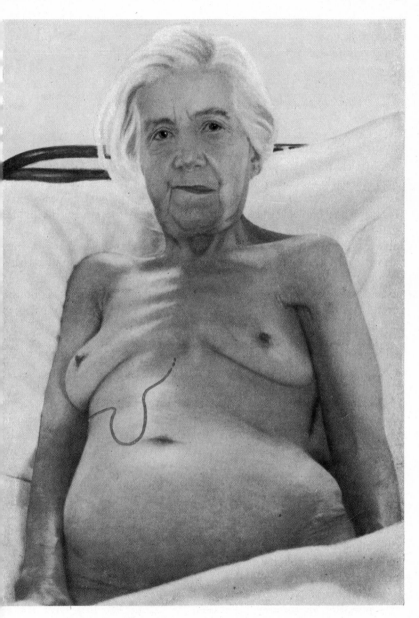

*Fig.* 388.—Profound jaundice. The outline of the enlarged gall-bladder
has been marked out with a skin pencil.

of the head of the pancreas, the onset of the jaundice is painless, apyrexial, and gradually becomes deeper and deeper.   In both conditions the patient wastes rapidly ;  therefore wasting is of no diagnostic importance.

I was once told by a clinician of the older school that jaundice following carcinoma of the pancreas never caused the patient to itch, but I have been able to disprove this statement on several occasions.  *All* jaundiced patients are liable to cutaneous irritation.

On examination of the abdomen shown in *Fig*. 388, the gallbladder could be felt to be enlarged enormously, and there is no doubt that this patient was an example of the truth of Courvoisier's law.   This law states that if in a jaundiced patient the gall-bladder is enlarged, it is *not* a case of stone impacted in the common bile-duct, for previous cholecystitis, which existed when the stone was in the gall-bladder, must have rendered the gall-bladder fibrotic and incapable of dilatation.   Courvoisier's law has much to be said for it, but, as with all laws in medicine, there are many exceptions, and on this account the law has fallen into disrepute.   The most notable of these exceptions are :  double impaction, when there is one stone in the cystic and another in the common bile-duct, and a pancreatic calculus causing obturation at the ampulla of Vater.

**Acholuric Jaundice.**—In a case where the signs point to cholecystitis, but the subject does not conform to type—for instance, supposing the patient is both young and slim—it is well to make it a rule to palpate carefully for an enlarged spleen. By doing this consistently I have been enabled to diagnose two or three cases of acholuric jaundice.

**Infective Hepatitis** (syn. catarrhal jaundice).—Again the patient does not always conform to type, and is usually young.   If there is an epidemic in the district, the diagnosis is not particularly difficult. Vomiting precedes the jaundice, which may affect the skin before the conjunctivæ (Leak).

When catarrhal jaundice does not clear up within a reasonable period, the diagnosis should be revised.   In the short space of a few months I encountered a case of stone impacted in the ampulla of Vater, another of stones in the common bile-duct, and a third of carcinoma of the head of the pancreas, all diagnosed and treated for long periods as catarrhal jaundice.   Warren Cole makes the following practical observation.   *No patient with catarrhal jaundice has an absence of bile in the stools (clay-coloured stool) for more than four days.*

**Jaundice in Infancy.**—Between the second and fifth days of life, more than half of all newly-born infants develop jaundice (*icterus neonatorum*).   Such jaundice reaches its zenith in three or four days,

LUDWIG COURVOISIER, 1843–1918, *Professor of Surgery, Basle, Switzerland.*
ABRAHAM VATER, 1684–1751, *Professor of Anatomy and Botany, Wittenburg, Germany.*
WALTER NORMAN LEAK, *Contemporary Surgeon, Albert Infirmary, Winsford, Cheshire, England.*
WARREN COLE, *Contemporary Professor of Surgery, University of Illinois College of Medicine, Chicago.*

and then fades gradually. The liver is not enlarged, neither are the stools clay-coloured nor is the urine deeply bile-stained. In *icterus gravis neonatorum* (*syn. erythroblastosis fœtalis*) the baby is born jaundiced, and the spleen is obviously enlarged. In *congenital atresia of the common bile-duct* or *the common hepatic duct*, the infant, exhibiting no more jaundice than one would expect in icterus neonatorum, instead of following the usual course, becomes more and more jaundiced (*Fig.* 389), and it is soon evident that the liver is enlarged.

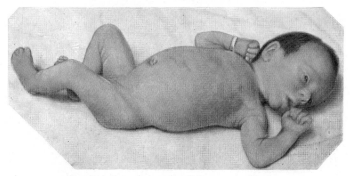

*Fig.* 389.—Congenital atresia of the common bile-duct.

## EXAMINATION OF THE LIVER FOR ENLARGEMENT

Inspection is not usually of great value, although, on occasions, the edge of a large liver can be seen to move downwards on inspiration. The normal liver cannot be felt. A general enlargement of the organ can be detected by palpating the free edge of the right lobe below the costal margin. A well-developed right rectus muscle hinders this palaption, and one should commence by attempting to feel for the liver edge to the right of this muscle. Lay the flat of the

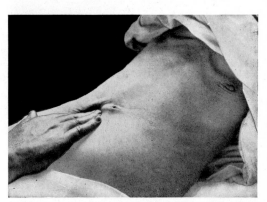

*Fig.* 390.—Examining the free edge of an enlarged liver. The fingers have just overridden the liver edge, which can be seen. In this case of secondary carcinoma the free edge felt irregular and was stony hard.

hand upon the abdomen, with the fingers directed upwards and slightly to the left. Gently work the hand about in such a way as to produce a loose fold of skin above the fingers. Ask the patient to take a deep breath, and whilst inspiration is in progress the finger tips may be felt to ride over the free edge of the liver (*Fig.* 390). Sometimes this manœuvre has to be repeated several times at slightly different levels before the liver edge is felt indisputably.

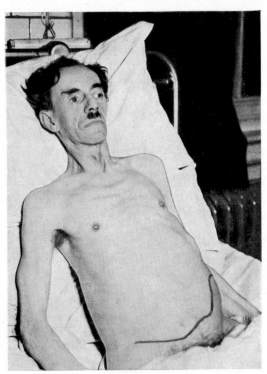

*Fig.* 391.—Gross enlargement of the liver and a glass eye (which has been worn for, maybe, many years) is practically pathognomonic of secondary melanoma, the primary growth having been in the uveal tract.

At the moment of impact of the fingers with the liver edge the character of the organ is noted ; for instance, very characteristic is the stony-hard irregular liver edge of secondary carcinoma. Once the liver edge has been felt distinctly, working from right to left, the lower border of the liver is defined as far as possible and outlined with a skin pencil (*Fig.* 391).

Attention is directed now to the upper surface of the organ. Commencing in the mid-axillary line at about the fourth interspace, percuss and obtain a clear resonant note. Then work downwards until the resonance is supplanted by dullness. Here mark the upper border of the liver. The anterior and posterior thoracic walls are examined in the same manner. It may be noted that hydatid cysts in particular often cause enlargement in an upward rather than a downward direction.

When the patient is obese and/or the transverse colon is distended, it is difficult to feel the lower edge of the liver. In such cases Cantlie's method is useful. The skin is very gently flicked while a stethoscope is applied to the abdomen. Auscultation is carried out from below upwards and there is a distinct difference in quality of the sound as soon as the lower edge of the liver is reached. By systematic examination in this manner over the relevant part of the abdomen, the lower edge of the liver can be marked out.

It should be more widely known that during infancy and until about the end of the third year the normal liver extends one or two finger-breadths below the costal margin (*Fig.* 392). During inspiration, at this period of life the extreme edge of the normal spleen is also palpable (Norman Capon).

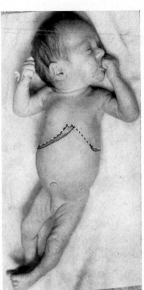

*Fig.* 392.—During infancy the edge of the normal liver can be palpated : it is also possible to feel the edge of the normal spleen during inspiration.

## ASCITES

A general fullness of the abdomen may be due to : (1) Fat ; (2) Fluid ; (3) Flatus ; (4) Fæces ; (5) Fœtus.

**Fluid Thrill.**—The orthodox method of testing for ascites is shown in *Fig.* 393. An assistant places the edge of his hand firmly on the centre of the abdomen in order to damp down a fat thrill. The abdominal wall on one side is flicked, and the thrill is felt by the hand on the other side of the abdomen. Shifting dullness (*see* Chapter XXIII)

SIR JAMES CANTLIE, 1851–1926, *Surgeon, Charing Cross Hospital, London ; later practised in Hong Kong.*
NORMAN BRANDON CAPON, *Contemporary Professor of Child Health, University of Liverpool.*

is a valuable sign when the quantity of fluid in the peritoneal
cavity is comparatively small.

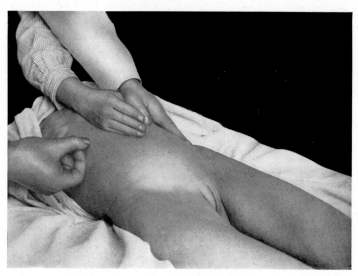

*Fig.* 393.—Testing for a ' fluid thrill ' in a case of tuberculous peritonitis.

'**Dipping**'.—A special technique is required to palpate organs
or tumours in cases of ascites. This is known as ' dipping '. The
pads of the fingers are placed on the abdomen, and then, by
a quick push, the abdominal wall is depressed. By this method
an enlarged liver is felt easily, and a tumour mass can usually be
defined.

**Differential Diagnosis between a Large Ovarian Cyst and
Ascites.**—A large ovarian tumour may be mistaken for ascites.
After the bladder has been emptied by a catheter the problem can
often be elucidated by percussion (*Fig.* 394). When the whole
abdomen is filled by a cystic swelling this differential diagnosis
becomes exceedingly difficult unless the following method is applied.
A flat ruler is laid upon the abdomen just above the level of the anterior
superior iliac spines. With the fingers of both hands this is pressed
firmly and steadily backwards towards the lumbar spine (*Fig.* 395).
In the case of an ovarian cyst the pulsations of the abdominal aorta
can be felt and—by the movements imparted to the ruler—seen.
This phenomenon is not present in ascites (Blaxland).

ATHELSTAN JASPER BLAXLAND, *Contemporary Surgeon, Norfolk and Norwich Hospital, England.*

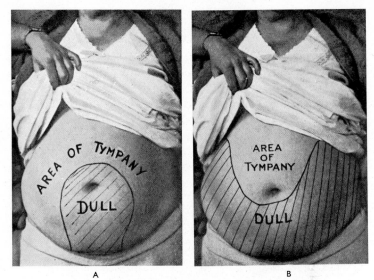

Fig. 394.—Differential diagnosis between ovarian cyst and ascites. A, Ovarian cyst. B, Ascites.

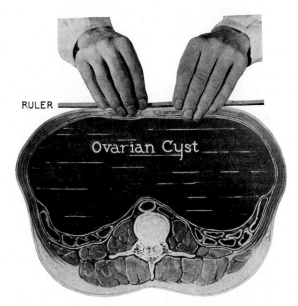

Fig. 395.—Differential diagnosis between ascites and an ovarian cyst filling the abdomen. If the swelling is due to a cyst, the pulsations of the aorta are transmitted to the fingers and can be demonstrated by the ruler.

## BIMANUAL PALPATION OF THE SPLEEN FOR MINOR ENLARGEMENT

The left hand is placed over the lateral aspect of the costal margin, and, whilst exerting a certain amount of even compression, at the same time it draws the skin and subcutaneous tissues downwards and forwards over the ribs towards the expectant fingers of the right hand. This leaves a loose fold of skin under the costal margin. The right hand lies on the abdominal wall just below the margin of the ribs, with the finger-tips pointing towards the spleen (*Fig.* 396). Keep the hands still, and do not expect to feel anything until near the end of inspiration. Just before the zenith of inspiration, draw the

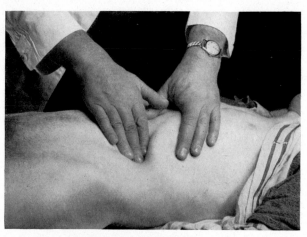

*Fig.* 396.—Bimanual palpation of the spleen.

hands slightly together and dip a mere trifle with the right finger-tips. If the spleen is palpable, the finger tips will be felt momentarily to ride over its edge. The spleen must be at least one-third as big again as normal before it can be detected by clinical methods.

On the whole, I am inclined to think that the most potent cause of the failure to detect a large spleen is that the organ is sought for more medially than it should be. In other words, the spleen lies more laterally than we are inclined to think when visualizing the position of the organ.

In order to facilitate palpation of the spleen, Middleton advises that the patient's left fist be inserted beneath his lower left ribs.

WILLIAM SHAINLINE MIDDLETON, *Contemporary Professor of Medicine and Dean, University of Winsconsin, U.S.A.*

Undoubtedly this expedient brings about anterior displacement of the lower ribs and helps to render the spleen more accessible. In cases of uncertainty further examination can be attempted in the manner shown in *Fig.* 397, where the examiner changes his position and stands on the left side of the patient's head.

**An Enlarged Spleen as an Abdominal Tumour.**—An enlarged spleen moves freely with respiration, and has a sharp anterior edge which always faces downwards and inwards. Often this edge is notched (*Fig.* 398), but not necessarily so. A splenic

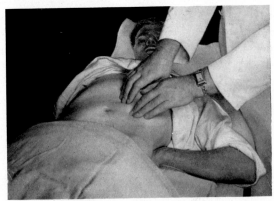

Fig. 397.—Middleton's method of palpating the spleen. Note the position of the patient's left forearm.

tumour is dull to percussion, and this dullness is continuous with the normal splenic dullness, which may also be increased upwards. In obscure cases of great enlargement of the spleen, examine the conjunctivæ. In Gaucher's disease there is a peculiar conjunctival thickening.

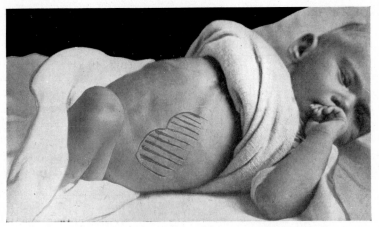

Fig. 398.—Massive enlargement of the spleen (splenic anæmia). Splenic notch easily palpable.

PHILIPPE CHARLES ERNEST GAUCHER, 1854–1918, *Physician, St. Louis Hospital, Paris.*

The usual difficulty in differential diagnosis is between a splenic and a left renal tumour.  In the case of the spleen there is always a small space between the posterior edge of the organ and the erector spinæ.

*Kenawy's sign* is sometimes useful in conditions where both the liver and the spleen are enlarged, e.g., Banti's disease ; Egyptian splenomegaly.  Auscultation over the liver reveals a hum which is louder during inspiration.  This phenomenon is probably due to engorgement of the splenic vein, and the hum is louder during inspiration because the spleen is then compressed.

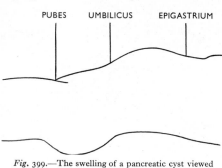

PUBES    UMBILICUS    EPIGASTRIUM

*Fig.* 399.—The swelling of a pancreatic cyst viewed from the side.  (*Grey Turner.*)

## PANCREATIC CYST

A pancreatic cyst usually gives rise to a swelling above the umbilicus, best seen when viewed laterally (*Fig.* 399).  The cyst is round, smooth, and usually tense.  It is almost always immovable.  A pseudo-pancreatic cyst is a collection of fluid in the lesser sac, and not infrequently follows a severe injury to the upper abdomen.

## THE UMBILICUS

Every time we examine an abdomen our eyes, almost instinctively, rest momentarily upon the umbilicus.  How innumerable are the variations of this structure !

**Exomphalos.**—The infant is born with a defect at the umbilicus, the protruding abdominal contents being covered only by a diaphanous membrane (*Fig.* 400).  Through this transparent veil the viscera are exposed to view, as if exhibited in a show-case (Ladd).

**Umbilical Hernia.**—The so-called umbilical hernia of adults (seen most often in obese females) is a *para*-umbilical hernia (*Fig.* 401), in that the umbilicus is either just above or, more commonly, just below the hernial protrusion.  An endeavour should be made to reduce the hernia by gentle pressure.  If the hernia has existed for any length of time, reduction is usually only partially successful, for omentum becomes adherent within the sac.

MOHAMMED RADWAN KENAWY, *Contemporary Medical Tutor, Fouad I University Hospital, Cairo, Egypt.*
WILLIAM EDWARD LADD, *Contemporary Chief of Surgical Service, Children's Hospital, Boston, U.S.A.*

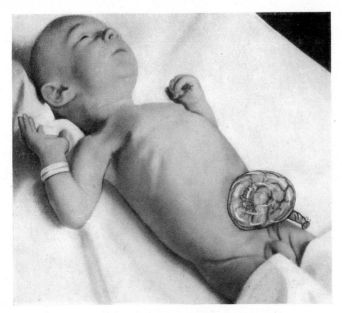

*Fig.* 400.—Exomphalos.

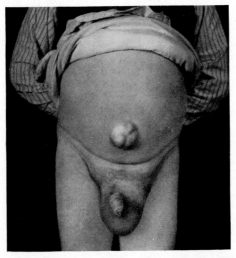

*Fig.* 401.—Para-umbilical hernia. The umbilicus lies beneath the protrusion and can be seen only by lifting it up. The patient has also a left inguinal hernia.

True umbilical hernia may be congenital (*Fig.* 402) or acquired the former is very common in infants the latter is due to the umbilicus, which is a scar, giving way, and is always secondary to some increase in intra-abdominal tension. Therefore search must be made for the cause—the commonest cause in a child is the ascitic form of tuberculous peritonitis (*Fig.* 403).

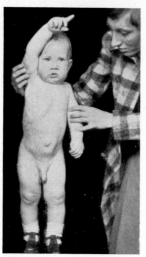

*Fig.* 402.—Congenital umbilical hernia.

**Unfolding of the Umbilicus.**—When the abdomen becomes distended the umbilicus tends partially to unfold (*Fig.* 403). I have found this a helpful sign in several early cases of intestinal obstruction.

**Enlargement of Veins around the Umbilicus.**—Engorged veins about the umbilicus suggest the presence of portal obstruction. In advanced cases of this condition the well-known caput Medusæ is seen (*see* p. 19).

**Umbilical Fistula.**—This may or may not be associated with an umbilical adenoma. Express and, if possible, collect some of the discharge, which may be urine (urachal fistula), fæcal (patent omphalo-mesenteric duct), or mucous.

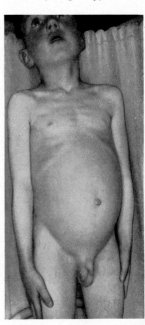

*Fig.* 403.—Tuberculous peritonitis. Note the unfolding of the umbilicus.

Local infective dermatitis usually accompanies any umbilical fistula.

**Umbilical Adenoma.**—This can very easily be diagnosed at sight. It is a pedunculated, raspberry-like mass (*Fig.* 404).

**Endometrioma of the Umbilicus.**—This condition should be suspected when there is a growth at the umbilicus simulating an umbilical adenoma in a woman between 25 and 50 years af age.

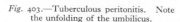

MEDUSA, *one of the three Gorgons whose fine hair was turned into snakes (Greek mythology).*

On inquiry, in the case illustrated (*Fig.* 405), the patient said bleeding occurred from the umbilicus at each menstrual period.

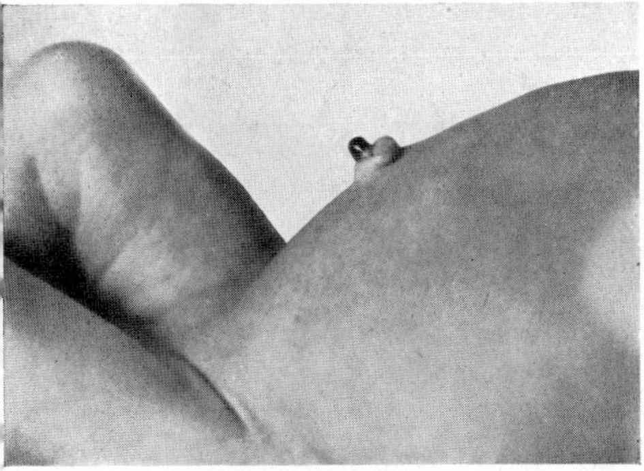

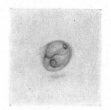

*Fig.* 404.—Umbilical adenoma.

*Fig.* 405.—Endometrioma of the umbilicus.

**Umbilical Carcinoma.**—In advanced intra-abdominal carcinoma a neoplastic nodule can sometimes be seen (*Fig.* 406) or felt at the umbilicus. This is known as Sister Joseph's nodule.*

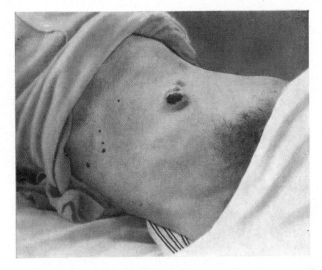

*Fig.* 406.—Secondary carcinomatous nodule at the umbilicus. The red spots near the costal margin are Campbell de Morgan spots. (*See* p. 39.)

---

* Sister Joseph of the Mayo Clinic imparted this clinical observation to Dr. William Mayo.

**Discoloration of the Umbilicus.**—Very occasionally, in certain acute abdominal conditions the umbilicus and surrounding skin become discoloured. If discoloration is suspected, gently clean the

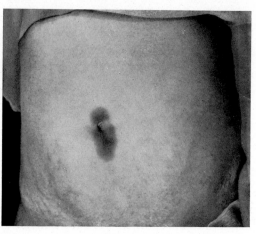

Fig. 407.—Cullen's sign.

area with a little ether and view again. Cullen has observed a bluish tinge in cases of ruptured ectopic gestation (*Fig.* 407). Johnston

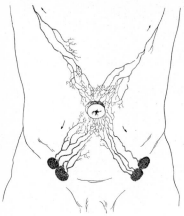

Fig. 408.—The lymphatic drainage of the umbilicus.

noted a yellow tinge around the umbilicus in a woman with acute pancreatitis. A dirty-greenish stain has been seen in cases of intra-peritoneal rupture of a hydatid cyst.

Regarding the lymphatic drainage of the umbilicus, it is recounted that the prince of surgical anatomists, Sir Frederick Treves, anxious to escape axillary lymphadenitis following vaccination, and believing that the umbilicus was relatively bereft of lymphatics, directed his medical attendant to scarify and apply the lymph to the skin in the immediate vicinity of his umbilicus. Two days later he was unable to attend the hospital, being incapacitated by tender swellings of both axillæ and both groins (*Fig.* 408).

THOMAS STEPHEN CULLEN, *Contemporary Professor Emeritus of Gynæcology, Johns Hopkins University, Baltimore, U.S.A.*

LLOYD B. JOHNSTON, *Contemporary Surgeon, Good Samaritan Hospital, Cincinnati, U.S.A.*

SIR FREDERICK TREVES, 1853–1923, *Surgeon, London Hospital. Operated on King Edward VII for an appendix abscess.*

## CHAPTER XX

# RECTAL AND VAGINAL EXAMINATION

## EXAMINATION OF THE RECTUM

MANY times the omission of a rectal examination has been a cause of regret. " If you don't put your finger in, you put your foot in it."

**Position of the Patient.**—The examination can be made in one of three positions, each having its advantages and special uses.

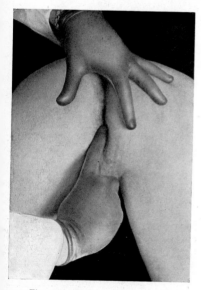

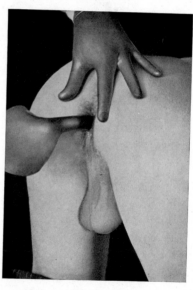

*Fig.* 409.—Rectal examination. Knee-elbow position. 1st stage : The pulp of the finger is laid on the anus.

*Fig.* 410.—Rectal examination. Knee-elbow position. 2nd stage : The finger is introduced with a rotary movement.

1. *The knee-elbow position* is the one that should be used as a general rule in the male (*Figs.* 409, 410). It is efficacious particularly when the prostate and seminal vesicles are to be palpated, and for a thorough general examination of the rectum it is unsurpassed.

15

2. *The left lateral (Sims') position (Fig.* 411) is employed as a routine in women, for the knee-elbow position would be indecorous. It is also used as a standard procedure in the male in many clinics.

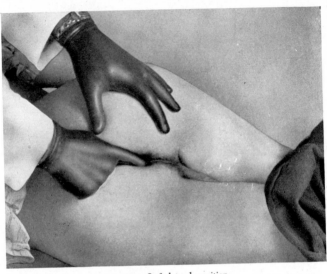

*Fig.* 411.—Left lateral position.

It is said that lesions high in the rectum can be detected more readily with the patient in the *right* lateral position and using the left index finger; there is much to be said in favour of this observation.

3. *The dorsal position,* with the right leg flexed, is invaluable in cases of an intra-abdominal catastrophe where alteration of the patient's posture is contra-indicated. The patient will be lying in bed in Fowler's position; he is instructed to draw up his right leg. The examiner passes his hand beneath the thigh, and his finger can then be made to enter the rectum, his other hand, meanwhile, resting above the pubes (*Fig.* 412). In this way fair access to the rectovesical pouch (the main point of the

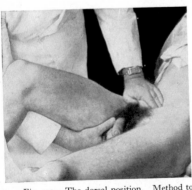

*Fig.* 412.—The dorsal position. Method to be adopted when the patient is too ill to be subjected to much movement.

examination) can be effected with minimal disturbance of the exhausted patient.

The dorsal position, with the patient lying flat on his back and his knees flexed and (preferably) with the pelvis raised on a small pillow, is the position to be chosen when it is desired to make a thorough examination of the interior of the pelvis. In this instance the hand does not pass under the patient's thigh, but the rectum is approached from between the legs. The index finger in the rectum is used in conjunction with the other hand upon the abdomen, for the size and other characteristics of a pelvic swelling can be estimated only by bimanual palpation.

I have noted repeatedly that a growth high in the rectum can sometimes be felt in this posture when other clinicians, no doubt employing other postures, have failed to detect it.

**General Principles in a Rectal Examination.**—Inspection must never be omitted. When a female is being examined disregard of this fundamental rule has many times led to a mistake, and the finger has been introduced into the wrong orifice. Furthermore, inspection often yields information of cardinal importance ; for instance, rectal prolapse (*Fig.* 413 ), prolapsed internal hæmorrhoids of the third degree, and pruritic* dermatitis, can be diagnosed at sight. External hæmorrhoids (*Figs.* 414, 415), which are covered with skin, are at once apparent. In relevant cases look for the external orifice of a fistula-in-ano (*Fig.* 416) or the sentinel tag of a fissure. Ask the patient to ' strain down ', observe the relaxation of the corrugator cutis ani of Ellis, followed by relaxation of the external sphincter, and, in a normal case, the very slightest protrusion of mucosa. As the patient strains, internal hæmorrhoids, which before were hidden from view, may now slowly protrude (*Fig.* 417). If the sphincter is tightly closed in spite of the patient straining down, be suspicious of a fissure-in-ano (*see* p. 234).

If both vaginal and rectal examinations are deemed necessary, do the vaginal first (*see also* p. 239). Inspection as outlined above may show that a vaginal examination is not contra-indicated on the grounds of supposed virgo intacta.

**Special Signs and Methods.**—

*Rectal Examination in Infancy.*—However small an infant, the index finger can be inserted in the usual way. Because of the relatively small size of the pelvis, a large part of the abdominal cavity

---

* *Pruritus.*   Latin, *prurire* = to itch.

SOME CONDITIONS REVEALED BY INSPECTION OF THE ANUS

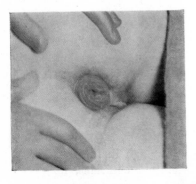

Fig. 413.—Prolapse of the rectum.

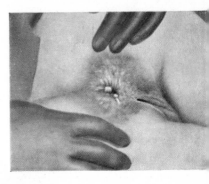

Fig. 414.—Pruritus ani with external hæmorrhoids (cutaneous tags) which are probably the irritating cause.

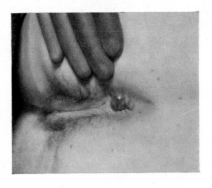

Fig. 415.—' Thrombotic pile '—subcutaneous rupture of an anal venule.

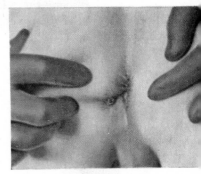

Fig. 416.—Fistula-in-ano.

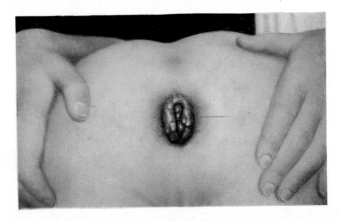

Fig. 417.—Internal hæmorrhoids can be seen coming into view as the patient strains. External hæmorrhoids are present also.

can be palpated per rectum. The apex of an intussusception feels like a cervix uteri.

When the finger is withdrawn, if a substance simulating red-currant jelly is seen upon the finger-stall, the diagnosis of intus-susception is very probable. On the other hand, if green stools are revealed in this manner, it is contributory evidence of enteritis (e.g., summer diarrhœa).

*Internal Hæmorrhoids.*—It should be especially noted that internal hæmorrhoids which are neither engorged nor thrombosed are so soft that they cannot be felt with the finger. The insertion of a speculum is necessary to detect their presence.

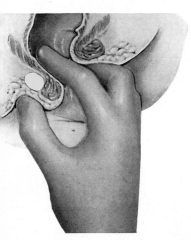
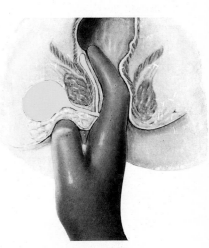
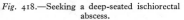

Fig. 418.—Seeking a deep-seated ischiorectal abscess.

Fig. 419.—An upward extension of the suppuration under the mucosa feels like a pencil.

*Carcinoma of the Rectum.*—First of all determine whether you can get above the growth. Next feel around the whole circumference of the bowel and determine the relationship of the growth to the circum-ference. In this way you will often be able to state whether the tumour is of the annular, ulcer, or cauliflower type. By trying to move the growth gently it is possible to ascertain whether it is fixed to the surrounding structures or tethered at any one point (e.g., to the sacrum).

*Ballooning of the Rectum* suggests obstruction to the lumen higher up (e.g., at the pelvirectal junction). This is not a sign of uniform reliability.

*Simple Stricture of the Rectum.*—One feels a diaphragm with a clean-cut hole in the centre. The sensation conveyed to the examining finger has been likened to palpating a hole in a turnip.

*Ischiorectal Abscess.*—Redness and swelling between the anal verge and the tuber ischii may make the diagnosis obvious. In earlier cases the palpating finger within the rectum in conjunction with the thumb resting over the base of the ischiorectal fossa may disclose the induration of a deep-seated abscess (*Fig.* 418). In other cases the palpating finger within the rectum detects a tender indurated swelling on one side over which the mucosa can be moved.

In such cases the pus may have tracked upwards under the mucous membrane and its track can be felt as a pencil-like induration (*Fig.* 419). From the point of view of correct treatment this is a most important clinical finding.

In all cases of ischiorectal abscess scrutinize the mucocutaneous junction for the internal orifice of a fistula-in-ano.

*Fissure-in-ano.*—The anal sphincter is in spasm; it is impossible to introduce the finger without causing excruciating pain. This is an occasion where rectal examination, as such, is contra-indicated, but the anal canal must be examined with especial care. With the

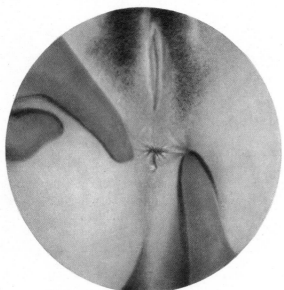

*Fig.* 420.—Method of displaying a fissure-in-ano. The patient is in the left lateral position.

pulps of the index fingers gently separate the folds of anal mucosa (*Fig.* 420) and look for the fissure, especially in the middle line posteriorly. A so-called sentinel* pile, which is usually nothing more than a cutaneous tag, sometimes marks the external limit of the fissure.

*Fistula-in-ano.*—When there is an external opening, search for an internal orifice. If present, this can be seen either at the muco-cutaneous junction or felt as a small elevation about half an inch from the anal verge ; it is a common mistake to search for the internal opening too high in the rectum. Palpate the tissues between the external opening and the anal margin between the forefinger and thumb. Except in the case of tuberculous fistulæ, the indurated track, whether straight or curving, can usually be felt.

A probe introduced into the fistula while the finger is within the rectum is always instructive.

*Pilonidal*† *Sinus.*—A large proportion of cases with this condition arrive at the out-patient department diagnosed as being ' fistula-in-ano ' or ' ischiorectal ' abscess. Regarding the first group : Observe the opening of the sinus. It is situated in the middle line, near the base of the coccyx. Purulent fluid and sometimes loose hairs can often be expressed by pressure over the last segment of the sacrum.

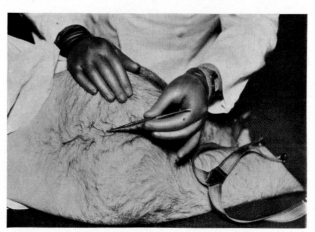

*Fig.* 421.—Pilonidal sinus. A probe has been introduced into the sinus. Note that the patient is a very ' hairy ' man.

---

* Sentinel—so called because it metaphorically watches over the fissure.
  † Pilonidal—so called because it contains a nest of hairs.

When the small mouth of the sinus becomes blocked, the contents become bottled up and a tender swelling is present ; often this overlies the sacrococcygeal area to one or other side of the middle line, usually the left. Patients with a pilonidal sinus are usually dark, hairy men (*Fig.* 421).

*Sphincter Relaxation.*—Loss of sphincter tone, as in cases of rectal prolapse, can be demonstrated by digital traction on the sphincter. If, by this means, the sphincter can be made to gape so that the rectal lumen is displayed, a subnormal sphincter tone is certainly present.

*Examination of a Case of Suspected Coccydynia.*—The index finger is introduced into the rectum in the usual way. It is then rotated so that the coccyx can be grasped between the finger and thumb (*Fig.* 422). Abnormal mobility and tenderness of the coccyx can be ascertained by this manœuvre.

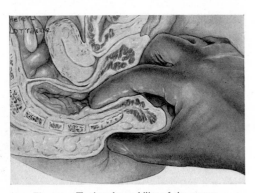

*Fig.* 422.—Testing the mobility of the coccyx.

*Massive œdema of the rectal wall* has been noted in volvulus of the pelvic colon. This is due to the inferior mesenteric vein becoming occluded by the torsion.

\*      \*      \*      \*      \*      \*      \*

When summoned to a case of supposed acute abdominal catastrophe I have been enabled to make a diagnosis of ' probably typhoid ' (which was later confirmed) by noting, in the course of a rectal examination, that the rectum was hot. This is not an infallible sign, but I have found it of great practical utility on several occasions.

*Rectal examination of the prostate* is discussed on p. 259.

## TECHNIQUE OF RECTAL PALPATION

One of the greatest factors in an efficient rectal palpation is that it should be a painless process. To a very large extent this can be achieved by correct technique. Always warn the patient what you are about to do. After you have him in the desired position, say : " I am now going to examine you by the bowel. It will not hurt you. Open your mouth and breathe quietly in and out, and keep on breathing."

The gloved finger should be anointed liberally with vaseline. Lay the pulp of the index flat upon the anal verge (*Fig.* 423), and exert firm pressure until the sphincter is felt to yield. Then, with a rotatory movement, the finger is introduced *slowly*. If the rectum

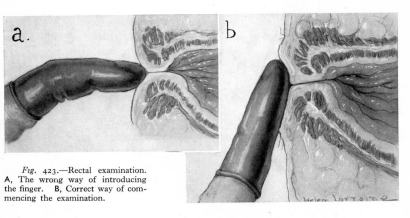

*Fig.* 423.—Rectal examination. A, The wrong way of introducing the finger.   B, Correct way of commencing the examination.

is found to be full of hard fæces, it will be wise to defer the examination (unless the case is urgent) and record this fact in your notes. Sometimes the question arises in the mind : " Is this a neoplasm or a mass of hard fæces ? " Fæces may be indented with the finger, and this clears up the doubt in many cases. There are instances in which the indentation cannot be performed, because the main mass lies just out of reach. In such a case re-examine the patient at a later date when the rectum has been emptied. It is sometimes a difficult matter to decide whether a particular lump is within or without the rectal wall. Pass the finger to one side of the lump and then slide it over the elevation. In this way one may be able to feel a continuity of the normal mucosa, and to move the mucosa on the lump—in the event of which the lump is outside the rectal wall.

The *pons asinorum* of a rectal examination is the cervix uteri, which can be felt projecting through the anterior rectal wall. Even after considerable experience the inconstant size and shape of the os may, in a given case, cause momentary bewilderment. So great is the pitfall of the cervix that, in making a rectal examination in the female, it should be the rule to find the os deliberately first, and take bearings from that structure. Mistakes from this cause are then impossible.

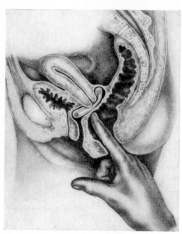

*Fig.* 424.—Make sure that a woman patient is not wearing a pessary before expressing an opinion on a lump that can be felt per rectum.

A pessary in the vagina can be felt per rectum (*Fig.* 424). It is astounding how often this seemingly obvious fact proves to be the cause of utter diagnostic confusion ; a typical example is as follows : Four keen and industrious Fellowship candidates each digitally examined the rectum of a woman of fifty who complained of abdominal pain and constipation. Two of them were satisfied that there was a growth in the ampulla of the rectum. Two of them looked puzzled ; they considered that the growth was in the muscular wall of the rectum, or even outside it, and that it was rather smooth. On requesting one of them to follow up the examination by inserting a finger into the vagina all agreed that the term ' pons asinorum ' was not inapt.

When one is engaged in an examination of the rectum, unless there is some striking abnormality, it is well to have in mind a routine, a kind of formula, which will synchronize the brain and finger. Proceed in order, palpating and thinking all the time of what you are doing.

### RECTAL EXAMINATION

*In the Male*
- Anterior Wall
  1. Prostate, right lobe, left lobe
  2. Seminal vesicles, position of left vesicle, position of right vesicle
  3. Rectovesical pouch
- Left lateral wall
- Right lateral wall
- Superiorly, as far as can be reached
- Posteriorly { Hollow of sacrum / Coccyx

*In the Female*
- Cervix
- Pouch of Douglas
- Left lateral wall
- Right lateral wall
- Superiorly, as far as can be reached
- Posteriorly { Hollow of sacrum / Coccyx

Having completed the routine palpation, look at your finger for blood, mucus, etc. : better still, wipe it on a gauze swab, which will show up the colour of the discharge.

JAMES DOUGLAS, 1675–1742, *Physician to Queen Caroline.*

## VAGINAL EXAMINATION

" Never insult the vagina by examining the rectum first " is an old axiom, which can be retained provided it does not convey to the clinician the impression that, having completed a vaginal examination, he is entitled to proceed with a rectal examination, using the same rubber glove without even cleansing it. Gonorrhœa of the rectum in women is more common and is more harmful than was realized in the heyday of this aphorism (Greenslade).

Actually it is immaterial which of these examinations is done first ; the important point is to *change the glove.*

Vaginal examination is dealt with so thoroughly by the gynæcological department that only a comparatively brief reference to this important method will be made here ; vaginal examination as it concerns clinical surgery is what I wish to portray.

**Position.**—In Britain Sims' position is usually adopted ; this is a legacy from the days of prudery. With the patient in Sims' position it is almost impossible to scrutinize the urethra and cervix ; moreover, Sims' position tends to carry the pelvic contents higher and more out of reach of the examining fingers. So great are the baneful repercussions that may result from pandering to this form of false modesty that Frank Kidd expostulated " Sims' position is the curse of British gynæcology ".

As Greenslade emphasizes, the only satisfactory position for a thorough examination of the female generative organs is the lithotomy position ; a consulting room without a lithotomy couch is insufficiently furnished.

When the lithotomy position is employed a sheet can be placed over the patient and draped around her legs. So long as the patient realizes that her body is covered, any objection to the lithotomy position is over-ruled (Connell).

**Technique.**—The hands are sterilized. The right hand should be gloved, and its index and middle fingers lubricated thoroughly. The labia are separated and the index finger is introduced into the vagina. This is followed, in women who have borne children, by the middle finger. First the cervix is located, and its characteristics are noted. The anterior, posterior, and lateral fornices are palpated in turn. It is important to remember that the bladder must be emptied, either naturally or by catheter, before a bimanual examination is performed.

CHARLES MILLS GREENSLADE, *Contemporary Surgeon, Dunedin Hospital, New Zealand.*
FRANCIS SEYMOUR KIDD, 1878–1934, *Surgeon, London Hospital.*
JOHN STEWART MARSHALL CONNELL, *Contemporary Gynæcologist, Midland Hospital, Birmingham.*

**Bimanual Examination.**—The fingers of the right hand are kept high in the vagina, while the left hand presses downwards and backwards. The size and other characteristics of the uterus can be ascertained by this method (*Fig.* 425). Normal ovaries may often be felt ; they are somewhat tender on pressure. Normal Fallopian tubes are not palpable. The size and other characteristics of a pelvic swelling, whether or not it is attached to the uterus (*Fig.* 426), whether it is cystic or solid, fixed or free, regular or irregular, can be ascertained by skilful bimanual palpation.

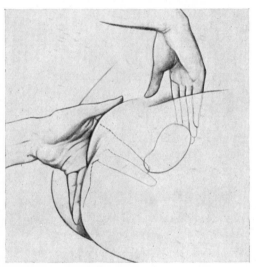

Fig. 425.—Bimanual palpation of the uterus. (*After Edward Martin.*)

In general, resistance or swelling anterior to the cervix denotes an affection of the pelvic connective tissue, while posteriorly anything abnormal is in the pouch of Douglas.

*Palpation of Bartholin's Glands.*—While a fully-formed abscess of a Bartholin's gland is obvious (*Fig.* 427), nevertheless, considerable enlargements of this gland can be missed unless they are searched for correctly. Palpate the posterior part of the labia majora between the finger and thumb (*Fig.* 428). The gland lies more deeply and more posteriorly than one would expect.

*Examination of the Female Urethra.*—The dorsal position is desirable ; indeed, it is almost essential. A urethral caruncle can be seen as a pouting of granulomatous-like tissue from the urinary

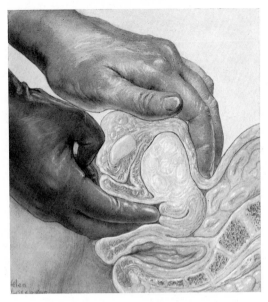

*Fig.* 426.—Bimanual palpation. There is a fibroid tumour of the uterus.

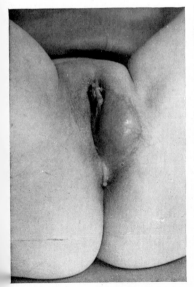

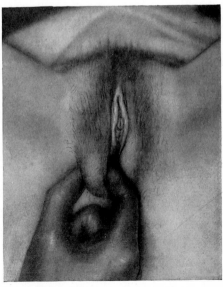

*z.* 427.—Abscess of the left Bartholin's gland.    *Fig.* 428.—Method of palpating Bartholin's gland.

meatus. When the patient strains, the urethral mucosa becomes more evident (*Fig.* 429).

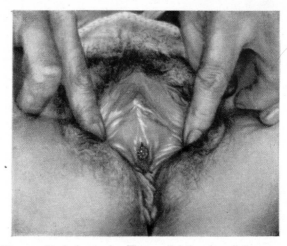

*Fig.* 429.—Urethral caruncle. The so-called " raspberry " tumour.

The urethra can be palpated through the anterior vaginal wall ; the meatus should first be swabbed. In cases of gonorrhœa, sometimes pus can be milked from the urethra. When Skene's tubules are infected, pus can be expressed from their openings, which lie on the dorsal edge of the urinary meatus or just within its orifice (*Fig.* 430).

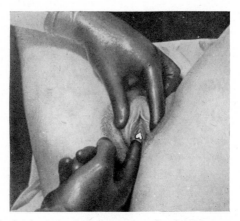

*Fig.* 430.—Palpating the urethra through the vagina.    In relevant cases pus can be milked from the urethra and expressed from Skene's tubules, which are shown exuding pus in this case.

ALEXANDER JOHNSTON CHALMERS SKENE, 1838–1900, *Surgeon, Long Island College Hospital, U.S.A.*

## CHAPTER XXI

## CLINICAL EXAMINATION OF THE URINARY ORGANS

DIAGNOSIS of urinary disease is to-day largely a matter of special investigation. With the advent of the cystoscope, the urethroscope, X-rays- and biochemistry, clinical methods occupy a comparatively unimportant place. Often the principal object of the preliminary clinical examination is to direct attention to the necessity of such an investigation and the exact form that it will take, and to exclude disease of other organs.

### HÆMATURIA

Hæmaturia, especially painless hæmaturia, is a signal that should stir the clinician to elucidate the cause. When, as is so usual, the bleeding proves transitory, sometimes, sad to relate, instead of receiving an appointment for a full urological investigation, the patient is seen returning to his home carrying a bottle of medicine.

As likely as not, the patient will bring with him a bottle of blood-stained urine. Pour the contents of the bottle into a glass, and observe whether there are any clots or sediment. More valuable is it to obtain a contemporary specimen, and if the patient is a male, to watch him pass some urine into one glass and the remainder into another. Is the blood integrally mixed with the urine ? Is it bright red ? Is there more or is there less blood in the terminal portion of the specimen ? Such are the data the clinician should collect and assemble. Nevertheless, in the whole realm of clinical surgery, the elucidation of the cause of hæmaturia stands unrivalled as an example where scientific methods (in this instance cystoscopy combined with radiography) have so bedwarfed physical signs as to render them puerile.

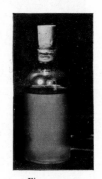

Fig. 431.—
" Beeturia."

Be that as it may, clinical acumen is never superfluous. Even in this instance it may come into its own ; for instance, when beetroot is in season. The shade of red given by urine containing blood certainly varies very greatly, but it never resembles the peculiar purplish hue of beeturia (*Fig.* 431), if that term be allowed.     Alex Roche likens this colour to that of cherry brandy.

## THE TWO-GLASS TEST

The patient is instructed to pass about two or three egg-cupfuls of urine into test glass No. 1, and the remainder of his urine into test glass No. 2.     If the contents of the first glass are turbid and those of the second clear, it suggests (but not with scientific certainty) that the patient has an anterior urethritis.     On the other hand, should the urine in the first glass be clear, and the second heavy with muco-pus and/or contain prostatic threads, it suggests a posterior urethritis (*Fig.* 432). Similarly, if the urine contains blood one can see whether it is mixed intimately with the urine or whether the bleeding tends to occur at the commencement or at the end of micturition.

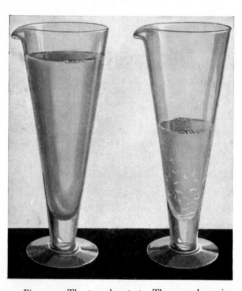

*Fig.* 432.—The two-glass test.   The second specimen shows muco-pus and prostatic threads, while the first specimen is clear.   Presumptive diagnosis—posterior urethritis.

The three-glass test is a little more accurate than the foregoing, and one can go on multiplying the number of glasses *ad libitum.*

Personally, I look on the two-glass test as a convenient method of obtaining a specimen of urine, and by collecting it in this way have sometimes stumbled upon useful information.

## CLINICAL EXAMINATION OF THE KIDNEYS

In order to be precise and accurate, it is best to discard the term ' renal colic ' and speak of ' renal pain ' and ' ureteric colic '. *Renal pain* is usually a dull ache situated mainly in the costovertebral angle, but also in the outer and upper quadrant of the upper abdomen. Often the patient indicates the site of this pain in the manner shown in *Fig.* 433 (Pelouze).

ALEXANDER ERNEST ROCHE, *Contemporary Surgeon-in-Charge, Genito-urinary Department, West London Hospital.*

PERCY STARR PELOUZE, *Contemporary Urologist, University Hospital, Philadelphia, U.S.A.*

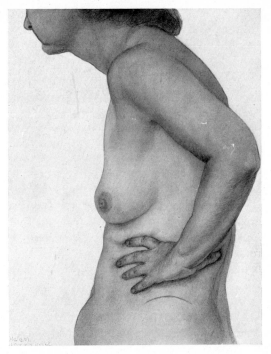

Fig. 433.—A usual position of the hand of a patient who is showing where she experiences renal pain.

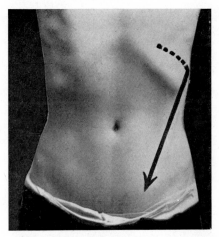

Fig. 434.—The pointing test in ureteric colic. The patient will map out the direction of the pain as passing from the loin to the groin.

16

*Ureteric colic* is nearly always characteristic—the pain passes from the loin to the groin, and in the male this radiation is frequently prolonged to the testicle. A patient attacked with ureteric colic can often accurately map the course of this pain for one's edification (*Fig.* 434).

In days gone by there was a sign known as Lucas's sign. The patient jumped on to the floor from an elevated position, and it was noted if this brought on an attack of renal colic. If the sign was positive, a diagnosis of renal calculus was made. More exact methods have rendered this painful process obsolete.

**The Reno-renal Reflex.**—Occasionally pain associated with a lesion of one kidney is referred to the contralateral (normal) side. Nevertheless, not every example of a seeming reno-renal reflex is genuine. When one kidney is undergoing gradual destruction, its fellow is usually undergoing compensatory hypertrophy, and during this process it is liable to be the seat of attacks of pain.

If the patient has passed a stone he will often bring it for your benefit. Try to guess its chemical composition by physical characteristics before sending it to the laboratory. When there is a history of recurrent urinary calculi never neglect to palpate the thyroid gland for the possible presence of a parathyroid tumour.

**Palpation of the Kidneys.**—The patient should lie on his back. The value of the examination is enhanced by placing a pillow under the patient's knees, and often it is advisable to have him rolled slightly toward the side that is being examined.

There are several variations in technique. The first, and probably the best, is the bimanual method, which is illustrated in *Fig.* 435.

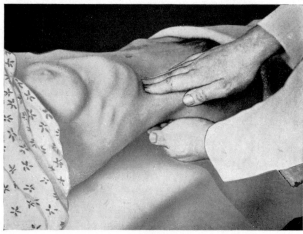

*Fig.* 435.—Bimanual palpation of the kidney.

RICHARD CLEMENT LUCAS, 1846–1915, *Surgeon, Guy's Hospital, London.*

After the hands are adjusted nicely in position, and the maximum amount of relaxation of the patient's musculature is ensured, he is asked to take a deep breath. The pulps of the fingers of the two hands are approximated as *expiration* is in progress. The second method, shown in *Fig.* 436, is used by a number of clinicians. It

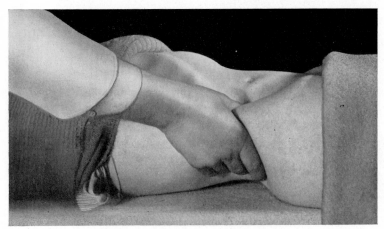

Fig. 436.—Another method of palpating the kidney.

is possible to endeavour to palpate both kidneys at one and the same time by this method, which is of service only in thin subjects and children. On occasions, especially in cases of difficulty, it is valuable to examine the kidney with the patient lying upon the sound side (*Fig.* 437).

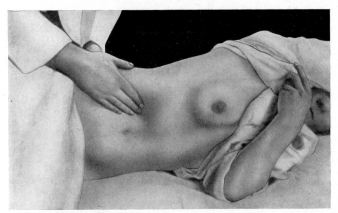

Fig. 437.—Examining the kidney with the patient on the sound side. A useful method of examining and determining the nature of a lump that *may* be the kidney.

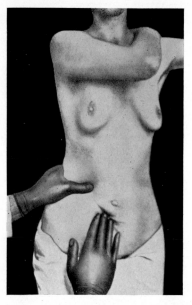

*Palpating the kidney with the patient in the erect position* is useful, not as a routine method, but as a confirmatory test in a doubtful case of nephroptosis. The patient stands with her weight resting on the sound

*Fig.* 438.—Method of palpating the kidney to confirm a diagnosis of nephroptosis. In this case the left hand is above the upper pole of the right kidney, and the right hand is palpating its inferior pole.

side. The leg on the affected side is flexed slightly and the body leans forward a little. The hands are placed as is shown in *Fig.* 438, and, while the patient takes a deep breath, the kidney is imprisoned by the left hand and palpated by the right.

Watkins maintained that the usual method of examining the kidneys by forcing them between the fingers is too crude to be of much value, and only gross abnormalities can be detected. He advocated bimanual palpation by light touch, the posterior hand being held quite still, whilst the anterior makes light vibratory movements.

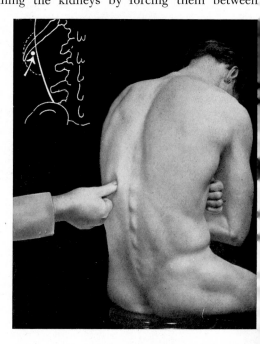

*Fig.* 439.—The renal angle test (Murphy's 'kidney punch'). The thumb is placed under the 12th rib and to the lateral side of the erector spinæ muscle, and sharp jabbing movements are made.

**The Renal Angle Test (Murphy's 'Kidney Punch').**—The patient sits up and folds his arms in front of him.

---

The thumb is then placed under the 12th rib, and short, jabbing movements are made (*Fig.* 439.) At first the movements are very gentle, but if pain is not experienced their strength is increased. This sign is of great value in determining deep-seated tenderness ; also, by this method, with practice and comparison of the two sides, it is possible to estimate relative muscular rigidity.

**Renal Tumour.**—A tumour of the kidney is said to possess these characteristics : (1) It lies in the loin, or can be moved into the loin ; (2) It is reniform in shape ; (3) It moves on respiration ; (4) There is a band of colonic resonance anteriorly ; (5) It is dull posteriorly.

This classical picture will seldom be seen in its entirety, e.g., it is frequently impossible to demonstrate the band of colonic resonance unless special methods are invoked.

*Baldwin's Method.*—The colon is inflated with air by means of a rubber catheter fixed to a Higginson's syringe. After the introduction of three or four syringefuls of air, the band of colonic resonance, formerly impossible to demonstrate, becomes evident. The method is of distinct value for tumours that occur on the left side, but is unreliable on the right owing to the difficulty of safely introducing sufficient air to inflate the ascending colon.

Neoplasms of the kidney tend to enlarge anteriorly (*Fig.* 440), whilst large abscesses and hydronephroses sometimes produce considerable posterior projection.

A varicocele that has appeared more or less suddenly in a man over thirty is indicative of malignant neoplasm of the kidney. Its presence does not necessarily imply that the renal tumour is inoperable.

It is well to bear in mind that an enlarged kidney may

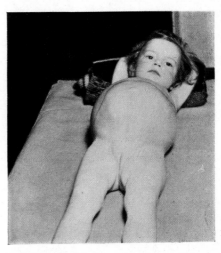

*Fig.* 440.—Wilms' tumour (malignant embryoma of the kidney), though rare, is the most frequent cause of abdominal enlargement due to a solid unilateral intra-abdominal tumour in childhood.

be the one healthy kidney, the enlargement being due to compensatory hypertrophy. Hypertrophy of the opposite kidney is unusual in neoplasm.

HUGH ALLEN BALDWIN, *Contemporary Surgeon, Grant Hospital, Columbus, Ohio, U.S.A.*
ALFRED HIGGINSON, 1808–1884, *Surgeon, Southern Hospital, Liverpool.*
MAX WILMS, 1867–1918, *Professor of Surgery, Heidelberg.*

When both kidneys are much enlarged and *nodular*, congenital cystic kidneys should be thought of, particularly if the symptoms are few (*Fig.* 441).

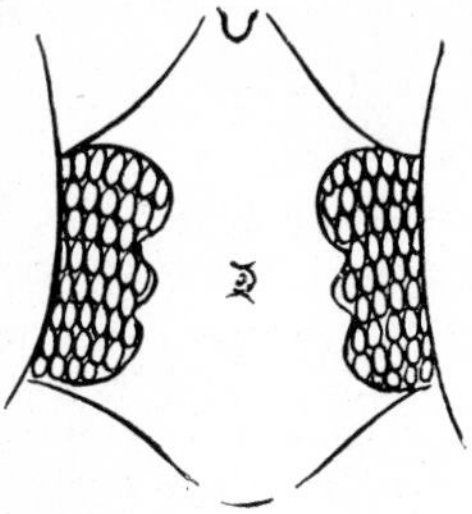

*Fig.* 441.—Congenital cystic kidneys. The physical signs recorded in the case of a woman of 28 who attended for an abdominal examination after the birth of her seventh child. The patient seemed in perfect health and had noticed nothing amiss with her abdomen.

## PERINEPHRIC ABSCESS

The diagnosis of perinephric abscess rests almost entirely on the clinical examination, and it is necessary to bear the condition constantly in mind when one is searching for an obscure focus of infection. It is sad to relate that too often the diagnosis of perinephric abscess (*Fig.* 442) is delayed unduly because the patient's *back* has never been examined.

**Inspection.**—First examine the patient in the sitting posture (*see Fig.* 439). The area immediately beneath the last rib and lateral to the erector spinæ is scrutinized ; it is compared with the opposite side. In this situation the merest fullness is often the indication of a large collection of deep-seated pus. Scoliosis of the lumbar spine with concavity towards the affected side is almost a constant sign, even in early cases, but it often requires an X-ray examination to reveal it (LeComte).

When an abscess in the perinephric fat is related to the lower pole of the kidney a swelling in the renal area may be present early (*Fig.* 442), but when, as is more usual, it is related to the upper

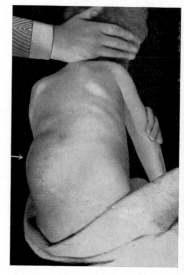

*Fig.* 442.—A large perinephric abscess. Seldom is a swelling like this apparent. It is to direct attention as to where to look for the faintest semblance of a fullness that this illustration is included.

pole or the posterior surface of the kidney, the mass is imperceptible, even in well-advanced cases, because the rigid lower part of the costal cage renders it inaccessible. Bending the trunk *away* from the side of the abscess may produce pain (*Fig.* 443),

Ralph Michael LeComte. *Contemporary, Professor of Urology, Georgetown University, Washington, D.C.*

whereas the patient can bend his body towards the lesion without much discomfort (Foulds).

**Palpation.**—The renal angle test (*see* p. 248) is now applied; it often yields valuable information. In cases where diagnosis is still in doubt, pillows should be removed, and the patient instructed to lie prone; it is important to ensure that he is lying quite straight. On the sound side the fingers can be dipped deeply towards the kidney; on the affected side, muscular resistance prevents this manœuvre. This difference on the two sides is obvious, and out of proportion to the resistance occasioned by tenderness. Indeed, tenderness is often surprisingly inconspicuous (Morrison.)

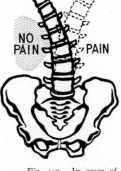

*Fig.* 443.—In cases of perinephritis and perinephric abscess, bending the trunk *away* from the side of a lesion is more likely to cause pain than the reverse manœuvre.

## PALPATION OF THE URETER

**Vaginal Palpation of the Ureter.**—The index finger is passed into the vagina and the position of the internal urinary meatus is sought. The finger is carried upwards and outwards until its pulp reaches the highest point it can touch; it is then carried downwards and inwards, stroking the pelvic wall and estimating the character of structures felt rolling beneath it. When the clinician believes that it is the ureter that is being felt, he again catches this structure with the hooked finger, and slides the finger, first towards the bladder, and then backwards and upwards as far as can be reached. By using this method, which was first described by Kelly, a ureteric calculus can be sometimes felt (*Fig.* 444); at other times the thickened ureter of tuberculosis or the tender ureter of a ureteritis can be discerned.

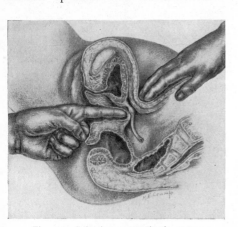

*Fig.* 444.—Palpating a stone in the ureter. via the vagina.

GEORGE SUTCLIFFE FOULDS. *Contemporary, Consulting Urologist, Women's Hospital, Toronto.*

JOHN TERTIUS MORRISON, *Contemporary Surgeon, Royal Southern Hospital, Liverpool.*

HOWARD A. KELLY, 1858–1943, *Professor of Gynæcology, Johns Hopkins University, Baltimore, U.S.A.*

**Trans-abdominal Palpation of the Ureter.**—The practical application of this measure is small. Stand on the same side as the ureter to be examined and place the hands flat upon the abdomen over the line of the ureter (*Fig.* 445). Ask the patient to respire slowly and deeply. With each expiration the fingers sink into the abdomen, and at each inspiration they hold the ground gained already. After two or three expirations, the fingers have sunk to the back of the abdomen. They are then drawn laterally, palpating the structures which roll beneath them (Sir John Thomson-Walker).

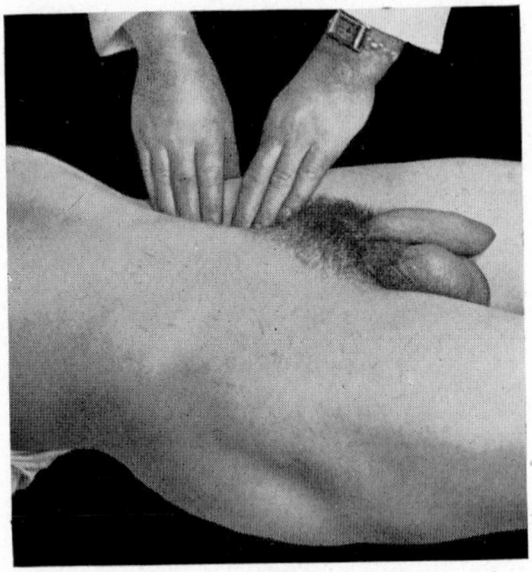

*Fig.* 445.—Trans-abdominal palpation of the ureter.

## THE BLADDER

The dome of an overfull bladder is usually rounded. In cases of long-standing chronic urinary obstruction, i.e., retention-with-overflow (a condition in which the patient makes but little or no complain of pain or dysuria), the swelling arising out of the pelvis is wont to be mistaken for some other condition. This frequent error reaches its zenith when the contour of the dome of the bladder is unorthodox (*Fig.* 446).

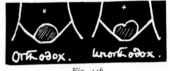

*Fig.* 446.

Not once, but scores of times, I have seen clinicians beguiled by this phenomenon. For instance, the patient illustrated in *Fig.* 447 came to my out-patient clinic bearing the following letter from an experienced practitioner :—" Mr. C. has a large tumour filling up the hypogastrium and extending to the left. The remarkable thing is that he looks and feels well."

An empty bladder cannot be felt. Occasionally a large vesical diverticulum surrounded by inflammatory thickening can be recognized by deep palpation above the pubes or per rectum. It is only when a neoplasm of the bladder is very advanced that it becomes palpable by ordinary methods ; on the other hand, bimanual palpation (*Fig.* 448), especially when performed under the relaxation afforded by anæsthesia, is often of inestimable diagnostic assistance in assessing the extent of a vesical neoplasm, the presence of which has been ascertained by cystoscopy.

So unusual is it for affections of the bladder, other than retention of urine, to provide any physical signs, that it is sometimes forgotten that a large stone in the bladder can be felt per rectum.

SIR JOHN THOMSON-WALKER, 1870–1937. *Surgeon, St. Peter's Hospital, London.*

In cases of prostatic enlargement it is useful to examine the base of the bladder per rectum *soon after the patient has passed urine.* By careful palpation a rough idea will be obtained of the amount of residual urine present in the bladder.

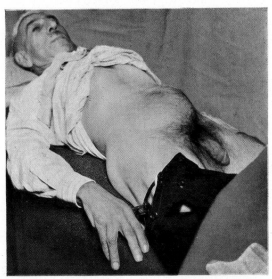

*Fig.* 447.—Retention with overflow. Note the contour of the dome of the overfull bladder. The patient made no complaint of pain or difficulty of micturition.

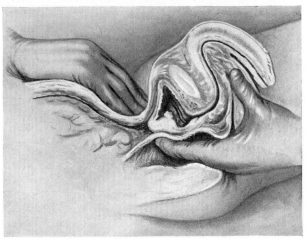

*Fig.* 448.—Assessing the size and extent of a carcinoma of the bladder, under general anæsthesia. (*After Jewett.*)

Once again opportunity is taken here to warn the reader never to express an opinion on a pelvic swelling until the bladder has been emptied by a catheter.

## ECTOPIA VESICÆ

In this condition the bladder mucosa (*Fig.* 449), with the ureteric orifices discharging urine, can be seen.

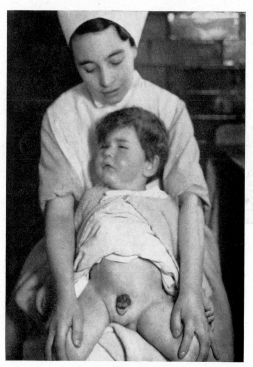

*Fig.* 449.—Ectopia vesicæ.

## ECTOPIC URETER

Any girl or woman who has dribbled for as long as she can remember, despite the fact that she has a normal desire to void, and indeed does urinate, has an ectopic ureteric orifice. In such a case, scrutinize the region of the vestibule for the opening of the ectopic ureter.

## CHAPTER XXII

## THE MALE GENERATIVE ORGANS

### EXAMINATION OF THE PENIS

WHEN the prepuce is present ask the patient to retract his foreskin. That this is a wise preliminary measure is shown by a perusal of the legends of *Figs.* 450 and 451.

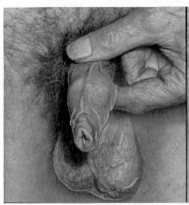 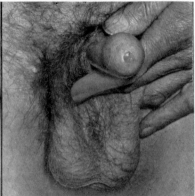

Fig. 450.—The patient is a man of 71, complaining of great difficulty in micturition. Two Fellowship candidates examined him and diagnosed enlargement of the middle lobe of the prostate. We see in this picture the patient's redundant foreskin, which shows nothing particularly unusual.

Fig. 451.—When an attempt is made to retract the prepuce it is evident at once that the patient has a most extreme phimosis—the orifice in his foreskin is no larger than that which could be made by a large pin. Circumcision cured him completely.

*Pinhole meatus*, as opposed to a pinhole opening in the foreskin, is often overlooked, both in infants and those of more mature years.

That thousands suffer from progressive urinary obstruction because their medical advisers fail to recognize a pinhole meatus early enough, has caused Campbell to call the condition the 'neglected step-child of serious urinary obstruction.' This is all the more regrettable because of the utter simplicity of the diagnosis. Pinch the glans between the finger and thumb, from before backwards; this opens the lips of the meatus (*Fig.* 452). Observe whether the orifice is adequate.

MEREDITH FAIRFAX CAMPBELL, *Contemporary Professor of Urology, New York University College of Medicine, New York.*

*Meatal ulcer* of infant boys is a clinical entity that is often imperfectly understood. It is rarely found in the uncircumcised. It is common after circumcision, although eighteen months may elapse

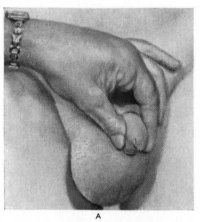
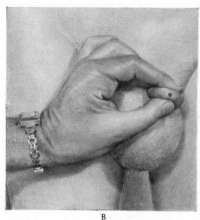

A            B

Fig. 452.—(A) Is the meatus adequate ?   (B) By compressing the tip of the penis between a finger and thumb anteroposteriorly the lips of the meatus are opened, and it can be observed at once whether the orifice is adequate.

between the operation and the onset of symptoms. The condition is probably due in the first place to abrasion of the delicate unprotected mucosa by napkins. Secondary urinary infection follows. The ulcer

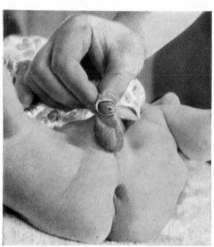

Fig. 453.—Meatal ulcer with scab formation.   The scab occludes the external urinary meatus.

at the external urinary meatus causes a scab to form (*Fig.* 453) ; this closes the meatus and the child can urinate only by bursting the scab. Such a process is accompanied by pain, screaming, and occasionally by hæmaturia. A spot of bright red blood on the diaper is often the first sign of meatal ulcer of infants that alarms the parents (Paul Freud). Ulceration and scab formation alternate. Untreated, cicatricial contracture of the meatus, in other words acquired pinhole meatus, is liable to ensue.

PAUL FREUD, *Contemporary Pediatrician, New York Medical College, New York.*

In the condition known as *hypospadias* there is an abnormal termination of the urethra, the external orifice of which lies at some point on the floor of the normal course of the anterior urethra (*Fig.* 454). The much rarer condition of *epispadias* is extremely obvious (*Fig.* 455).

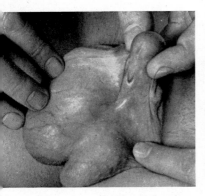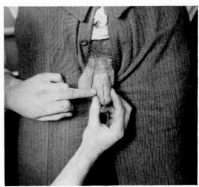

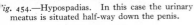

*ig.* 454.—Hypospadias. In this case the urinary meatus is situated half-way down the penis.

*Fig.* 455.—Epispadias

It is remarkable that *paraphimosis*, especially when it has been present for several days, is overlooked so often; seldom a month goes by without my having cause to reflect on the accuracy of this statement, which rarely fails to surprise listeners. If a suspicion arises as to whether the foreskin has been imprisoned in a retracted position, obviously the first thing to do is to ask the patient if he has been circumcised. It is amazing how often the reply is inconclusive; some seemingly intelligent men do not appear to know whether they have, or have not, been circumcised. In a case of paraphimosis, if the skin of the penis is drawn

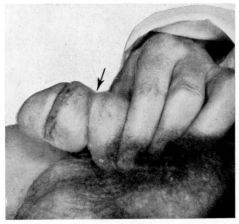

*Fig.* 456.—Paraphimosis. The constricting band is often inconspicuous until the skin of the shaft of the penis has been put on the stretch.

towards the pubis, and the first inch behind the corona scrutinized, an area of œdema limited abruptly by a constricting band (*Fig.* 456) can be seen. This leaves no doubt as to the diagnosis.

Palpation of the floor of the urethra (*Fig.* 457) in cases of suspected urethral stricture is a much neglected method of examination. Quite often a stricture can be felt from without, and a favourite site is the penoscrotal junction.

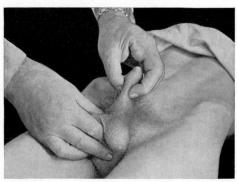

*Fig.* 457.—Palpating the floor of the urethra. This should be done systematically from the bulb, downwards. Note that for the deep urethra it is necessary to invaginate the scrotum.

A *penile periurethral abscess* first manifests itself as an indurated swelling in the floor of the urethra. Later it becomes rounded, tender and fluctuant. It is often situated about the middle of the penile urethra.

A localized, painless induration about half-way down the dependent part of one or both corpora cavernosa is pathognomonic of *induratio penis plastica*. When the area is rolled between the finger and thumb the impression gained is that the spongy tissue has been converted into soft cartilage.

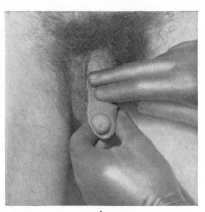
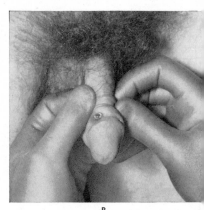

A                                         B

*Fig.* 458.—**A**, Palpation of the dorsum of the shaft of the penis reveals an indurated subcutaneous cord ; **B**, On retracting the prepuce a typical Hunterian chancre is displayed. Case of thrombosis of the dorsal vein.

*Thrombosis of the dorsal vein of the penis* gives rise to a physical sign that is absolutely characteristic. On palpation (*Fig.* 458A), in the subcutaneous tissues of the middle line of the dorsum of the penis, there is what feels like a ' pipe cleaner ' as a patient graphically described it. Unless the clinician knows of the existence of this condition, he will be puzzled. Retraction of the prepuce, if such be present, usually reveals the cause of the thrombosis at once (*Fig.* 458B).

When confronted with a case of *persistent priapism* palpate the spleen before undertaking an elaborate neurological examination ; thrombosis of the pelvi-prostatic venous plexus (the usual cause of persistent priapism) is not very unusual in myelogenous leukæmia. However, in most instances the thrombosis is idiopathic.

## EXAMINATION OF THE PROSTATE AND ITS ADNEXA

The routine examination of the prostate is performed best with the patient in the knee-elbow position. The finger, well anointed, is introduced slowly into the rectum in the manner indicated already in the section on rectal examination (p. 229).

**Visualizing the Parts to be Palpated.**—It is essential to have in mind a clear conception of the relationship of structures about the prostate to the palpating finger, and to know what can be felt (*Fig.* 459) in a normal case. The normal prostate feels firm and elastic. Each of its lateral lobes, which are separated by a median furrow, is about the size of the distal segment of the thumb.

Passing the finger *downwards* along this median furrow, as the prostate is left one comes to a soft area—here lies the membranous urethra. On each side of the middle line at this point Cowper's glands are situated. Sliding the finger *upwards* along the median furrow—a little to each side of the top of the prostate lie the seminal vesicles, which are well within the

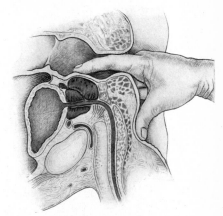

*Fig.* 459.—Palpation of the prostate. Each lateral lobe is palpated, paying particular attention to its consistency.

reach of the finger. A normal vesicle cannot be felt unless it is distended with seminal fluid. Between the vesicle and the prostate on each side there is a sulcus which is traversed by the lymphatics

WILLIAM COWPER, 1666–1709, *Surgeon, London.*

leaving the prostate. These points must be grasped clearly and *Fig.* 460 visualized before diagnosis of the abnormal is attempted.

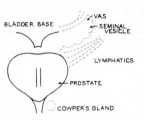

Fig. 460.—Diagram of the prostate and its adnexa in relation to rectal palpation. The parts in *black* are felt normally, those in *green* only when they are diseased.
(*After Sir John Thomson-Walker.*)

Before expressing an opinion on the size of the prostate, it is necessary to be certain that the bladder is empty. In acute retention the posterior surface of the full bladder can be mistaken for a large prostate ; I have seen this mistake made on many occasions.

**Palpating the Prostate.**—The common affections of the prostate, translated into terms of palpation, may be summarized as follows :—

1. *Chronic Inflammation* is suggested by small, firm nodules. An inflammatory process is usually gonococcal, but may be tuberculous in origin.

2. *The Common Condition ; So-called Senile Enlargement.*—There is a general hypertrophy of the gland, perhaps with a large nodule here and there. The impression gained is that the enlargement is firmly elastic.

3. *The Small Fibrous Prostate* is hard and smooth.

4. *Carcinoma of the Prostate.*—In the early stages the prostate feels normal in size, but one lobe is considerably harder than the other and the impression gained is that there is a hard central nodule covered by a layer of softer tissue (Swift Joly). Somewhat later the vertical median furrow between the lateral lobes (*see Fig.* 460) becomes obliterated. Later still, the whole gland is indurated and its mobility is impaired. If the sulcus between the vesicle and the prostate is filled up, it suggests that the periprostatic lymphatics are involved.

5. *Prostatic Calculi.*—When these small stones are near enough to the periphery to be detected by palpation, they are so embedded in the fibrous stroma as to simulate the irregular hardness of a carcinoma. Very occasionally the stones are comparatively free, and they impart to the palpating finger an impression described so aptly by Erichsen as of ' beads in a bag '.

**Examination of the Seminal Vesicles.**—There is probably no method of physical examination that is more dependent upon the clinician's physical attributes than that required for the detection of disease of the seminal vesicles. If the examiner is endowed with a

JOHN SWIFT JOLY, 1876–1943, *Surgeon, St. Peter's Hospital, London.*
SIR JOHN ERIC ERICHSEN, 1818–1896, *Surgeon, University College Hospital, London.*

long finger, these structures can be palpated per rectum readily. It seems probable, however, that a short index finger is not the chief reason why vesiculitis is overlooked; rather is it because so often no attempt is made to discover it. Usually the knee-elbow position is adopted for the examination of the seminal vesicles, but when the patient is obese or the prostate is enlarged, the Picker position (*Fig.* 461) is more practicable. The patient stands and leans forward, grasping a low chair or stool. The Picker position is advantageous when a specimen of the contents of the seminal vesicles is required.

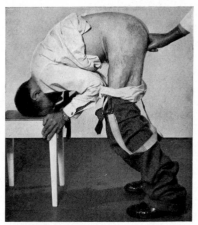

*Fig.* 461.—The Picker position for examining the seminal vesicles.

Guiteras advocated bimanual palpation. The left hand is placed above the spine of the pubis parallel with the inguinal canal. This hand exerts pressure downwards and inwards. Guiteras's method is a distinct improvement on that of employing the finger unopposed.

A seminal vesicle may be enlarged and fibrous as a result of chronic inflammation, which is usually gonococcal in origin. A tuberculous vesicle gives to the palpating finger a very characteristic sensation, which is best described as 'craggy'.

*Fig.* 462.—Bidigital palpation of Cowper's glands. The index finger is placed in the rectum, and the thumb in the perineum to one side of the middle line. An enlarged gland of Cowper can be felt between the finger and thumb.

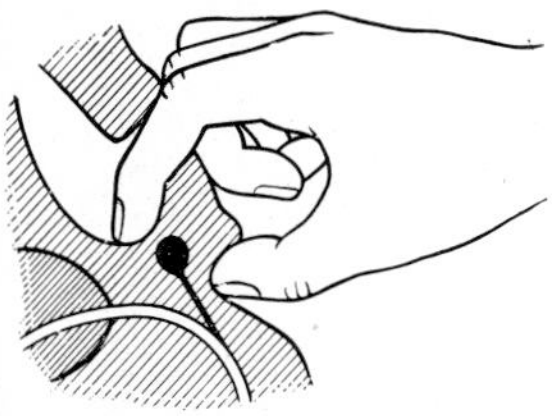

**Palpation of Cowper's Glands.**—Cowperitis, both acute and chronic, is often mistaken for prostatitis or vesiculitis. The diagnosis of Cowperitis is often missed for lack of a simple examination. On passing the forefinger into the rectum and placing the thumb first on one side and then on the other of the median raphe of the perineum Cowper's glands can be palpated (*Fig.* 462). In acute cases the least pressure causes excruciating pain—in chronic cases the enlarged gland can be felt. It varies in size from a pea to a hazelnut, is hard, and feels not unlike a malignant gland (Harkness).

RUDOLF PICKER, *Contemporary Urologist, Budapest.*

RAMÓN GUITERAS, 1860–1917, *Professor of Genito-urinary Surgery, New York Post-Graduate Medical School.*

ARTHUR HERBERT HARKNESS, *Contemporary Medical Officer-in-Charge of Venereal Department, St. Peter's Hospital, London.*

**Prostatic Massage as a Test of Posterior Urethritis.**—The prostate is massaged as shown in *Fig.* 463, the patient being in the knee-elbow position. The penile urethra is milked down. The urinary meatus is examined for a bead (*Fig.* 464), and the macroscopical characters of the bead noted ; these are unreliable, therefore microscopical examination of the specimen is essential.

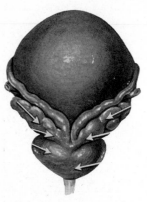

*Fig.* 463.—Directions in which to massage the prostate and vesicles.

*Vesicular Massage.*—The diagnosis of chronic vesiculitis rests upon the examination of the secretion expressed by massage of the seminal vesicles, and collected in a glass filled with water. In some cases a perfect cast of the vesicles can be expressed. Microscopical examination of the material expressed will be required.

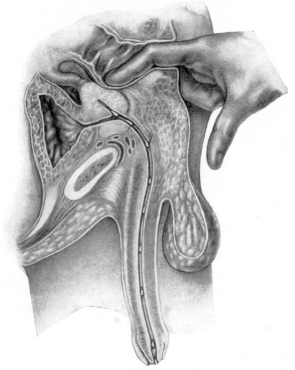

*Fig.* 464.—Prostato-vesicular massage. Expressing beads of the contents of these structures for macroscopical and microscopical scrutiny.

## EXAMINATION OF THE MALE PERINEUM

The male perineum, being hidden by the scrotum, is liable to escape scrutiny. Conditions in which cardinal diagnostic assistance is derived from displacing the scrotum upwards are depicted in *Figs.* 465–468, and a fifth is illustrated in *Fig.* 533, p. 314.

### EXAMINATION OF THE MALE PERINEUM

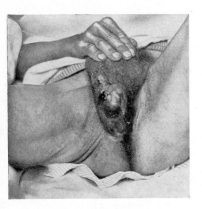

*Fig.* 465.—Periurethral abscess.

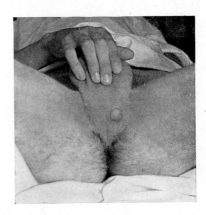

*Fig.* 466.—Abscess of left Cowper's gland.

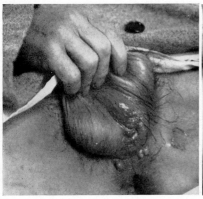

*Fig.* 467.—' Watering-can ' scrotum and perineum. A case of neglected stricture of the urethra.

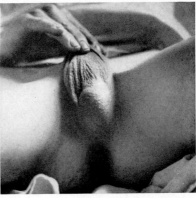

*Fig.* 468.—Perineal testis.

## EXAMINATION OF THE TESTICLE

The patient should (at least) let down his trousers completely, and roll up his shirt to the nipple line. Whilst he is getting ready for the examination he is told to micturate into two glasses (the two-glass test—*see* p. 244). The patient stands before the seated surgeon.

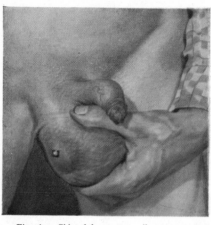

Fig. 469.—Skin of the scrotum adherent posteriorly where a sinus has developed. Case of tuberculous epididymo-orchitis.

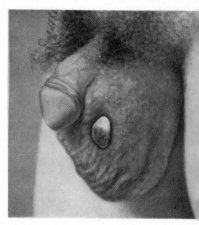

Fig. 470.—Gumma of testis commencing to ulcerate.

**The Skin of the Scrotum.**—First of all investigate the condition of the scrotal skin. Especially note if it is anchored to the underlying testis at any point (*Fig.* 469). If it is fixed anteriorly, it is slight contributory evidence of gumma (*Fig.* 470); if posteriorly, of tuberculosis; whilst a new growth may invade any portion of the overlying skin, the anterolateral aspect being the site of election. By the time the scrotum is visibly implicated, underlying testicular disease is far advanced.

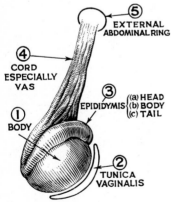

Fig. 471.—Order in which the constituent parts of the testis are palpated.

**Palpation.**—In order to carry out a thorough examination of the testis, it is useful to palpate its constituent parts in a definite order (*Fig.* 471).

1. Palpate the body of the testis and compare it with the unaffected side.

2. Whilst doing this, bear in mind the relationship of the tunica vaginalis. It is blended intimately with the anterior surface of the body of the testis.

3. Palpate the epididymis, body, globus major, and globus minor.

4. Palpate the vas. The technique has been described accurately by Lockwood : " Pass the index finger under the neck of the scrotum, pinch the thumb down upon it, and slip the constituents of the scrotum through your fingers from within outwards. You ought to feel the vas, which is like hard whipcord. You will feel a number of other small cords and strings and fibres, which you cannot define. You may possibly be able to feel the nerves of the cord, more especially the genitocrural and branches of the ilio-inguinal, but I think the fibres which you feel are probably the fibres of the cremaster muscle. Unless you feel these things clearly and accurately, you are not feeling a normal spermatic cord."

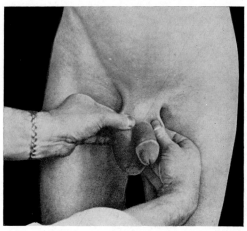

Fig. 472.—Palpating the vasa. Compare the size of the vas on each side.

*Testing for a Minor Degree of Thickening of the Vas.*—Using both hands, both vasa should be palpated simultaneously, and as these whipcord-like structures pass through the fingers, their relative sizes are estimated (*Fig.* 472).

*Test for Translucency.*—Anyone who is in close touch with clinical surgery will have seen scores of cases where the diagnosis has been vitiated, occasionally with disastrous results, by failure to carry out the test for translucency, or by carrying it out inefficiently. In the case of an intrascrotal swelling the first essential is to make the swelling tense by grasping the neck of the scrotum between the fingers and thumb. A pocket-torch is applied to the distal side of the swelling (*Fig.* 473), and most hydroceles and cysts of the epididymis can be irrefutably diagnosed at once because of their translucency. There

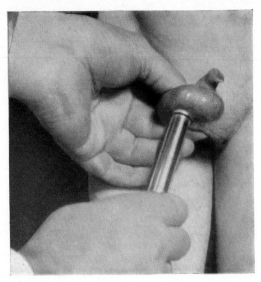

*Fig.* 473.—Testing for translucency (vaginal hydrocele).

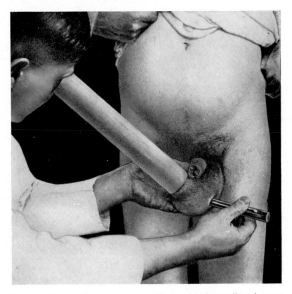

*Fig.* 474.—Testing for translucency with the aid of a cardboard carton.

are cases in which the sign is doubtful, especially in sunlight.    To instruct the patient to hold the front flap of his shirt in such a way as to form a screen, or to go to the trouble of pulling down a window blind, diminishes doubt in a large percentage of cases where it exists. Another expedient is to take advantage of a hollow cylinder (*Fig.* 474). My pocket transilluminoscope (*Fig.* 475) makes errors connected with

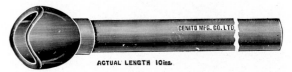

GENITO MFG. CO. LTD.

ACTUAL LENGTH 10 ins.

*Fig.* 475.—The author's pocket transilluminoscope.

transillumination improbable.    The fallacies of efficient transillumination in the diagnosis of hydrocele are few.    Obviously, if the walls are thick or calcareous the sign will be negative.    A hernia of a child, if it contains gut distended with gas, is likely to be translucent.

**Testicular    Sensation.—** The normal testis is squeezed gently between the finger and thumb (*Fig.* 476).    The patient experiences a peculiar ' sickening pain '.    Testicular sensation is lost early in syphilitic affections of the testis, but late in neoplasms.

The grave objection to the use of this sign is that, should the case be one of new growth, neoplastic cells are squeezed into venous or lymphatic channels.    Consequently, it is better to eschew this sign when there is any possibility of a doubtful

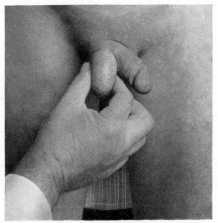

*Fig.* 476.—Testing testicular sensation.  This sign should not be attempted unless a testicular neoplasm cannot be excluded by other means.

swelling being a neoplasm.    If syphilitic orchitis has to be excluded, a Wassermann reaction will give the necessary information.

**Weighing the Testis.—**It is traditional that many years ago a house surgeon at the London Hospital, who had never been known to teach his dressers, suddenly remarked " Gentlemen, there are two varieties of tumours of the testicle, the light and the heavy ".    It was considered afterwards that this was a differential sign of some value. The affected organ is balanced on the palm of the hand, and its weight estimated (*Fig.* 477).

*a.* A testis relatively heavy is in favour of neoplasm (or old hæmatocele).

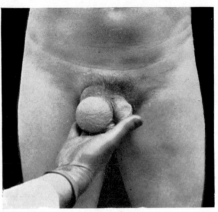

*b.* A testis relatively light is in favour of gumma.★

**Rectal Examination.**— With the sole exception of a simple hydrocele, a rectal examination should never be omitted as part and parcel of the routine examination of a case of testicular disease.

**Examination of the Regional Lymph-glands.**— In selected cases it is necessary to endeavour to palpate the regional lymph-glands.

Fig. 477.—' Weighing ' the testis.

Three sets of lymphatic vessels pass up the spermatic cord ; in order of importance these are :

*a. Those following the spermatic artery*, which pass to the para-aortic glands just below the origin of the renal arteries.

*b. Those following the artery of the vas*, which pass to the internal iliac glands.

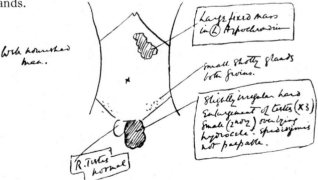

Fig. 478.—Facsimile of a record of the physical signs elicited in the case of a policeman, aged 28, with a malignant left testis.

---

★ Professor Dew, of Sydney, a great authority on the subject, considers this sign of doubtful value.

*c. Those following the cremasteric artery*, which pass to the super-ficial inguinal glands.

If the testis is the seat of an advanced neoplasm, secondary deposits are to be expected in the para-aortic glands above the level of the umbilicus (*Fig.* 478). Advantage may be taken of the knee-elbow position to seek for enlargement of these glands.

**Maldescended Testis.**—Certainly many patients with a mal-descended testis have a superadded inguinal hernia, but it should not require the peculiar talents of a Sherlock Holmes to detect that there is but a solitary testicle in the scrotum. Nevertheless, over and over again, I have marvelled that the type of maldescended testicle shown in *Fig.* 479 has been diagnosed as an inguinal hernia without the location of the testicle being questioned.

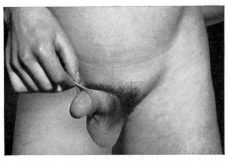

Fig. 479.—Maldescended testis at the left external abdominal ring.

If both testes fail to reach their destination and the patient is approaching, or has attained, years of maturity, the fact that the scrotum is empty and undeveloped (*Fig.* 480) is too arresting to escape notice.

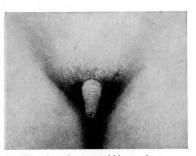

Fig. 480.—A cryptorchid at puberty, showing rudimentary scrotum.

When seeking a retained testis a light touch over the upper part of the inguinal canal, especially when the patient is examined in the upright position, sometimes reveals a mobile tell-tale swelling which up to that time had defied definition.

In infant boys intermittent contraction of the cremaster muscle pulls the testis into the inguinal canal, or, as Denis Browne would have it, the testis retracts into the superficial inguinal pouch, a space filled with loose areolar tissue lying between the fascia of Scarpa and the external oblique (*Fig.* 481). These disappearing testes have beguiled clinicians times without number. I have encountered a

DENIS BROWNE, *Contemporary Surgeon, Hospital for Sick Children, Great Ormond Street, London.*
ANTONIO SCARPA, 1747–1832, *Professor of Surgery, Modena, and Professor of Anatomy, Pavia, Italy.*

large number of male children with active cremaster muscles sent up as suffering from maldescended testes by competent practitioners. In unilateral cases scrutiny of the scrotum is sometimes of value. When the scrotal skin of the affected side is less rugosed than the normal side, it is probable that the half of the scrotum never contained a testis (Macrosson.)

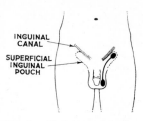

*Fig.* 481.—Mechanism of the disappearing testis (*after Browne*).

Coax the child, who is standing, to cough. This sometimes dislodges the organ from its resting place. Employing the pulp of the index finger, exert moderate pressure over the internal abdominal ring, and slide the finger down the whole length of the inguinal canal. If the testis is of the retractile type, it may be pushed into the scrotum, where it can be grasped between the finger and thumb of the other hand, and made to touch the bottom of the scrotum. When it is impossible to manipulate the testis into the scrotum, the little patient should be examined immediately after, or during, a warm bath, which regularly clears up doubt.

## THE DIFFERENTIAL DIAGNOSIS OF INTRASCROTAL SWELLINGS

Separated from the examining fingers by little more than a covering of loose integument, the testicle is unrivalled amongst organs of accessibility. Taking this into consideration, one would suppose the diagnosis of intrascrotal swellings to be a comparatively simple matter ; on the contrary, some testicular swellings are most difficult to diagnose with confidence. It is, however, evident that many more are misdiagnosed, not because of inherent difficulties, but rather for want of a careful clinical examination and the application of straightforward commonsense principles in the interpretation of the physical signs elicited.

I have reason to hope that, providing the reader is mindful of the fundamental necessity for carrying out conscientiously the routine examination described already, the short pictorial description that follows will enable him to diagnose a large percentage of testicular swellings with precision and to segregate those in which no time should be lost in advising that the swelling in question be displayed to the light of day. (*See Fig.* 484.)

### Traps for the Unwary—

*a.* Because there is a swelling within the scrotum, it does not signify that it arises in connexion with the testicular mechanism. The first question should always be, " Can I get above the swelling ? " (*Fig.* 482).

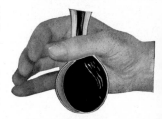

*Fig.* 482.—As shown, it is possible to get above an intrascrotal swelling when that swelling arises from the testicular apparatus.

KENNETH I. MACROSSON, *Contemporary Surgeon to Out-Patients, Royal Infirmary, Glasgow.*

*b.* A secondary hydrocele may mask underlying testicular disease. If doubt exists as to the condition of the underlying parts, it is advisable to aspirate the fluid there and then and to palpate the unmasked organ. The fluid withdrawn from a cyst connected with the testis may throw considerable light on the diagnosis (*Fig.* 483). A secondary hydrocele is present : (1) Almost always in acute and sub-acute epididymo-orchitis ; (2) In nearly all cases of syphilis of the testis ; (3) In 30 per cent of cases of testicular tuberculosis ; (4) Rarely in neoplasm.

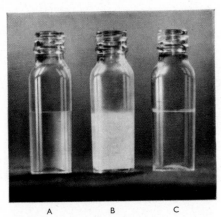

A          B          C

*Fig.* 483.—A, The fluid withdrawn from a vaginal hydrocele resembles normal urine ; B, That from a spermatocele is like barley water ; C, That from a cyst of the epididymis is crystal clear, like water.

*c.* In a small percentage of cases the testicle is anteverted ; this means that the epididymis is in front instead of behind. Unless the possibility of this anatomical variation is recognized, the physical signs elicited are difficult to interpret and much confusion can be caused.

**The Swelling is Translucent.**—Determine the relation of the transluscent swelling to the testicle. Sometimes the dark shadow of the body of the testis can be seen contrasted against the brilliantly illuminated area. Another reliable method that is often possible is to identify the testis by palpation. A vaginal hydrocele lies in front and to a variable degree above the body of the testis (*Fig.* 484, **2**). If the transluscent swelling is behind the body of the testis, it is most probably a cyst of the epididymis (*Fig.* 484, **3**). This is more common than a spermatocele (*Fig.* 484, **4**).

## THE DIFFERENTIAL DIAGNOSIS OF TESTICULAR SWELLINGS

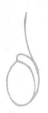

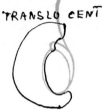

**1.**—If, on this simple outline, the physical signs elicited are recorded a reasoned diagnosis will be probable.

**2.**—Vaginal hydrocele.

**3.**—Cyst of the epididymis. Swelling tense. Often somewhat lobulated. May be in any part of the epididymis.

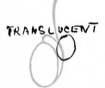

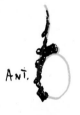

**4.**—Spermatocele. Same as **3**, but not so lobulated, not so tense, and not so brilliantly translucent.

**5.**—Cyst of the hydatid of Morgagni perched on the upper and anterior surface of the testicle. Diagnosis irrefutable.

**6.**—In an anteverted testis a vaginal hydrocele simulates a cyst of the epididymis. Largely an academic problem.

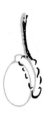

**7.**—Epididymo-orchitis. Epididymis enlarged and tender. Vas may be thickened.

**8.**—Tuberculous epididymitis. Epididymis craggy. Vas considerably thickened.

**9.**—Tuberculosis in an anteverted testis. Although rare, it is a source of diagnostic confusion.

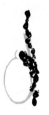

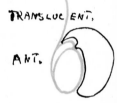

**10.**—Advanced neoplasm. Body of the testis enlarged and irregular. Epididymis cannot be felt. Old clotted hæmatocele gives rise to same signs.

**11.**—Early neoplasm. Any painless nodule in the body or even in the epididymis should be displayed to the light of day.

**12.**—Syphilis of the testis. Smooth, painless enlargement of the body.

*Fig. 484.*

GIOVANNI BATTISTA MORGAGNI, 1682-1771, *Professor of Anatomy at Padua. He held the chair for fifty-six years.*

**Non-translucent Swellings.—**

**Tuberculosis.—**Except in the rare subacute and acute forms, the comparative absence of tenderness helps to differentiate tuberculosis from other forms of epididymitis. When the condition is fully established physical signs are characteristic (*Fig.* 484, **8**). In early testicular tuberculosis there is often a loss of cutaneous elasticity as shown by smoothing out of the rugæ consequent upon wasting of the cellular tissues beneath the dermis (Morson). Normally the testis can be moved freely within its coverings, particularly in an upward and downward direction. This movement is often restricted in tuberculosis.

**Syphilis** of the testis is encountered principally in three forms :—

*Orchitis of Congenital Syphilis.* Should a congenital syphilitic boy be fortunate enough—if, indeed, he can ever be called fortunate—to reach puberty, certain ills are liable to befall him. He tends to become lame, deaf, blind, and impotent. *Lame* because of Clutton's joints, *deaf* because of neuro-labyrinthitis, *blind* because of interstitial keratitis (*Fig.* 485), and

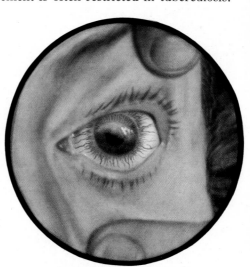

*Fig.* 485.—Interstitial keratitis.

*impotent* because of diffuse fibrosis and atrophy of the testes. The reason for the testicular changes is a previous attack of bilateral interstitial orchitis. Usually this occurs between the third and tenth months and gives rise to what are known as the ' pigeon-egg testicles of syphilitic infants '.

*Tertiary Interstitial Orchitis.* When the condition is fully established, the testicle is rounded, densely hard, completely insensitive, and freely movable in its scrotal coverings. What better name could be given to it than the ' billiard-ball ' testicle ?

*Gumma of the Testis.* In its early stages a gumma (*Fig.* 484, **12**) gives rise to signs somewhat like those of chronic interstitial orchitis, but also much the same as those of neoplasm of the testis.

ALBERT CLIFFORD MORSON, *Contemporary Surgeon, St. Peter's Hospital, London.*
HENRY HUGH CLUTTON, 1850–1909, *Surgeon, St. Thomas's Hospital, London.*

Considerable diminution of testicular sensation favours a diagnosis of testicular syphilis, but as pointed out already, this may be a dangerous manipulation.

Another point in the differential diagnosis is that a gumma of the testis is relatively light. A positive Wassermann reaction is, of course, most suggestive, but it should be remembered that it is possible for malignant disease to appear in a syphilitic patient.

**Malignant Disease** of the testis is not by any means the hopeless proposition that many think, provided an early diagnosis is made. When there is just a hardness of the body of the testis or an unexplained nodule (*Fig.* 484, **11**), even if that nodule is in the epididymis, it should be exposed to the light of day. Should this course be followed the clinician will, from time to time, suffer from humiliation, for an old clotted hæmatocele (*see Fig.* 484, **10**), an atypical tuberculous lesion (*Fig.* 484, **9**), or even a gumma of the testis will be removed unnecessarily. With reasonable clinical acumen such mistakes, if one can call them mistakes, are few and are relatively unimportant.

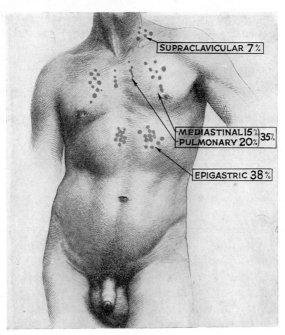

*Fig.* 486.—Showing the distribution of metastases from malignant disease of the testis.

AUGUST VON WASSERMANN, 1866–1925, *Director of the Institute for Experimental Therapy, Berlin.*

The necessity of searching for secondary deposits in cases of established or suspected malignant disease of the testicle has been emphasized already (p. 268). In this connexion the diagram (*Fig.* 486) showing the distribution of metastases is useful.

*Varicocele.*—The enlarged veins of the pampiniform plexus are so obvious that it is unlikely that a varicocele will be confused with any other condition. The condition is nearly always left-sided. After the examination in the erect position is concluded, the patient should lie down ; when the testis is elevated the veins will empty. In cases of long standing the body of the left testis will be found to be smaller than that of the right.

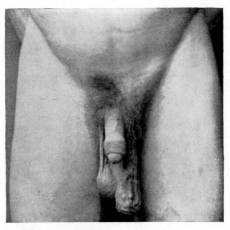

Fig. 487.—Varicocele. The impression conveyed on light palpation has been well likened to that of feeling a bag of worms.

Much academic attention has been given to a rapidly oncoming varicocele as a sign of malignant disease of the kidney. I have not found this sign of material value ; in those cases in which it has been present there has been an easily palpable kidney tumour.

What I have found to be a reliable, though depressing, sign is when a congenital *hydrocele* appears in a man past forty. On several occasions the excess fluid in the peritoneal cavity, manifesting itself by way of the funicular process, has been the first sign of an intra-abdominal carcinoma, notably of the stomach.

## EXAMINATION OF A CASE OF URETHRITIS
### (SUSPECTED VENEREAL DISEASE)

Adequate exposure of the lower abdomen, external genitalia, and upper portion of the thighs, and a good light are essential.

Commence by palpating the inguinal glands.

In *gonorrhœa* the glands on both sides are moderately enlarged and slightly tender.

In *soft sore* (chancroid) unilateral, tender, adenitis occurs early.

In *syphilis* adenitis occurs later than in the two previous conditions ; the glands are painless, elastic, and, in the absence of secondary infection, freely movable under the skin. The whole group from the saphenous opening upwards, and along the under surface of Poupart's ligament (*see Fig.* 352, p. 174), are usually involved.

Next the penis is examined. An external sore may be obvious, or a dorsal lymphangitis may be noted—hot and tender in gonorrhœa and chancroid, painless and indolent in syphilis (McLachlan).

The prepuce is retracted. Observe whether any discharge comes from the sub-preputial sac or from the urethra. A sub-preputial discharge, which is frequently confused with gonorrhœa, may be due to one of many causes, e.g., chancre, chancroid (*Fig.* 488), balanitis, or smegma accumulation.

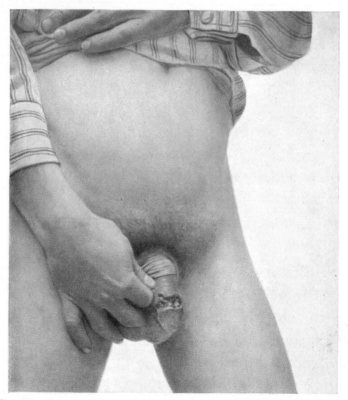

*Fig.* 488.—Chancroid (soft sore) with suppurating left-sided inguinal glands (bubo).

FRANÇOIS POUPART, 1616–1708, *Surgeon Hôtel-Dieu, Paris.*
ANGUS ELRICK WILLIAM MCLACHLAN, *Contemporary Lecturer in Venereal Diseases, University of Bristol.*

After thorough cleansing with cotton-wool moistened with saline, the glans is carefully inspected for the presence of a sore ; then the lips of the meatus are separated so that a meatal chancre is not overlooked. The urethra is now massaged to bring any discharge to the meatus. The characters of the discharge are classified as purulent, mucopurulent, or gleet. A " two-glass " urine test (*see* p. 244) is now carried out.

When contemplating the treatment of a patient with urethritis it is valuable to pay particular attention to the external urinary meatus. " The normal urethra is a good hose, and a good hose has a small nozzle. But an inflamed urethra is a drain, and a good drain has a wide mouth." (Keyes.)

Before concluding the examination the testes must be palpated and a rectal examination with prostatic massage carried out.

For examination of Suspected Urethritis in the Female *see* p. 240.

18

EDWARD L. KEYES, *Contemporary (retired) Professor of Urology, Cornell University, New York.*

## CHAPTER XXIII

# COMMON ACUTE ABDOMINAL CONDITIONS

*" Happy is he who has no serious consequences of his erroneous diagnosis to regret."*
*—Howard Marsh.*

PHYSICAL signs and their interpretation reach a high pinnacle of importance in the diagnosis of acute abdominal disease. Frequently an urgent and all-important diagnosis has to be formulated by their aid alone. It is for this reason that this section is considered somewhat fully.

In deciding the momentous question, " Is this an acute abdominal condition ? " there are two signs that may prove helpful in a general way :—

1. *The Rising Test.*—The patient is instructed to place his arms by his sides and then to raise himself in bed by means of the abdominal muscles alone. The sign is positive when the patient fails to rise or complains of great pain on attempting to do so (Granville Chapman).

2. *Altered Abdomino-thoracic Rhythm.*—Normally, during inspiration, when the chest comes out the abdomen comes out. If, however, when the chest comes out the abdomen goes in, it is highly probable that a diffuse leak is present and general peritonitis is imminent. It should be remembered that the first three or four respirations must be disregarded in order to allow the patient to overcome his self-consciousness. (Jeans.)

When called upon to examine the abdomen of a patient who has been placed in Fowler's position, have the bed placed flat for the time being, unless there is some contra-indication. It is impossible to examine the abdomen thoroughly when a patient is in Fowler's position.

## EXAMINATION OF AN EARLY CASE OF ACUTE APPENDICITIS

Take the pulse and temperature. These show but little alteration in the early stages of this disease. An acceleration of the pulse-rate usually signifies the onset of peritonitis.

FREDERICK HOWARD MARSH, 1839–1915, *Surgeon, St. Bartholomew's Hospital, London.*
CHARLES LEOPOLD GRANVILLE CHAPMAN, *Contemporary Surgeon, Grimsby and District Hospital.*
FRANK JEANS, 1878–1933, *Surgeon, Liverpool Royal Infirmary.*
GEO. RYERSON FOWLER, 1848–1906, *Surgeon-in-Chief, Brooklyn Hospital, New York.*

The pain of acute appendicitis rarely begins in the right iliac fossa. Ask the patient where the pain *began*; he usually places a finger near the umbilicus (*Fig.* 489). Now ask where the pain is *now*; the pointing finger passes to the right iliac fossa (*Fig.* 490). The pointing test, when positive, is of the greatest possible diagnostic significance.

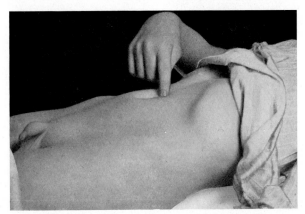

*Fig.* 489.—The pointing test in appendicitis. I. The answer to the question
" Where did the pain begin ? "

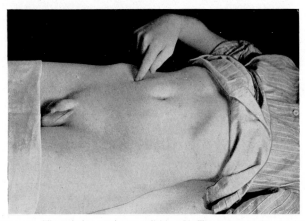

*Fig.* 490.—The pointing test in appendicitis. II. The answer to the question
" Where is the pain now ? "

**Inspection.**—Unless the appendix has perforated, we do not expect to see any alteration in the contour of the abdomen or in the movements of respiration.

**Epicritic Hyperæsthesia.**—Take a pin and pass its point vertically down the *left* lower half of the abdominal wall, exerting very

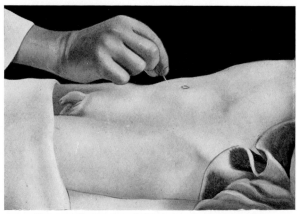

*Fig.* 491.—Testing for epicritic hyperæsthesia with a pin.

slight but even pressure.   Again, pass the pin down the *left* side a
little more medially, but parallel to the first line.   Proceed in the same
manner on the *right* side (*Fig.* 491).   If epicritic hyperæsthesia is

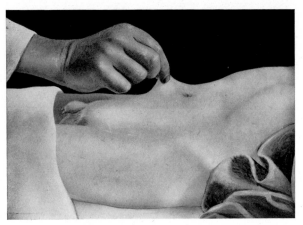

*Fig.* 492.—Testing for hyperæsthesia by Ligat's method.

present, the patient will experience pain when the pin reaches the
hyperæsthetic area.   There is no need to ask the patient any questions ;
one can discern at once the onset of pain by the facial expression.

DAVID LIGAT, *Contemporary Consulting Surgeon, Buchanan Hospital, St. Leonards-on-sea, England.*

This hyperæsthesia signifies that the appendix is, as yet, unperforated ; when perforation occurs, hyperæsthesia passes off immediately.

Sir James Walton has made a study of the exact situation of this hyperæsthetic area, and finds that it is a relatively narrow band about one and a half inches wide, running from the anterior superior iliac spine to the spine of the pubis.

Hyperæsthesia can also be demonstrated by Ligat's method.   This consists of picking up between the finger and thumb a portion of skin and subcutaneous tissue and lifting it off the abdominal musculature (*Fig.* 492).   The portion of skin is picked up as in pinching, but it should be noted carefully that the skin is *not* pinched.   In order to elicit hyperæsthesia by Ligat's method, we begin in the left iliac fossa, pass to the left and then the right hypochondrium, ultimately picking up the skin in Sherren's triangle (*Fig.* 493). Again there is no need to question the patient ; rely entirely upon facial expression. Well-marked hyperæsthesia is one of the best single signs of early acute appendicitis.

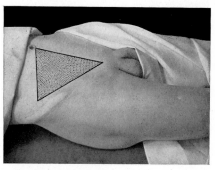

*Fig.* 493.—Sherren's skin triangle for appendicitis, formed by : (1) The highest point of the iliac crest ; (2) The right pubic spine ;   (3) The umbilicus.

Tested by Ligat's method Livingston found it positive in 86 per cent of 428 consecutive cases of appendicitis.   I have used Ligat's method for a long time, and consider it to be the method of choice.

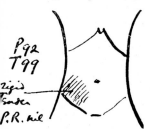

*Fig.* 494.—Signs recorded in a typical case of acute appendicitis of ten hours' duration.

**Palpation.**—Commence palpation diagonally opposite the point where pain is or was experienced, viz., lay the hand upon the left hypochondrium.   Next palpate the right hypochondrium, then the left iliac fossa, leaving the right iliac fossa until last.   In typical cases there is rigidity and tenderness in this area, the extent of which should be recorded (*Fig.* 494).

When the diagnosis is doubtful (and in about one out of four cases the history and physical signs are atypical) further examination is required.   At this juncture it is useful to apply Rovsing's and Blumberg's signs.

Sir James Walton, *Contemporary Consulting Surgeon, London Hospital.*
James Sherren, 1872–1945, *Surgeon, London Hospital.*
Edward Meakin Livingston, *Contemporary Professor of Clinical Surgery, New York College of Medicine.*

**Rovsing's Sign.**—Even pressure is exerted over the descending colon. This forces gas into the cæcum (*Fig.* 495). If, when the left iliac fossa is pressed, pain is appreciated in the right iliac fossa, the case is probably one of acute appendicitis.

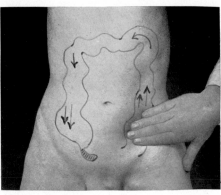

*Fig.* 495.—Rovsing's sign. Pressure on the left iliac fossa produces pain in the right iliac fossa when the sign is positive.

I constantly employ Rovsing's sign when the diagnosis of acute appendicitis is not perfectly evident, and I have found it valuable, especially when used in conjunction with the following :—

**Blumberg's Sign.**—Deep pressure is exerted in the left iliac fossa, as for Rovsing's sign. The hand is then removed suddenly. The patient experiences sudden pain in the lower abdomen.

**McBurney's Sign.**—Finger-tip pressure is made over McBurney's point (*Fig.* 496), which, if the sign is positive, registers the maximum abdominal tenderness. This sign is sometimes useful in very early or subacute cases of appendicitis.

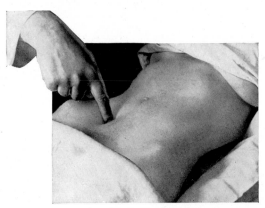

*Fig.* 496.—Finger-tip pressure over McBurney's point.

**Signs in Retrocæcal Appendicitis.**—Rigidity is inclined to be ill-defined in front, but it is sometimes present in the flank, which

THORKILD ROVSING, 1862–1927, *Professor of Surgery, Copenhagen.*

MORIR BLUMBERG, *Contemporary, formerly a Practitioner-Surgeon in Berlin.*

CHARLES McBURNEY, 1845–1913, *Surgeon, Roosevelt Hospital, New York. Described a point between* 1½ *in. and* 2 *in. from the right anterior superior iliac spine upon a line joining the spine and the umbilicus* may be the seat of greatest tenderness. The flank should be palpated with particular care. In many instances maximum tenderness will be found just medial to the anterior superior iliac spine (*Fig.* 497). In cases of high retrocæcal appendicitis the point of greatest tenderness to deep pressure is in the same plane, but higher, even as high as the level of the umbilicus.

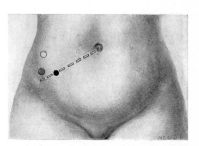

**Testicular Retraction.**—In cases of *gangrenous* appendicitis, if even pressure is exerted over McBurney's point the right testis is drawn upwards. As long as the pressure is maintained the retraction commonly persists. When the pressure is released the testis drops back into its usual position. La Roque has found the sign positive in 500 cases of gangrenous appendicitis.

*Fig.* 497.—*Black*: McBurney's point. *Red*: Point of maximum tenderness in retrocæcal appendicitis. *Green*: In cases of maldescent of the cæcum, this point may be as high as the level of the umbilicus.

**Rectal Examination.**—Take particular care to insinuate the finger slowly with a rotatory movement. When the finger can be placed within the rectum without causing pain, not only can a more

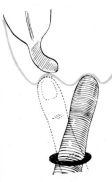

thorough examination be made, but the discovery of a tender area becomes of real diagnostic significance. The best method of procedure is as follows. Palpate the left side of the rectovesical pouch ; then palpate the right side (*Fig.* 498). If there is any doubt as to the relative tenderness, repeat the process, at the same time asking the patient, " Is there any difference in the two sides ? " In early cases of pelvic appendicitis tenderness on the right is often the crucial point in an all-important diagnosis. In later cases the finding of a tender lump, or cystic swelling (pelvic abscess) when

*Fig.* 498.—Differential rectal palpation.

perhaps there are few, if any, signs on abdominal examination, brings home the cardinal importance of rectal examination in cases of pelvic appendicitis.

**Differential Diagnosis.**—Manifestly it is impossible here to enter at length into the differential diagnosis of acute appendicitis, and it must suffice to urge the examiner to bear in mind the old maxim : " Always examine the right lung and the right kidney (urine)." To this may be added an examination of the pelvic organs in the female.

George Paul La Roque, 1876–1934, *Professor of Surgery, Richmond, Virginia, U.S.A.*

In this connexion attention is drawn to the fact that abdominal rigidity in acute salpingitis is inclined to be less evident than in a case of acute appendicitis with a corresponding elevation of pulse and temperature.

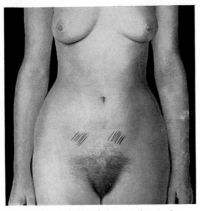

Fig. 499.—Areas of deep tenderness in acute salpingitis.

In salpingitis there are often two symmetrical points of deep tenderness, as shown in *Fig.* 499.

Perhaps the most confusing differential diagnosis is between acute appendicitis and stone in the right ureter. In this connexion Ben-Asher's cough sign is helpful. The pulps of two fingers are placed immediately below the left costal margin, i.e. over the region of the spleen. The patient is told to (*a*) breathe in, (*b*) breathe out, (*c*) cough. While (*b*) and (*c*) are in progress, deep upward and backward pressure is exerted by the fingers (*Fig.* 500). When the patient volunteers the information that the manœuvre causes him pain, *not* where he is being pressed but in the right iliac fossa, the vermiform appendix is acutely inflamed. This sign is sometimes useful, but *if the diagnosis of stone in the ureter cannot be confirmed by scientific methods within an hour, and the case is an early one, it is safer to remove the appendix.*

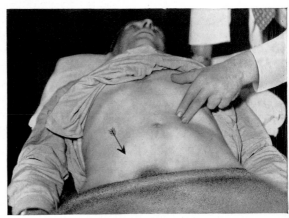

Fig. 500.—Eliciting Ben-Asher's sign.

**Atypical Acute Appendicitis.—** Lengthy experience shows that the atypical case of acute appendicitis is the most difficult of all the abdominal emergencies to diagnose. The stage of illusion is really worthy of the name; it occurs a few minutes after an obstructed appendix has perforated. The patient may say that he feels better; the hyperæsthesia goes; the rigidity to a large extent passes off; but fortunately the pulse-rate begins to rise, or probably we should be mistaken more often than we are.

For the real case of doubt and difficulty there are yet a few special physical signs that sometimes prove helpful.

1. *A Confirmatory Test for Retrocæcal Appendicitis.*—The finger locates the most tender spot in the flank.  Pressing lightly, but just enough to produce a little pain, ask the patient to lift his right leg a few inches off the bed, keeping the knee stiff. If the patient promptly complains of an increase in pain, or drops the leg with a distinct outcry, the test is positive.  (Baldwin.)

2. *The Psoas Test.*—Extend the hip-joint.  If the psoas muscle is in a state of irritation from its proximity to an inflamed appendix, the manœuvre brings on pain.

3. *The Obturator Test.*—Flex the right thigh, rotate the hip-joint internally. This puts the obturator internus on the stretch.  An inflamed appendix in contact with and adherent to this muscle will be irritated by this movement and pain will be experienced in the hypogastrium.  (Z. Cope.)

**Special Points in the Examination of a Young Child.**—Screaming children, too young to co-operate in the search for physical signs, sometimes can be placated by the following expedient. The abdomen is palpated with the child's own hand (*Fig.* 501). When the point of maximum tenderness is approached, the child pulls its hand away, and commences crying.  This sim-

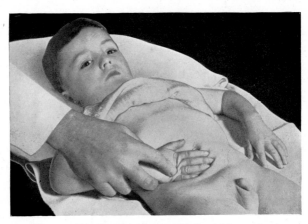

Fig. 501.—Palpating the abdomen with the child's own hand.

ple method will often succeed, if carried out patiently, in elucidating the area of maximum tenderness when other methods are inconclusive. (R. Grainger.)

*The Thoracic Compression Test.*—When it is difficult to decide whether a young child has acute appendicitis or basal lung involvement, compression of the lower thorax from side to side elicits obvious distress when the lesion is above the diaphragm, whereas in appendicitis it has no effect.  (N. M. Dott.)

HUGH ALLEN BALDWIN, 1851–1937, *Surgeon, St. Francis Hospital, Columbus, Ohio.*
VINCENT ZACHARY COPE, *Contemporary Consulting Surgeon, St. Mary's Hospital, London.*
ROBERT GRAINGER, *Contemporary Surgeon, Berkhampsted, England.*
NORMAN MCOMISH DOTT, *Professor of Neurological Surgery, University of Edinburgh.*

## APPENDIX ABSCESS

Palpate the lump gently. It is very helpful to mark out the limits of the mass with a skin pencil. Marking the limits of the swelling is almost essential if the case is going to be treated by the Ochsner-Sherren method (Fowler's position, and giving only water by mouth). The general signs are watched by keeping a two-hourly pulse- and temperature-chart. The local signs can be kept under observation by noting the increase or decrease of the limits of the lump, which have been marked on the skin (*Fig.* 502).

*Mapping out the Lump.*— Take an ordinary indelible pencil,* and a glass containing a little water. After moistening the tip of the pencil in the water, try marking your own wrist. Ensure that the skin of the abdomen is not greasy, for it may be that antiphlogistine, or some other substance, has been applied. Palpate the lump, with special reference to its periphery, before starting the marking. The best method of ascertaining the periphery is by deep index-finger-tip pressure. Little by little, pressing, then marking, the periphery is outlined (*Fig.* 503). Explain to the patient the importance

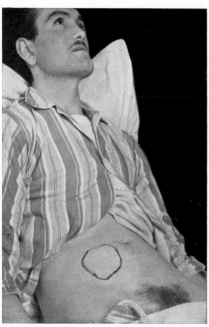

Fig. 502.—Appendix abscess. The extent of the lump has been marked on the skin.

of the procedure, and, should the lump be tender, ask him to bear the pain and, if possible, not to contract his abdominal muscles. When overlying rigidity makes the exact outlining uncertain, and assuredly this will occur quite often, on no account should one lull oneself into completing a hypothetical periphery ; the uncertain zone is left uncompleted.

Rectal examination is essential, for only by this method can it be ascertained whether the abscess is invading the pelvis. It should be noted that diarrhœa, accompanied by the passage of mucus, in a

---

* The recently introduced Biro pen (Great Britain) or the Eversharp 'CA' (U.S.A.) pen are admirable for marking the skin.

ALBERT JOHN OCHSNER, 1858–1925, *Surgeon, Augustana Hospital, Chicago.*
JAMES SHERREN, 1872–1945, *Surgeon, London Hospital.*

patient who has not had dysentery or mucous colitis, is proof positive of a pelvic abscess. This is a sign of the highest diagnostic importance and one that is absolutely reliable.

*     *     *     *     *

One is called to see a patient some days or even weeks after an operation for acute appendicitis or appendix abscess because his condition is unsatisfactory ; the temperature is swinging and the pulse is elevated—signs that foretell the pocketing of pus. The clinical investigation of such a case is carried out as follows :—

1. Examine the wound and the adjacent abdominal wall for an abscess thereof.

2. Consider the possibility of a pelvic abscess (*see above*).

3. Palpate the left iliac fossa for an abscess in this situation.

4. Examine the loin for a perinephric abscess (p. 250).

5. Look at the legs to exclude the possibility of phlebitis.

6. Examine the conjunctivæ for an icteric tinge and the liver for enlargement. Also inquire if the patient has had rigors—signs that denote pylephlebitis.

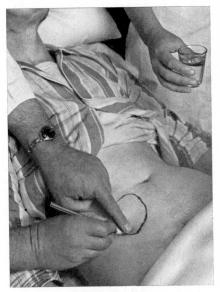

Fig. 503.—Method of marking out the periphery of the lump with an indelible pencil.

7. Examine the lungs—pneumonia or empyema.

8. Examine the urine for pus (pyelitis) and the fæces for blood and pus (enteritis).

9. Lastly, concentrate diagnostic endeavour upon the possibility of a subdiaphragmatic abscess (p. 149).

## THE SIGNS ELICITED IN A CASE OF PERFORATED GASTRIC OR DUODENAL ULCER

**Pulse.**—*For the first six hours the pulse-rate is often practically unaltered.* This basic fact should be borne in mind constantly.

Over and over again the diagnosis of perforated peptic ulcer has been delayed *on one sign alone*, with fatal results, ' because the pulse-rate was only 75 '. So great is the importance of recognizing this trap, that it can be said with truth that the gravity of the prognosis varies directly with the pulse-rate ; for the majority of patients operated upon while the pulse is still under 100 recover, while almost all those who are delayed until their pulse-rate has risen to 120 or more, die, no matter what is done.

One must strive to discriminate between the rapid pulse-rate of shock and the rising pulse-rate of peritonitis. Of 122 consecutive cases of perforated peptic ulcer examined by me only sixty-nine arrived in under eight hours from the time of perforation. In these sixty-nine comparatively early cases, the pulse-rate was under 100, except in twelve instances. Some of the exceptions were very early cases (i.e., under two hours) ; obviously the fast pulse was due to the shock of sudden perforation. Experience shows that there is a tendency to spontaneous recovery from this early shock unless the perforation is a very large one.

**Temperature.**—The temperature is likely to be subnormal, for the patient has lost heat owing to shock. There are but few exceptions to this rule.

**Inspection.**—*Retraction of the Epigastrium.* In an early case of perforation, especially if the subject is a spare, muscular man, retraction of the epigastrium is a characteristic sign. In well-marked examples, when they are viewed laterally, the appearance is as if an invisible rope were constricting the abdomen at the level indicated in *Fig.* 504. This is due to muscular contraction of the diaphragm and anterior abdominal wall (Willan). As time passes this sign is lost.

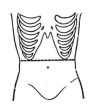

*Fig.* 504. Retraction of the epigastrium is maximal at the level indicated by the dotted line. (*R. J. Willan.*)

Carefully inspect the abdomen for respiratory movement (*Fig.* 505). The patient should be placed between the light and the examiner. In perforated ulcer the abdominal muscles are held so rigidly that respiration is almost entirely of the thoracic type. The respirations are often of a peculiar grunting character, and altered abdomino-thoracic rhythm, already referred to, may be noted (p. 278).

" *Point to the place where it hurts you now.*" This is not a sign of great value in perforated ulcer. It should not, however, be omitted.

" *Point to the place where the pain started.*" Quite frequently there is a finger pointing to the epigastrium.

The abdomen is now palpated sytematically, beginning with the left iliac fossa. *Board-like rigidity* is characteristic, and the

ROBERT JOSEPH WILLAN, *Contemporary Emeritus Professor of Surgery, University of Durham, Newcastle-upon-Tyne.*

cardinal sign of the condition.   With the onset of general peritonitis and consequent distension, the rigidity (and to a great extent the agonizing pain) passes off to a varying degree.

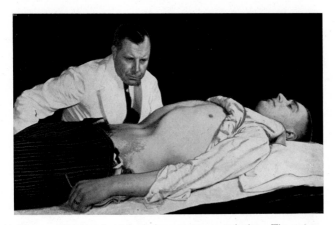

*Fig.* 505.—Watching for abdominal movement on respiration.   The patient is placed between the light and the examiner.

*Liver Dullness.*—The absence of liver dullness in the mid-axillary line is very fair evidence of gas in the peritoneal cavity (*Fig.* 506).   Usually it is only in late cases of perforation that sufficient gas collects to give a tympanitic note.   However, when sought for carefully, provided the examiner is experienced in percussing the

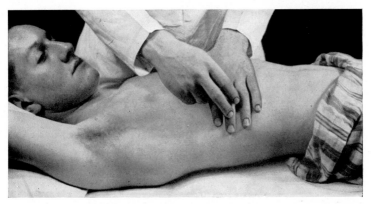

*Fig.* 506.—Percussing the liver dullness.  Ir should be noted that this is reliable only in the mid-axillary line.   If the sign is doubtful the patient should turn on to his left side and the area is percussed again.

liver, this sign proves helpful in making the diagnosis. To summarize : liver dullness is usually not obliterated ; it is of value only if tested in the mid-axillary line, and we should remember that we may be deceived by overlying emphysema of the lung.

Percuss the abdomen. In perforated gastric ulcer there is a dull note over most of the abdomen. In the early case this cannot be made to shift satisfactorily, but as time goes on the amount of fluid becomes so considerable that shifting dullness can be demonstrated with ease. In order to demonstrate shifting dullness ask the patient to turn somewhat on to his left side. Wait for a minute in order to allow the fluid to gravitate. Commence percussion from the right side to the left, noting where the resonant area becomes dull and marking the spot on the abdominal wall. Then the patient is asked to turn slightly on to his right side, and after a reasonable interval, if shifting dullness is present, the dull area will have become resonant, and vice versa (*Fig.* 507).

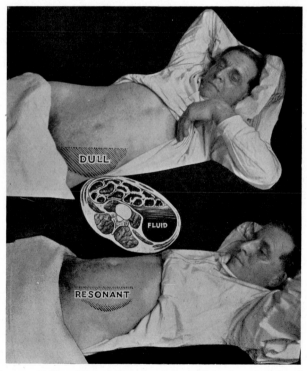

*Fig.* 507.—Shifting dullness. The sign of free fluid in the peritoneal cavity.

If board-like rigidity is present, shifting dullness is not usually demonstrable ; indeed it is not prudent to attempt to elicit it, for the necessary turning causes the patient much pain.   As the pain and rigidity pass off it is a method that can be applied justifiably, and may yield most valuable information.

**Rectal Examination.**—When the patient is in great pain, rectal examination should be undertaken in the dorsal position.   Sometimes tenderness can be detected in the rectovesical pouch, especially if the patient is in Fowler's position.

**Reflexes.**—The examination may well be concluded by testing the knee-jerks and the reaction of the pupils to light.   If this is not carried out in every case of suspected perforated ulcer, sooner or later a gastric crisis of tabes will be confounded with a perforation.

The diagnosis of perforated *gastric* ulcer is seldom really difficult. Diaphragmatic pleurisy (*see* p. 292) and an acute cardiac attack, particularly coronary thrombosis, are the conditions with which it is most likely to be confused.

## SPECIAL FEATURES OF PERFORATED DUODENAL ULCER

Perforated duodenal ulcer is more common than perforated gastric ulcer.   The features already enumerated in connexion with perforated gastric ulcer are identical with those of perforated duodenal ulcer.   There is one pitfall in the diagnosis of the latter that I have noted time and again.   When a duodenal ulcer perforates, the ascending colon acts as a watershed and directs the escaping fluid to the right iliac fossa (*Fig.* 508).   Thus the diagnosis between a perforated duodenal ulcer and appendicitis becomes difficult.   If it is a perforated duodenal ulcer the rigidity tends to be more extensive, but it is often admittedly a problem to decide which of

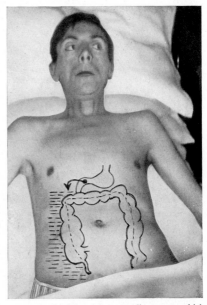

Fig. 508.—The right paracolic gutter, which explains how the symptoms and signs of a perforated duodenal ulcer can be referred to the right iliac fossa.

two organs is at fault.    In this connexion Rovsing's sign (*see* p. 282) is sometimes useful.

*Differential Diagnosis between Diaphragmatic Pleurisy and Perforated Peptic Ulcer.*—When there are no physical signs to be found in the chest, as may happen in diaphragmatic pleurisy, differential diagnosis becomes exceedingly difficult.    A patient with diaphragmatic pleurisy prefers to be propped or sitting up in bed, whilst if the lesion is below the diaphragm he prefers to lie flat (Black).    Unfortunately, there are occasionally exceptions to this rule and a patient with a perforated peptic ulcer may beg to remain in a sitting posture.    In pneumonia with abdominal pain the skin is hyperæsthetic, but pressure affords relief and there is little, if any, restriction of respiratory movements of the abdominal wall (Birch).

When rigidity is of thoracic origin it will often be found that there is some relaxation of the upper abdominal wall when the patient is told to hold his breath, with his mouth open, at the end of expiration (Raw).

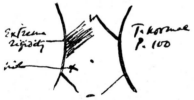

Fig. 509.—Physical signs recorded in a case of perforated duodenal ulcer partially sealed by omentum, colloquially known as 'dry perforation'.

*Perforated Duodenal Ulcer Partially Sealed by Omentum.*—This is a clinical entity that is well worth bearing in mind. The patient can move about surprisingly well ; indeed, he may walk to hospital. Vomiting is absent, which is against appendicitis or cholecystitis.    Rigidity is very high, *i.e.*, just beneath the costal margin.    Fig. 509 is a record of the physical signs of an example of this condition.

## ACUTE CHOLECYSTITIS

The methods employed in the examination of the *acute* gall-bladder case differ not at all from those already described on p. 211.

The differential diagnosis between a maldescended acutely inflamed appendix and an acute cholecystitis may be exceedingly difficult.    The radiation of the pain to the back in cholecystitis sometimes proves helpful.    Boas's test (*see* p. 213) should be tried, and the urine examined for traces of bile.

## EXAMINATION OF A CASE OF INTESTINAL OBSTRUCTION

Vomiting occurs early in obstruction of the small intestine, but when the large gut is obstructed vomiting is often absent until late.

If any vomit has been saved, observe its character—whether it is undigested food, bile-stained, or fæcal.    " Fæcal vomiting is not to

KENNETH BLACK, *Contemporary Surgeon, formerly Professor of Surgery, Singapore.*
CHARLES ALLAN BIRCH, *Contemporary Physician, Chase Farm Hospital, Enfield, London.*
STANLEY C. RAW, *Surgeon, St. Helier County Hospital, Carshalton, Surrey.*
ISMAR ISIDOR BOAS, 1858–1938, *Gastro-enterologist, Berlin.*

be regarded as a sign of intestinal obstruction, but as a herald of approaching death" (Sampson Handley). Look at the patient's tongue. In late intestinal obstruction it is brown, furred, and dried.

When one is about to make a physical examination in a case of acute intestinal obstruction, the first duty should be to *examine the hernial sites, inguinal, femoral, and umbilical.* This axiom is an old one, but one that can still bear much repetition.

An umbilical hernia can hardly be missed ; a strangulated inguinal hernia is usually obvious ; it is the small unobtrusive femoral

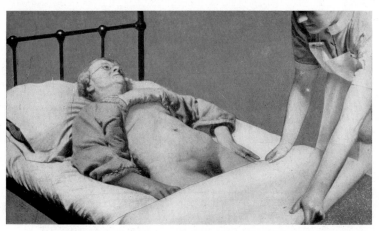

*Fig.* 510.—In every case where the history suggests intestinal obstruction, the abdomen should be uncovered from the nipple to the apex of Scarpa's triangle. Only in this way will small strangulated herniæ cease to be overlooked.

hernia that is the stumbling-block. It is not an exaggeration to state that never have six consecutive months of my surgical lifetime elapsed without my encountering at least one case of a small strangulated femoral hernia (frequently the Richter type) being overlooked. The patient is usually an old lady. Occasionally the attending practitioner has seen and felt the lump, but has considered it to be an enlarged lymphatic gland. Far more frequently, pandering to the false modesty of his patient brought up in the Victorian era, he has failed to draw down the bedclothes far enough (*Fig.* 510). The tell-tale lump is usually perfectly evident. The omission to draw down the bedclothes can be truly designated as the *chef d'œuvre* of acute abdominal diagnostic disasters.

WILLIAM SAMPSON HANDLEY, *Contemporary Consulting Surgeon, Middlesex Hospital, London.*
AUGUST GOTTLIEB RICHTER, 1742–1812, *Surgeon, Göttingen, Germany, in* 1777 *described strangulation of a portion only of the gut wall.*
QUEEN VICTORIA, 1819–1901. *During the* 19th *century fashionable practitioners were wont to confine abdominal examination of the female to palpation beneath the bedclothes.*

Thus it must be our unwavering rule in every case of intestinal obstruction to examine *all* the hernial sites before attempting to elicit other physical signs. We will assume that this has been done with a negative result.

**Inspection.**—Look at the abdomen. Obstruction to the large gut gives early abdominal distension. Conversely, obstruction to the smaller intestine rarely shows more than perhaps a suggestive fullness in those early stages when it is imperative to make a correct diagnosis if the life of the patient is to be saved. Ladder patterns are very characteristic (*Fig.* 511) but are not commonly seen, and, for that matter, should not be seen, for their presence indicates a

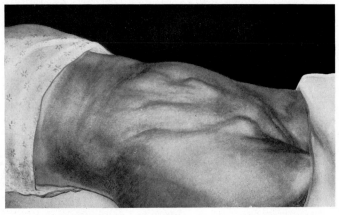

Fig. 511.—Visible peristalsis, showing the characteristic ladder pattern, Case of strangulated right femoral hernia which can be seen also.

late diagnosis. Visible peristalsis more often requires patient watchfulness. Sit down beside the bed and watch the abdomen. Sometimes gentle flicking of the abdominal wall will initiate visible peristalsis. A drop of ether allowed to fall upon the skin may initiate a peristaltic wave when other methods have failed (*Fig.* 512).

Wherever the obstruction in the large intestine may be—it matters not whether it is in the ascending, transverse, descending, or pelvic colon, or rectum—the brunt of the obstruction will be seen at the cæcum. Occasionally the cæcum can be seen momentarily rising up with each wave of peristalsis, like a small balloon. Very aptly this phenomenon has been likened to a gun backfiring into its own breech. The lesson to be learnt is that, in every suspected case of colonic obstruction, particular attention should be paid to the right iliac fossa.

**Auscultation.**—All the time we have been watching, we should at the same time have been listening for borborygmi.

"Auscultation is a much neglected method of investigation, and one to which I attach much value," said Professor Burgess, when speaking of acute intestinal obstruction. "After a little experience one gets to recognize certain sounds associated with distended intestine, and the contrast between the turbulent gurgling sounds of mechanical obstruction and the death-like silence of paralytic ileus is very marked."

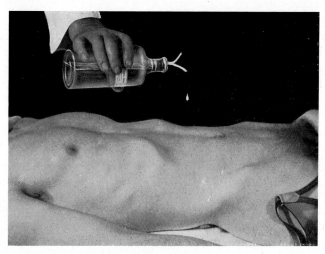

*Fig.* 512.—Inciting visible peristalsis by dropping ether upon the abdominal wall.

In cases of intestinal obstruction, Greig Smith recommended that the abdomen should be examined with a stethoscope *for no less than five minutes.* If, during the whole of that time, no gurgling is heard, it can safely be concluded that the jejunum, ileum, and large intestine have ceased to transmit peristaltic waves. (*See* also p. 325).

**Palpation.**—Even when peristalsis is not visible, it may be palpable ; if the hand is kept flat upon the abdomen the underlying coil may be felt to harden and soften alternately, much like a pregnant uterus (Burgess).

**Percussion** over the cæcum may yield a hyper-resonant note, which is additional and very useful evidence of large-gut obstruction.

ARTHUR HENRY BURGESS, 1864–1948, *Surgeon, Manchester Royal Infirmary.*
AMES GREIG SMITH, 1854–1897, *Surgeon, Royal Infirmary, Bristol.*

*Shifting dullness* may be tried ; but it should here be noted that quite often a shifting note can be demonstrated in the flanks, yet subsequently when the abdomen is opened, very little, if any, free fluid is present. I feel certain that dilated coils of small intestine reacting to the law of gravity can bring about a positive result in the test for shifting dullness.

**Rectal Examination.**—This may reveal the cause of the obstruction, e.g., a carcinomatous stricture. If the rectum is completely empty it is at least suggestive, and useful contributory evidence of obstruction. Occasionally one may be able to make out a distended coil of small intestine in the rectovesical pouch.

**Other Methods of Examination.—**

In doubtful cases an *enema* should be given, but it should be remembered that it is the second enema which yields the more useful information. By absolute constipation is meant that after the *second* enema no fæces and, above all, no flatus is passed.

Suppose the case is one of an old lady. The two enemata have been given, and the second has yielded just a small result. We are disinclined to operate if it can possibly be avoided, and it is hardly fair to exhaust the patient by giving a third enema just yet. Then take a *tape measure* and place it round the abdomen at the level of the umbilicus (*Fig.* 513). Note the measurement. Leave the tape measure in place behind the patient, and measure again in a few hours. This accurate measurement of the patient's girth is more reliable than an impression as to whether she is more distended than at a previous examination. Useful as this method is, it should, nevertheless, seldom be resorted to, for delay in intestinal obstruction is fraught with dangers. Doubtful cases should, as a rule, be submitted to laparotomy, for the risk of a laparotomy is a hundred times less than that of leaving a case of intestinal obstruction for even a few hours.

Perhaps the most elusive form of intestinal obstruction arises from obturation of the small intestine by a gall-stone. Usually the subjects are elderly, and the obstruction in the early stages is of an intermittent character. The possibility of this supremely remediable condition should be before us in every doubtful case of obstruction occurring in the evening of life.

Before leaving the subject of intestinal obstruction it is necessary to warn the reader to keep a sharp look-out for *uræmia*, which on occasions simulates intestinal obstruction closely. The examination of the urine is often helpful, but not necessarily so, for in both conditions the urine tends to be scanty.

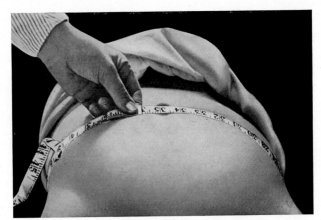

*Fig.* 513.—Suspected intestinal obstruction. Measurement of the girth of the abdomen at frequent intervals.

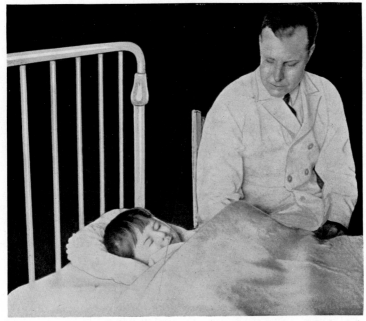

*Fig.* 514.—Examination of the abdomen of an infant for an intussusception. Palpation under the bedclothes between the spasms. The clinician must be seated.

## EXAMINATION OF AN INFANT FOR AN INTUSSUSCEPTION

Almost invariably the nurse will start to pull down the bed-clothes in order to expose the child's abdomen. Tell her not to do so. If the child is asleep, so much the better, but we are rarely so favoured. Take a chair and sit beside the bed—wait, and warm the right hand. Slip the warm hand under the bedclothes, place it upon the abdomen, and go on waiting until the child stops crying (*Fig.* 514). One cannot

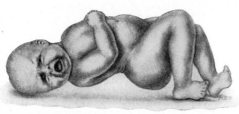

expect to feel anything when the child is screaming ; its abdominal muscles are contracted rigidly (*Fig.* 515). When the crying has ceased—palpate. Pay particular attention to the right hypochondrium. Sometimes the swelling will

*Fig.* 515.—Attitude of the infant during a spasm of colic that characterizes intussusception. (*After Farr.*)

be felt to harden as a wave of peristalsis commences, and the diagnosis is certain. When the bowel is flaccid, and the lump is small, it cannot be felt. Mere infolding of the gut does not render it palpable unless effusion has stiffened it (Fitzwilliams). In the splenic region the lump may pass under the costal margin, thus eluding the examiner (*Fig.* 516). It is pulled into this inaccessible position by the phrenico-colic ligament.

All the time we have been palpating the abdomen our eyes should be observing intently the patient's face. When crying has ceased, the colour of its cheeks are

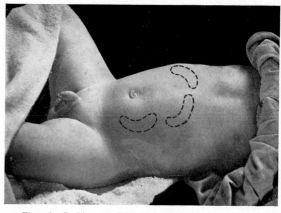

*Fig.* 516.—Positions at which the lump of an intussusception may be felt. In the left hypochondrium it may sometimes be difficult to feel, for it becomes sheltered by the costal margin.

noted—does the child become perceptibly paler : paler than it should be ? In this connexion, it is worth bearing in mind that a child suffering from intussusception never smiles, and in fully established cases there is often a sunken condition of the eyes suggestive of hydrocephalus (Anderson).   One most important piece of information to be gleaned from the face is, is the baby getting spasms of colic ?   If the abdominal muscles harden simultaneously with a fleeting expression of pain that is a prelude to an attack of crying, there can be no doubt about one important piece of information.   The little patient *is* experiencing colic.

The ' signe de Dance '—a feeling of emptiness in the right iliac fossa—is not of much help.   In saying this, I am in agreement with the majority of clinicians with whom I have worked.

Examination under anæsthesia is advisable in doubtful cases. With the additional muscular relaxation obtained by the anæsthesia the lump may be felt.

**Rectal Examination.**—Left lateral position.   If the lump is low enough in the colon, it will be felt.   The apex of an intussusception feels exactly like a cervix uteri.   Be careful to look at the examining finger afterwards—a ' red-currant jelly ' exudate is pathognomonic. Ask to see the baby's soiled napkin and scrutinize the discharge. When, as is probable, the stool is composed mainly of blood and mucus, look, in a good light, for evidences of bile.   If bile is absent, Barnard considered it proof of an intussusception.

*Intussusception Protruding from the Anus.*—The differential diagnosis between prolapse of the rectum and intussusception may cause much confusion, for in both conditions there is a large rosette of inflamed mucosa presenting externally.   The differential diagnosis should be simple if we really think about it.   In rectal prolapse the projecting mucosa will be felt continuous with the perianal skin, whereas in intussusception the finger passes *ad infinitum* into the depths of the sulcus (*Fig.* 517).

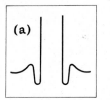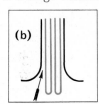

Fig. 517.—The differential diagnosis between rectal prolapse (*a*) and intussusception protruding from the anus (*b*).   In rectal prolapse the projecting mucosa will be felt continuous with the perianal skin, whereas in intussusception the finger passes *ad infinitum* into the depths of the sulcus.

**Intussusception and Purpura.**—In older children and adults purpura with intestinal symptoms may simulate intussusception ; indeed, an intussusception may follow a submucosal hæmorrhage occurring in this condition.   At first sight, especially in an artificial light, the multiple small hæmorrhages in the skin that characterize purpura are mistaken for flea-bites.   If the whole body is examined, larger hæmorrhages or bruises will be found, especially in the buttocks and the lobules of the ears. In doubtful cases the tourniquet test should be applied.

*The Tourniquet Test.*—If a rubber catheter is tied fairly tightly around the arm of a patient suffering from purpura, petechial hæmorrhages occur distal to the constricted area.   The tourniquet should be left in position for three minutes, and the arm examined a minute after its removal.

ROBERT ANDERSON, *Contemporary General Practitioner, Birmingham.*

JEAN BAPTISTE HIPPOLYTE DANCE, 1797–1832, *Physician, Hôpital Cochin, Paris.*

HAROLD LESLIE BARNARD, 1868–1908, *Surgeon, London Hospital.*

**Intestinal Obstruction in the New-born.**—When a new-born baby continues to vomit, there are only three explanations—intracranial hæmorrhage, severe infection (e.g., omphalitis) and intestinal obstruction. The first and second conditions show such special characteristics that their identification is assured (Sir John Fraser). What a pity it is that the last condition frequently remains undiagnosed for many days, for the various congenital bands, septa, and anomalies of rotation of the colon that cause it are so often supremely remediable.

## INTERNAL HÆMORRHAGE

**Signs.**—The classical signs of internal hæmorrhage are : (1) *Increasing* pallor ; (2) *Increasing* pulse-rate ; (3) Restlessness ; (4) Air hunger. Towards the closing stages, flashes of light before the eyes and attacks of blindness may be experienced, but the patient is usually conscious until the end. All of these signs are unreliable. The classical picture presents so many anomalies that one suspects that it was drawn from observations on the dying.

*Increasing Pallor and Increasing Pulse-rate.*—Pay particular attention to the increase. One can rarely diagnose early internal hæmorrhage on general signs by seeing the case once, but if it has been seen at intervals of half an hour, it may be possible to state definitely that the patient is paler than at a previous examination. The half-hourly pulse-reading (see p. 16) may be of signal service. On other occasions the patient's vasomotor system compensates for the gradual decrease in the total volume of blood until a point is reached when it suddenly gives out, as shown by a sudden *great* increase in the pulse-rate, with correspondingly grave outlook.

*Restlessness and air hunger* are seldom present, even in a severe internal hæmorrhage.

Sometimes help in a difficult diagnosis can be derived from examining the conjunctivæ and the finger-nails for blanching. When still in doubt an immediate hæmoglobin estimation may be helpful.

## ECTOPIC GESTATION

The commonest form of internal hæmorrhage arises in connexion with ectopic pregnancy. Probably because the condition is common and has thus been fully observed and worked out, the diagnosis is usually by no means difficult.

Ectopic gestation terminates in two ways : in each case it is abrupt, and consequently the symptoms come on suddenly. The ovum may be aborted through the abdominal ostium of the Fallopian tube, or the tube may rupture. In the latter, which is the rarer, the bleeding into the peritoneal cavity is of a violent character, and produces signs of internal hæmorrhage so severe and sudden that they approach the classical picture. In tubal abortion there is a series of smaller bleedings, each accompanied by a recrudescence of pain, and often a feeling of faintness, which tend to pass off as the vaso-motor system adjusts the blood-pressure. Physical signs will vary

greatly according to the stage at which the patient is examined. We will as-sume that the patient has had two or three attacks of pain, that the lower abdominal viscera are bathed in blood, but the general signs such as pallor and rapid pulse are not in evidence.

*The pain*, often sharp and stabbing (the so-called ' lavatory sign '), frequently radiates to the rectum.

*The temperature* may be normal, but quite often it is raised a little. In 6 per cent of cases it is subnormal.

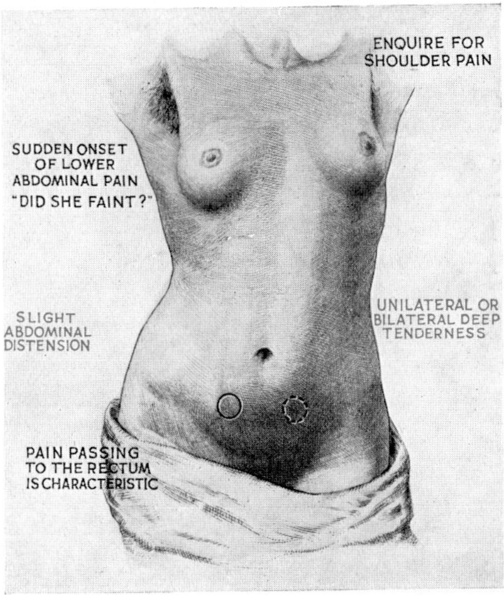

*Observe the abdomen.*

Fig. 518.—Only when a clinician becomes ectopic-minded are cases of tubal abortion and tubal rupture likely to be diagnosed early. Of cardinal significance, the history of a missed period is too often lacking to be a sheet anchor.

Slight distension is often in evidence. It is due to meteorism, which comes on early when there is blood in the peritoneal cavity. The abdomen moves well with respiration. On palpation there is usually absence of rigidity, but deep tenderness in one or both hypogastric areas is invariably present (*Fig.* 518). Cullen noted a blue dis-coloration of the umbilicus ; this is a most exceptional phenomenon, but it should be looked for in passing.

*Shoulder-pain* does not usually come on until the hæmorrhage is considerable and it occurs in about 30 per cent of cases. It is a common mistake to believe that the pain is referred only to the left

GABRIELE FALLOPIO, 1523–1562, *Professor of Anatomy, Surgery, and Botany, University of Padua, Italy.*
THOMAS STEPHEN CULLEN, *Contemporary Professor Emeritus of Gynæcology, Johns Hopkins University, Baltimore, U.S.A.*

shoulder. Stanley Way found that of 24 patients showing this sign the pain was referred to the right shoulder in 13, to the left shoulder in 4, and to both shoulders in 7. The side of the pain bore no relation to the side of the gestation. On two occasions I observed that the patient complained of shoulder pain after the foot of the bed had been raised on blocks. This fully substantiates the theory that the phenomenon is due to irritation of branches of the phrenic nerve on the under-surface of the diaphragm by blood.

*Shifting dullness* should be sought (*see Fig.* 507). If sufficient fluid blood is in the peritoneal cavity the sign will be positive.

*Vaginal examination.* In over half the cases there is loss of blood per vaginam; this is sometimes darker and thicker than the normal menstrual flow ('prune juice blood'). In 50 per cent of cases the cervix feels softer than usual. All the fornices are tender, and this is of considerable importance, as in inflammatory conditions tenderness is present only in the posterior and lateral fornices (Connell).

*Rectal examination.* Usually a tender swelling is present in the pouch of Douglas.

The patient should be questioned about the dates of her monthly periods. The history of a missed period is of the greatest possible significance, but it is by no means always obtainable.

If 'ruptured ectopic', as it is called, is doubtful, re-examine the patient in half an hour. *Remain ectopic-minded* (Johnson).

## ACUTE RETENTION OF URINE

**Distension of the Bladder.**—The distended bladder can be seen in the subject illustrated in *Fig.* 519 as a rounded swelling arising out of the pelvis. The full bladder, when it cannot be seen, may often be felt. One of the few instances when percussion applied to the abdomen is reliable is in determining the extent

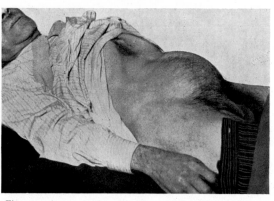

Fig. 519.—Acute retention. Bladder extending to the umbilicus.

STANLEY WAY, *Contemporary Associate Surgeon, Dept. of Gynæcology, Royal Victoria Infirmary Newcastle-on-Tyne.*

JAMES STEWART MARSHALL CONNELL, *Contemporary Gynæcologist, Midland Hospital, Birmingham.*

JAMES DOUGLAS, 1675-1742, *Physician to Queen Caroline.*

WILLIAM OSCAR JOHNSON, *Contemporary Associate Professor of Gynæcology, Louisville University, U.S.A.*

of distension of the bladder.  This percussion should be carried out from above downwards—that is, from the resonant area to the dull (*Fig.* 520).

**Cause of the Retention.**—Having determined that the bladder is distended, seek the cause of the obstruction.  The meatus should be examined for atresia or a urethral discharge ;  the perineum observed for signs of peri-urethral abscess.  Palpation along the course of the urethra, particularly in the neighbourhood of the penoscrotal junction, may reveal the induration of a stricture ;  occasionally an impacted urethral calculus can be felt.  The prostate should next be palpated by rectal examination (p. 259).

If the cause of the obstruction is not evident, the integrity of the central nervous system is investigated by testing the knee-jerks and the reaction of the pupils.

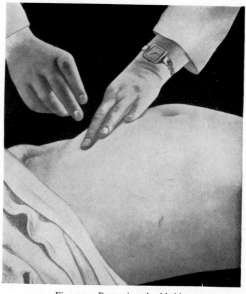

*Fig.* 520.—Percussing the bladder.

The final elucidation of the cause of obstruction sometimes necessitates refined methods of diagnosis, such as urethroscopy, with which we are not concerned here.

For practical clinical purposes, allow me to recall to the reader's memory the ' Seven Ages of Man ' from *As You Like it.*

*Jaques.*           All the world's a stage,
And all the men and women merely players :
They have their exits and their entrances ;
And one man in his time plays many parts,
His acts being seven ages.  At first the infant,
Mewling and puking in the nurse's arms.
And then the whining schoolboy, with his satchel
And shining morning face, creeping like snail
Unwillingly to school.  And then the lover,
Sighing like furnace, with a woeful ballad
Made to his mistress' eyebrow.  Then a soldier,
Full of strange oaths, and bearded like the pard,
Jealous in honour, sudden and quick in quarrel,

Seeking the bubble reputation
Even in the cannon's mouth. And then the justice,
In fair round belly with good capon lin'd,
With eyes severe, and beard of formal cut,
Full of wise saws and modern instances
And so he plays his part. The sixth age shifts
Into the lean and slipper'd pantaloon,
With spectacles on nose, and pouch on side ;
His youthful hose, well sav'd, a world too wide
For his shrunk shank ; and his big manly voice,
Turning again towards childish treble, pipes
And whistles in his sound. Last scene of all,
That ends this strange eventful history,
Is second childishness, and mere oblivion—
Sans teeth, sans eyes, sans taste, sans everything.

Apply these seven ages to the cause of acute retention :—

1. " The infant, mewling and puking in the nurse's arms." The cause of his retention is undoubtedly either extreme phimosis or atresia of the meatus.

2. " The whining schoolboy with his satchel " probably has a stone in his bladder.

3. " The lover sighing like furnace " is likely to be a case of retention following acute urethritis.

4. " The soldier, full of strange oaths," has almost certainly a urethral stricture.

5. " The justice, in fair round belly with good capon lin'd," is highly probably a case of prostatic enlargement.

6. When " the sixth age shifts into the lean and slipper'd pantaloon," a common cause of acute retention is cystitis complicated by ropy mucus.

7. And the last age " that ends this strange eventful history " is atony of his bladder.

This dismisses the common causes of acute retention in the male.

In the female, acute retention is comparatively uncommon, the three most usual causes being a retroverted gravid uterus, disseminated sclerosis, and hysteria. Therefore, when confronted with a female with acute retention of urine, palpate the uterus bimanually, and examine the central nervous system thoroughly.

## CHAPTER XXIV

## ABDOMINAL AND PELVIC INJURIES

WE are considering here ' closed ' injuries, as opposed to wounds. When a patient has received an injury to his trunk, as often as not there is little to guide us in the matter of external bruising. The problem before us is to decide, and decide as quickly as possible, whether or not he has sustained an intra-abdominal lesion. This is often a difficult matter, particularly when the patient is suffering from severe shock. In such circumstances the correct method of procedure is to treat the shock, and to examine and re-examine the patient at frequent intervals while this treatment is in progress.

### RUPTURED BLADDER

The prelude to the examination of an injury of the trunk should be an inquiry whether the patient has passed urine since the accident. For obvious reasons the importance of the rule reaches its zenith in injuries to the pelvis.

*Surgeons agree in saying that, except in utter smashes and perforation by fragments of bone, no rupture is possible unless the bladder is full* (Houel). Rupture of the bladder may be intraperitoneal, extra-peritoneal, or both.

**Intraperitoneal Rupture.**—There may be no physical signs until general peritonitis supervenes. So it comes about that no examination of a patient who has had an injury to the trunk is complete until one has observed that urine has been voided, or until a sterile catheter has been passed with withdrawal of a quantity of normal urine consistent with the history. If, after the passage of a catheter, doubt as to the integrity of the bladder exists, the introduction of a measured quantity of sterile saline solution into the bladder, with the patient in Fowler's position (to prevent dissemination to the upper abdomen if a tear exists), should be undertaken, whenever possible in the operating theatre.

**Extraperitoneal Rupture.**—The signs are identical with those of intrapelvic rupture of the urethra (*see* p. 312).

20

CHARLES NICOLAS HOUEL, 1815–1881, *Surgeon, Paris.*
GEORGE RYERSON FOWLER, 1848–1906, *Professor of Surgery, New York Polyclinic.*

## TRAUMATIC RUPTURE OF THE NORMAL SPLEEN

Cases of rupture of the spleen are divided conveniently into three groups : (1) The patient rapidly succumbs, never rallying from the initial shock ; (2) Initial shock—recovery from shock—signs of ruptured spleen ; (3) The signs of an intra-abdominal disaster are delayed.

**1. Rapid Succumbing of Patient.**—A comparatively rare result. Complete avulsion of the spleen from its pedicle is the type of accident that is most likely to give rise to the symptoms characterizing this group.

**2. Shock—Signs of Rupture.**—This is by far the largest group —more than three-quarters of all cases belong to it. After the initial shock has passed off, there are signs that point to an abdominal disaster.   It is not always possible to state precisely which organ is damaged, but in the majority of instances the physical signs point clearly to the spleen as the site of injury.

GENERAL SIGNS are those of internal hæmorrhage. The half-hourly pulse reading may be of value.   Attention has been directed already to the unreliability of the general signs of internal hæmorrhage (p. 300) ; the local signs of a ruptured spleen therefore become increasingly important.

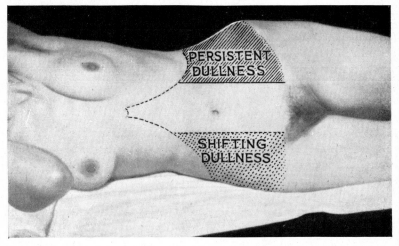

*Fig.* 521.—Ballance's sign (ruptured spleen).   Dullness in both flanks, *but the right alone shifts* when the posture is changed.

LOCAL SIGNS.—

*Abdominal rigidity* is variable, but it is present in more than half he total cases. Often most pronounced over the left upper abdomen.

*Local tenderness* is found very :onstantly in the same region.

*Shifting dullness in the flanks* s present fairly regularly. It was lemonstrable in six out of eight :onsecutive cases that I examined. *Ballance's sign* (*Fig.* 521) is said :o be pathognomonic of splenic :upture: there is a dull note in ɔoth flanks, but on the right side t can be made to shift, whereas ɔn the left it is constant. The nterpretation of the sign is that :here is blood in the peritoneal :avity, but the blood in the neighɔourhood of the lacerated spleen ɿas coagulated. There are many ·eferences to this sign in the literature, but the consensus of opinion ɿppears to be that it is present so rarely it is almost valueless.

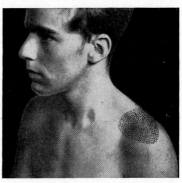

*Fig.* 522.—Kehr's sign. Often pain is referred via the phrenic nerve to the left shoulder when blood is in contact with the under-surface of the diaphragm. The sign is of especial significance after abdominal accidents, and should be inquired for and the test for hyperæsthesia applied.

*Abdominal distension* begins to appear about three or four hours after the accident, and is due, probably, to paralytic ileus.

*Referred pain at the left shoulder* (*Fig.* 522). There may be hyperæsthesia in this area (Kehr's sign). This is a most valuable sign and it should always be looked for in cases of abdominal injury.

*Fig.* 523.—The splenic point. Saegesser's sign.

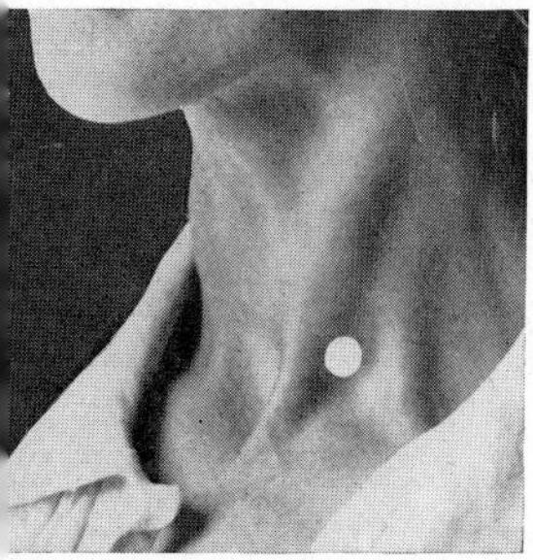

*Saegesser's Sign.* Deep finger-point pressure is made between the sternomastoid and the scalenus medius on the left side. This Saegesser calls *the splenic point* (*Fig.* 23) and in cases of ruptured spleen the pressure causes violent ɔain, even in cases of intracapsular hæmorrhage.

**3. The Delayed Type of Case.**—To quote an example that ypifies this group: A navvy, age 40, was hit in the upper bdomen by a pole. He fainted, but soon recovered sufficiently to valk to hospital, where he was examined and told to report the next

IR CHARLES BALLANCE, 1856–1936, *Surgeon, St. Thomas's Hospital, London.*
ANS KEHR, 1862–1916, *Professor of Surgery, Halberstadt, Saxony.*
IAX SAEGESSER, *Contemporary Surgeon, Berne, Switzerland.*

day. On the morrow he felt better, and stayed at home. Five days later he was brought in with well-marked signs of internal hæmorrhage, having collapsed at home a few hours before admission. Recovery followed splenectomy.

Delay of serious bleeding may be explained in three ways: (1) The great omentum, performing its well-known constabulary duties, shuts off that portion of the general peritoneal cavity in the immediate vicinity of the spleen; (2) A bloody coagulum temporarily seals the rent; (3) A subcapsular hæmatoma forms, and later bursts. It is probable that each of these three factors, at one time or another, temporarily arrests serious hæmorrhage.

**Ruptured Liver and a Tear of the Mesentery** also give rise to internal hæmorrhage, but the exact source of the hæmorrhage is uncertain until the abdomen has been opened.

**Injury to the Pancreas** is very difficult to diagnose. A pseudo-pancreatic cyst (a large collection of fluid in the lesser sac) may be the first intimation that the pancreas has been injured. (*See* p. 224.)

## RUPTURED INTESTINE

In traumatic ruptured intestine, before the onset of general peritonitis, the *rigidity* is like that of an early perforated gastric ulcer.

**Pointing Test.**—There is one sign of great value in ruptured intestine, and that is the pointing test. Ask the patient to point with one finger to where the pain is most acute. In two cases under my observation the patient has located accurately the site of the perforation. In the first case the patient pointed to the left iliac fossa. At operation a perforation of the ileum was found under the place the patient had pointed out. In the second case the patient pointed to the left hypochondrium and when the abdomen was opened a rupture of the jejunum near the duodenojejunal flexure was demonstrated. The pointing test, used in conjunction with Monks's method of intestinal localization (*Fig.* 524), is of signal value.

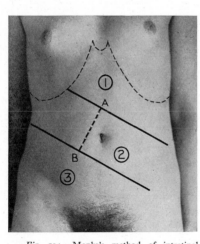

*Fig.* 524.—Monks's method of intestinal localization. A, B, Line of mesenteric root. Parallel lines are drawn at right angles to the extremities of this line, dividing the abdomen into three parts. Upper, middle, and lower compartments, indicated (1, 2, 3), contain, in most cases, the upper, middle, and lower thirds of the small intestine respectively.

GEORGE HOWARD MONKS, 1853–1933, *Surgeon-in-Chief, City Hospital, Boston, U.S.A.*

**Shifting Dullness** should be tried, but usually in an early case it s absent until general peritonitis is unmistakably present.

**The Sign of Transmitted Sound.**—The heart and respiratory sounds can be heard with a stethoscope all over the abdomen as clearly as they can be heard over the chest. The transmission of sound is due to the presence of peritoneal exudate (Claybrook).

\*          \*          \*          \*          \*

Before leaving the subject of the diagnosis of intraperitoneal injuries, it is well to bear in mind that acute abdominal pain and rigidity can be due to irritation of the lower intercostal nerves by fractured ribs. Still another pitfall is the presence of an unsuspected lesion of the spinal cord. There may be the most excruciating pain from such a lesion (Schrire).

## INJURIES TO THE KIDNEYS

The absence of superficial bruising counts for nothing ; it is present in only a small proportion of cases. The same may be said of the classical ' swelling in the loin ' when the posterior aspect of the patient is inspected. Of greater general utility, as an early sign, is a flattening of the normal contour of the affected side when viewed from the front, provided the patient is spare (*Fig. 525*). A dullness of the percussion note lateral to the outer border of the rectus, as compared with the opposite side, is often a sign of value, whilst rigidity of the anterior abdominal wall on the affected side is present constantly in cases of ruptured kidney.

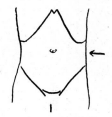

Fig. 525.—Injury to the kidney. Showing the flattening of the normal contour on the affected side.

If, after the initial examination, it is decided that no immediate operation is necessary, put the patient at rest between sandbags, and, in even moderately severe cases, arrange to have the pulse taken every half-hour.

**Hæmaturia.**—This cardinal sign of damaged kidney may not make its first appearance until some hours after the accident. In quite a large proportion of cases the urine voided soon after the accident is clear. The second sample, however, shows blood and urine intimately mixed.

EDWIN B. CLAYBROOK, 1871-1931, *Surgeon, Alleghany Hospital, Cumberland, U.S.A.*
THEODORE SCHRIRE, *Contemporary Surgeon, Groote Schuur Hospital, Capetown.*

In all cases the urine should be saved and placed in glasses bearing a label indicating the time of voiding (*Fig.* 526). It is then possible to compare one sample of urine with a later specimen, and thus to estimate whether the external bleeding is progressive or not. In comparing two samples—especially in an artificial light—it is helpful to dip a strip of white blotting-paper into each specimen after it has been stirred. For purposes of comparison, the concentration of blood in the urine is seen more readily in the absorbent paper. The presence of clots in one sample would of, course, vitiate the result.

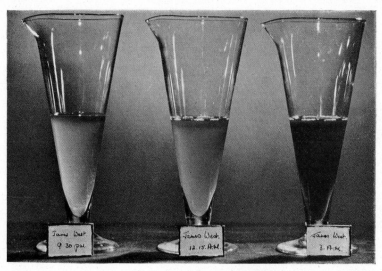

*Fig.* 526.—Injury to a kidney. The urine is saved, and placed in glasses labelled with the time of passing. In this way one sample of urine may be compared with a later specimen, and an estimation can be formed as to whether the bleeding is progressive or not.

Exceptionally, the hæmaturia is not noticed for some days ; this, however, occurs after slight injuries, and it is highly probable that the blood escapes notice in the earlier stages.

**Clot Colic.**—Two different clinical conditions are included under this heading :—

1. *Ureteric colic* is not very common, and when seen usually occurs within forty-eight hours of the accident. The passage of clots down the ureter gives rise to pain radiating from the loin to the groin.

2. *Bladder colic* is a much more frequent complication. It occurs generally between the third and fifth days. The pain is considerable, and referred to the glans penis.

**Severe Delayed Hæmaturia.**—A sudden profuse hæmaturia may occur (usually between the third and the fifth days) in a patient who appeared to be progressing favourably up to that time. The determining factor is probably some movement on the part of the patient which dislodges a clot in the renal pelvis. Under the title of *hæmaturie tardive*, Tuffier describes the passage of large quantities of dark, altered blood occurring several days after the accident.

**Residual Hæmaturia** may be the cause of some anxiety after nephrectomy has been performed for ruptured kidney. In spite of the fact that a damaged kidney has been removed, blood-stained urine continues to be passed. In such instances one might well wonder whether the remaining kidney is injured also. The explanation is that urine becomes stained by washing over clots that are present in the bladder. Doubtless this is the explanation of many cases of prolonged hæmaturia following renal injury.

**Meteorism.**—In many cases of severe renal injury abdominal distension is seen, and may give rise to difficulty in precise diagnosis. De Quervain suggested that abdominal distension, following a renal injury, was due to interference with the blood-supply of that portion of the colon overlying the kidney.

**Perinephric Hæmatoma** is frequently encountered in cases of renal injury. The hæmatoma sometimes causes a bulging in the loin, but this is somewhat exceptional ; more often it tracks retroperitoneally to the iliac fossa.

It is stated that the hæmatoma may follow the course of the spermatic vessels, and after a few days ecchymoses appear in the skin of the scrotum and around the external abdominal ring. Concerning this phenomenon, Sir Henry Morris pointed out that most of the cases in which it had been observed were complicated by a fractured pelvis. Not unnaturally, therefore, some scepticism exists as to the relationship of the perinephric hæmatoma and this remote bruising.

## FRACTURE OF THE PELVIS

When a fracture is present transverse compression (*Fig.* 527) and distraction (*Fig.* 528) of the pelvis are likely to produce acute pain. The genitocrural fold is explored by following the bony margin of the obturator foramen (*Fig.* 529).

A rectal examination may yield valuable information, particularly in cases of fracture of the coccyx. *Fig.* 530 shows the technique of examining for this fracture.

THEODORE TUFFIER, 1857–1929, *Professor of Surgery, University of Paris.*
FRITZ DE QUERVAIN, 1868–1940, *Professor of Surgery, University of Berne.*
SIR HENRY MORRIS, 1844–1926, *Surgeon, Middlesex Hospital, London.*

## IS THE PELVIS FRACTURED?

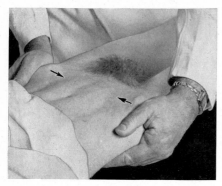

*Fig.* 527.—Compression.

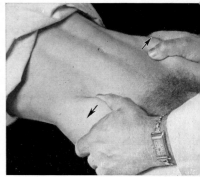

*Fig.* 528.—Distraction.

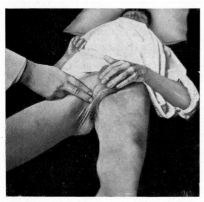

*Fig.* 529.—Palpating the ischio-pubic ramus.

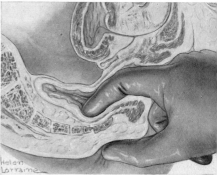

*Fig.* 530.—Examining for a fractured coccyx.

## INTRAPELVIC RUPTURE OF THE URETHRA

Usually signs of a fractured pelvis are evident. The patient has not passed urine since the accident, and the escape of blood via the meatus is a common occurrence. In intrapelvic rupture, as opposed to rupture of the bulbous urethra, there is no perineal swelling, but ecchymoses may be present. Abdominal examination may show a swelling in the hypogastrium. Extravasation into the pelvic fascia occurs early, and, curiously, it usually proceeds more on one side than on the other (*Fig.* 531); I have noticed this on a number of occasions. Unless the rounded dome of the bladder can be palpated distinctly from the rest of the swelling (the extravasation), it is impossible to arrive at a differential diagnosis between extraperitoneal rupture of the bladder and intrapelvic rupture of the urethra unless a rectal examination is made (*Fig. 532*). If the case is one of intrapelvic rupture of the urethra, the prostate is displaced posteriorly out of reach, and in its place there is a soft mass, no doubt blood and blood-clot (Hutchinson).

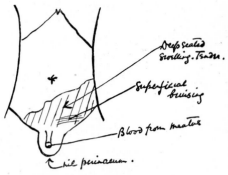

*Fig.* 531.—The physical signs recorded in a case of intrapelvic rupture of the urethra complicating a fractured pelvis. There was grating on compressing the iliac crests.

It cannot be emphasized too strongly that when, by a clinical examination, a ruptured urethra or bladder is suspected, further investigation, such as an attempt to pass a catheter, should, whenever possible, be

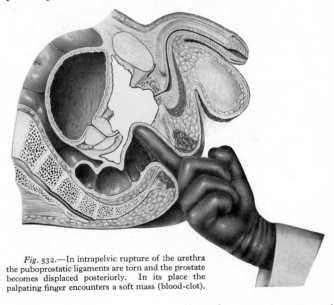

*Fig.* 532.—In intrapelvic rupture of the urethra the puboprostatic ligaments are torn and the prostate becomes displaced posteriorly. In its place the palpating finger encounters a soft mass (blood-clot).

carried out in the operating theatre, where sterility can be ensured and adequate operative treatment can follow immediately in necessary cases.

C. H. HUTCHINSON, *Contemporary Medical Officer, Transvaal Mines, South Africa.*

In cases of intrapelvic rupture of the urethra, the tip of the catheter can be felt per rectum protruding from the urethral tear as a longitudinal cord lying beneath the anal sphincter (Graham).

## RUPTURE OF THE BULBOUS URETHRA

*Fig.* 533 shows a patient who had sustained a complete rupture of the bulbous urethra three hours before the photograph was taken. There is a swelling in the perineum that is obviously a hæmatoma.

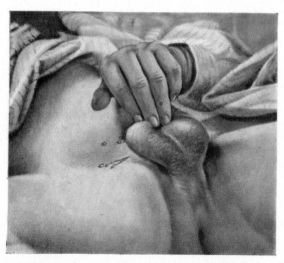

Fig. 533.—Rupture of the bulbous urethra after a fall astride on to a beam. The hæmatoma in the perineum is plainly visible. Blood is trickling out of the meatus. At operation the urethra was found completely divided.

The external urinary meatus was examined, and showed a few drops of bright red blood escaping. The bladder was percussed, and it was found to be moderately distended, for, in order to prevent extravasation (*see* p. 320), the patient, before being sent to hospital, was rightly warned *not even to try* to pass urine.

Rupture of the bulbous urethra is almost always the result of a fall astride.

WALLACE HARRY GRAHAM, *President Truman's personal physician, and Lecturer on Surgery, George Washington University, U.S.A.*

*CHAPTER XXV*

# SOME RARER ACUTE ABDOMINAL CONDITIONS

*Once again early correct diagnosis, the handmaiden of successful treatment, holds aloft her lamp of understanding.*—HAMILTON BAILEY.

## ACUTE PANCREATITIS

THE following signs should be noted : (1) *Frequently the subjects of this catastrophe are obese* ; (2) *The pain is severe, and passes to the back* ; (3) *Cyanosis may be present, particularly about the face.* The absence of general rigidity on abdominal palpation is a sign of considerable importance. As with every dogmatic statement in medicine, there are exceptions, but in most of the cases of acute pancreatitis that I have examined, the comparative absence of general rigidity has been a notable feature. When acute pancreatitis is suspected the left costovertebral angle should be palpated. Tenderness here, due to inflammation of the tail of the pancreas, has been noted by several observers.

**The Mydriatic Test.**—In order to get reliable results, the technique laid down by Otto Loewi must be carried out. Examine the pupils ; into one conjunctival sac instil 4 drops of fresh 1–1000 adrenaline solution ; wait five minutes ; then instil another 4 drops, and wait half an hour. Adrenaline of course, has no effect upon the pupil of a healthy subject, but in acute pancreatitis one often gets

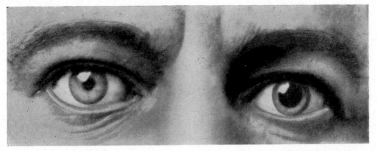

*Fig.* 534.—The mydriatic test : a positive reaction. (Photograph taken twenty hours after an operation for acute pancreatitis.)

OTTO LOEWI, *Contemporary Professor of Pharmacology (retired), Graz, Austria.*

a positive reaction, namely, dilatation of the pupil (*Fig.* 534). The dilatation is not infrequently slightly eccentric, and often conspicuously oval in form. A negative result implies nothing, but a positive result in an acute abdominal case is highly suggestive of acute pancreatitis. In a consecutive series of 13 cases of acute pancreatitis under my care this test has been tried in 10; of these, the test was positive in 8, negative in 1, and unreliable in 1 because the patient had had an iridectomy performed. The mydriatic test had been positive or doubtful in two or three cases that were not acute pancreatitis, notably on one occasion in acute pulmonary œdema.

### Local Discoloration of the Skin.—

*In the Loin* (*Fig.* 535).—The patches have the appearance of the skin in late extravasation of urine. It is seen only in cases of some two or three days' standing. Clearly the condition is due to the direct action of the pancreatic juice, which escapes via the retroperitoneal tissues and passes by the most direct route to the surface. (Grey Turner.)

*At the Umbilicus.*—A yellow discoloration for $1\frac{1}{2}$ in. around the umbilicus was seen in a case of acute pancreatitis by L. B. Johnston.

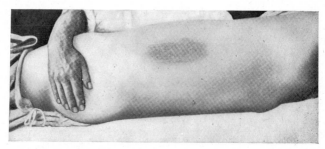

*Fig.* 535.—Photograph of a case of acute pancreatitis, showing the area of discoloration.
(*Grey Turner.*)

## ACUTE COLONIC DIVERTICULITIS

The patient is rarely under 35. Generally the pelvic colon is affected, and physical signs resemble, in some respects, those of left-sided appendicitis. When this condition is suspected, lay the hand over the cæcum and exert gentle, but increasing, pressure so as to force gas from the right-hand side into the left-hand side of the large intestine. Pressure on the right causing pain on the left may prove a significant feature. In 30 per cent of cases a lump is present in the left iliac fossa, but it may be difficult to feel because of overlying rigidity or excessive fat. Bimanual palpation with the right index finger in the rectum and the left hand over the left iliac

GEORGE GREY TURNER, *Contemporary Professor of Surgery (retired), Post-Graduate Medical School, London.*
LLOYD B. JOHNSTON, *Contemporary Surgeon, Good Samaritan Hospital, Cincinnati, Ohio, U.S.A.*

fossa (*see Fig.* 412, p. 230) sometimes proves helpful. If the peritonitis spreads, diagnosis becomes increasingly difficult.

## TWISTED OVARIAN CYST

A very sudden onset of abdominal pain, followed by attacks of lower abdominal pain of a colicky nature recurring at frequent intervals, together with repeated vomiting, is the usual history. If a lump is present (*Fig.* 536), the diagnosis is tolerably simple. Overlying rigidity tends to mask the lump, which, if small, is situated entirely within the pelvis.

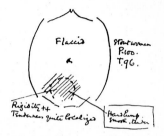

Fig. 536.—Signs recorded in a case of twisted ovarian cyst.

Before examining the patient bi-manually, either per vaginam or per rectum according to circumstances, always have the bladder emptied by a catheter.

## RUPTURED LUTEIN CYST

The patient is an unmarried, or recently married, woman. Particularly when right-sided, a ruptured lutein cyst is extremely difficult to differentiate from appendicitis. Unlike the latter, the pain *commences* in the iliac fossa. In exceptional cases intraperitoneal hæmorrhage is considerable, and the signs simulate those of a tubal abortion (p. 301).

## PNEUMOCOCCAL PERITONITIS

Pneumococcal peritonitis may occur primarily or as a complication of pneumonia. The signs closely resemble acute appendicitis with pelvic peritonitis, the only distinguishing features being :—

1. The type of individual. Usually a poorly nourished female child.

2. Rigidity is less marked than in appendicitis of corresponding severity—as judged by pulse, temperature, and general appearance of the patient.

3. Considerable meteorism is often an early feature.

4. Even in the primary variety, the alæ nasi may move as actively as in pneumonia.

## MESENTERIC EMBOLISM

The symptoms are those of intestinal obstruction. In three cases that I examined, a somewhat ill-defined soft lump could be felt which reacted to the law of gravity when the patient was placed on her side. This lump was shown by laparotomy to be congested œdematous coils of intestine. Blood is passed per rectum in a few instances. Mesenteric embolus should be suspected when a patient with intestinal obstruction is known to have heart disease.

## PYLEPHLEBITIS (PORTAL PYÆMIA)

In the early stages pylephlebitis is difficult to differentiate from subdiaphragmatic abscess (*see* p. 149). Both lesions arise as a complication of inflammatory conditions of organs, notably the appendix, that drain their venous blood into the portal system, and both give rise to a swinging temperature.

In pylephlebitis the patient soon develops a slightly jaundiced tinge. If the liver is examined it will be found to be enlarged and often tender. When there is no known focus of infection the rectum should be examined for inflamed hæmorrhoids.

## SUPPURATING DEEP ILIAC GLANDS

Suppurating deep iliac glands are a diagnostic Waterloo to many. Psoas spasm is often in evidence ; the thigh is flexed (*Fig.* 537). This, combined with pain and tenderness in the *right* iliac fossa, often leads to a diagnosis of appendicitis, whilst on either side purulent arthritis of the hip or osteomyelitis of the upper end of the femur may be suspected. The superficial inguinal glands may be enlarged, but this is not essential. Hip-joint disease can be eliminated by careful examination, the ' anvil test ' (p. 344) being particularly

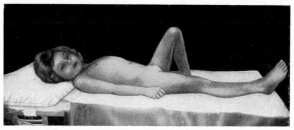

*Fig.* 537.—A case of suppurating deep iliac glands. Photograph taken in the operating theatre just prior to anæsthetization of the patient. The amount of flexion of the hip is not exaggerated.

useful in this instance. Deep pressure over the upper end of the femur does not cause pain. On abdominal examination a fullness may be seen above Poupart's ligament, or (more often) a tender lump will be felt in this situation, tending to be rather nearer the anterior superior iliac spine than to the pubic spine. On the right side, the differential diagnosis from appendix abscess can be extremely difficult. The lower limb should be scrutinized for a focus of infection.

## TORSION OF THE SPERMATIC CORD

If a boy or young man complains of sudden, intense pain in the inguinal region and vomits, and upon examination the testis on that side is found to be enlarged and tender, torsion of the spermatic cord should be the first thing to cross the clinician's mind. In early cases the spermatic cord will be found thickened, and on one occasion I could feel four twists distinctly.

It is true that it is the spermatic cord that is twisted, and correctly speaking one should refer to the condition as torsion of the spermatic cord. However to employ the less accurate but more generally accepted term ' torsion of the testis ' has so many advantages in giving a pen picture of the clinical phenomenon occasioned by the axial rotation that I have decided to employ it.

**Torsion occurring in an Incompletely Descended Testis** is almost impossible to distinguish by physical methods from a strangulated

inguinal hernia ; indeed, there is no reliable sign by which the diagnosis of torsion of a maldescended testis can be rendered even highly probable. All that is required of the clinician is to note the absence of the testis in the scrotum of the affected side, and arrange that the painful swelling in the inguinal canal be displayed to the light of day as soon as possible. In most early cases an indecisive pre-operative diagnosis of ? torsion of a maldescended testis, ? strangulated inguinal hernia, bespeaks clinical acumen.

**Torsion occurring in a Completely Descended Testis.**—One would imagine that this is a simple diagnostic problem, but as time goes on many revise their opinion. Torsion of a fully descended testis must be distinguished particularly

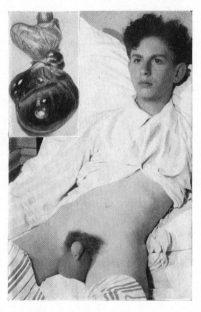

Fig. 538.—Torsion of the spermatic cord of twenty-four hours' duration in a boy aged 15. The inflamed acutely tender testis and scrotum simulate acute epididymo-orchitis exactly.

from acute epididymo-orchitis. The frequency with which epididymo-orchitis is mistaken for torsion of the testis is revealed by the fact that each and all of seven consecutive cases of torsion of a fully descended testis I was called upon to see had been diagnosed and treated as epididymo-orchitis for varying periods from twenty-four hours to ten days. Although the local signs may simulate exactly those of acute epididymo-orchitis (*Fig.* 538), and regularly the temperature registers 99°F., because so often the patient is a boy between the ages of 10 and 15 it is reasonable to expect the clinician, before pronouncing the diagnosis of epididymo-orchitis, to catechise himself thus : Here is a boy who has no signs of urethritis—no history of dysuria, and his urine looks perfectly normal.   There have been no cases of mumps at his school or in the district.   No swelling or tenderness of the prostate detected on rectal examination, and the seminal vesicles are impalpable. Why on earth should this boy be suffering from a *bacterial inflammation* of the testis ?

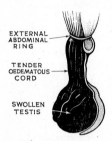

EXTERNAL
ABDOMINAL
RING

TENDER
OEDEMATOUS
CORD

SWOLLEN
TESTIS

Fig. 539.—Explanation of how a small strangulated hernia may cause testicular symptoms by pressure on the cord.

*Prehn's Sign.*—Elevation and support of the scrotum for an hour will relieve the pain in epididymo-orchitis, but will not relieve it, or will make it worse, in torsion.

Another difficulty, but a far less common one, is that when the sac is small, very tense, and situated in the upper part of the inguinal canal, the signs of torsion of a completely descended testis can be mimicked by a strangulated inguinal hernia which brings about compression of the veins of the spermatic cord, and swelling and tenderness of the testis result (*Fig.* 539).

**Torsion of an Appendage of the Testis.**—The appendage to undergo axial rotation is usually the pedunculated hydatid of Morgagni (*Fig.* 540).

Again, the signs are those which lead the unwary to diagnose acute epididymo-orchitis.   Again the temper-

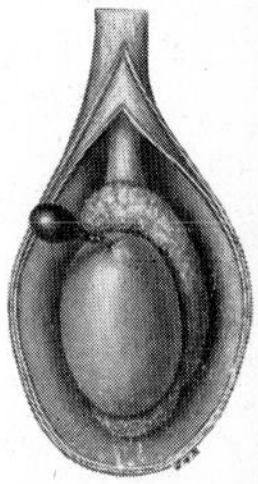

Fig. 540.—Torsion of the pedunculated hydatid of Morgagni.
(*After Foshee.*)

ature is slightly elevated (usually 98·8°F.) and, as might be expected, other signs and symptoms are milder.   My aphorism (and it has never let me down) is : If the patient is able to walk to seek advice, he has a torsion of the hydatid of Morgagni, whereas in the case of torsion of the spermatic cord, the symptoms are such that the clinician is summoned to the bedside.

## EXTRAVASATION OF URINE

**Deep Extravasation of Urine** usually takes place into planes of pelvic fascia (*Fig.* 541).   It occurs in intrapelvic rupture of the urethra and extraperitoneal rupture or perforation of the bladder.

DOUGLAS T. PREHN, *Contemporary Captain U. S. Navy, Chelsea Naval Hospital, Massachusetts, U.S.A*
GIOVANNI BATTISTA MORGAGNI, 1682–1771, *Professor of Anatomy, Padua.   He held the Chair for fifty-six years.*

The extravasated urine gives rise to a swelling that is difficult to distinguish from a full bladder, but, unlike the latter, the swelling is not always rounded (*see also* p. 312).

**Subcutaneous Extravasation of Urine** may follow a complete rupture of the bulbous urethra or acute retention complicating a periurethral abscess.

*The extravasated urine cannot pass* : (1) Behind the middle perineal point, because of the fusion of Colles's* fascia with the anterior layer of the triangular ligament (*Fig.* 542) ; (2) Into the thighs, for Scarpa's fascia blends with the fascia lata just distal to Poupart's ligament ; (3) Into the inguinal canal, because of the intercolumnar fibres and fascia of the external oblique.

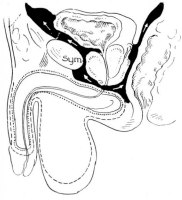

Fig. 541.—Deep extravasation of urine following intrapelvic rupture of the urethra.

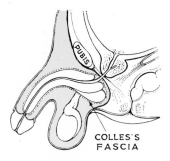

Fig. 542.—Superficial extravasation. The fusion of Colles's fascia with the anterior layer of the triangular ligament prevents extravasated urine from passing backwards beyond the middle perineal point.

*It therefore must pass* : (1) Into the scrotum ; (2) Into the subcutaneous tissues of the penis ; (3) Up the abdominal wall in the subcutaneous planes. (*Fig.* 543.)

In extravasation a black patch on the glans penis is a harbinger of death (Sir Benjamin Brodie).

Superficial extravasation may be simulated very closely by anasarca complicating a failing heart (*Fig.* 544). The differential diagnosis can be made readily by *examining the ankles*. In anasarca the legs will be found to be swollen, and pitting on pressure can be demonstrated (*see* p. 6).

---

* Colles's fascia is known in the U.S.A. as Buck's fascia.

21

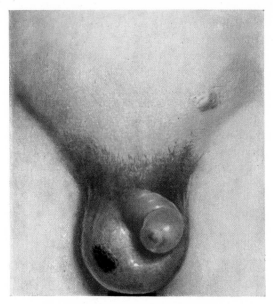

*Fig.* 543.—Subcutaneous extravasation of urine.

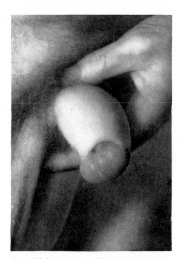

*Fig.* 544.—Obvious œdema of the prepuce with palpable scrotal œdema.  The patient was admitted as a case of extravasation of urine.  Examination of the perineum showed no peri-urethral abscess or induration of a stricture.  This aroused suspicion.  Examination of the ankles revealed pitting on pressure.  The cause of the œdema was a failing heart.

# SOME ACUTE POST-OPERATIVE ABDOMINAL CONDITIONS

## ACUTE DILATATION OF THE STOMACH

Acute dilatation of the stomach comes on very suddenly, sometimes after operations, particularly upper abdominal, pelvic, and prostatic operations accompanied by a fall of blood-pressure, but sometimes after no operation at all ; for instance, on two occasions I have seen the condition arise as a complication of fracture of the

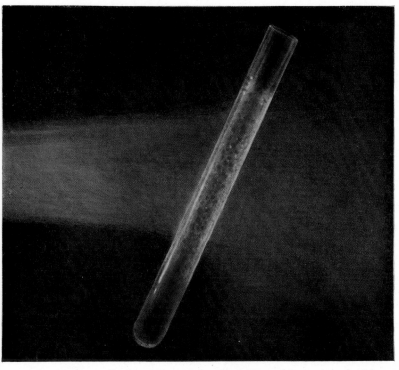

Fig. 545.—Acute dilatation of the stomach. If a specimen of the vomit is placed in a test-tube and held in a strong light, its characteristic colour will become evident and myriads of small particles may be discerned suspended in the fluid.

femur. Typically the patient vomits—usually a very large amount— and soon exhibits signs of shock. He continues to vomit enormous quantities ; one wonders where it has all come from. The character of the vomit should bring the condition to mind at once. The very large quantity of brownish-black fluid, which may be likened to the storm water of a peat-laden stream, is pathognomonic.

If some of the vomit, after having been stirred, is placed in a test-tube and held in a strong light (*Fig.* 545), one can see the characteristic colour and the myriads of small particles suspended in the fluid.

*Early Diagnosis.*—Acute dilatation of the stomach can be diagnosed before the patient vomits. The day should have passed when the condition remains unsuspected until an enormous quantity of the characteristic fluid is ejected.

Early symptoms and signs are far from being stereotyped. We are summoned to the bedside because there is something amiss. The pulse is rising. The patient need not look gravely ill. He is not in any pain, but he usually says that he feels uncomfortable. It is of paramount importance to realize that vomiting occurs relatively late. At this stage he does not necessarily experience even nausea, let alone vomiting, but an occasional hiccup is not uncommon. The output of urine is invariably scanty, although during the first few hours this fact cannot be gauged with accuracy. Careful observation of the upper abdomen may show slight fullness in the hypochondria ; the characteristic sign is the obliteration of that normal sulcus immediately beneath the costal margin (*Fig.* 546), but in obese subjects this is difficult to assess, if not entirely unreliable.

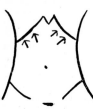

Fig. 546.—Obliteration of the normal concavity beneath the costal margin is seen in some cases of acute dilatation of the stomach.

Occasionally when the abdomen is examined a dilated stomach can be made out, but as the greater curvature may be so low as to be hidden in the pelvis (a post-mortem observation), usually a general fullness is all that can be seen. In any case this is not the time to palpate and percuss. If acute dilatation of the stomach is even suspected a small gastric aspiration tube should be passed, preferably through the nose, and the contents of the stomach aspirated.

## PARALYTIC ILEUS

A certain amount of distension and flatulence are only too frequent after abdominal operations. These symptoms are due to what may be termed intestinal paresis. Paralytic ileus can be looked upon as a much more serious and widespread inhibition of the peristaltic wave. On inspection the abdomen is obviously distended. It is tympanitic, and in the more severe forms one notices, as in the case of acute dilatation of the stomach, that the normal slight concavity below the costal margin is converted into a convexity, which indicates that the jejunum is distended also.

The differentiation of paralytic ileus from intestinal obstruction is often difficult. At times it is well-nigh impossible; indeed, both conditions may be present.

**Auscultation of the Abdomen** is of cardinal importance in the diagnosis of paralytic ileus. Take a chair, and sit beside the right side of the patient's abdomen. Exhort those in attendance to make every effort to be quiet. It is, I consider, essential to be seated, for the cup of the stethoscope must be kept still, perhaps for five full minutes; this is a more exacting undertaking than might be imagined. One often sees the stethoscope applied here and there to the surface of the abdomen for a matter of seconds; this is useless when an all-important diagnosis of paralytic ileus is at stake. Apply the stethoscope firmly to the skin just below and to the right of the umbilicus (*Fig.* 547), and keep it

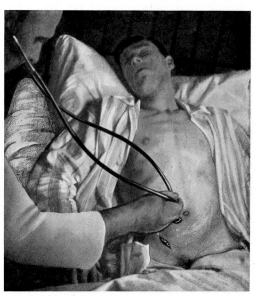

*Fig.* 547.—The cup of the stethoscope should be kept immobile at a central listening point for, if necessary, five minutes, before pronouncing that peristalsis has ceased.

absolutely still. If there is a gurgle in any part of the abdomen, assuredly it will be heard at this central 'listening post'. It must be clearly understood we are not concerned here with tumultuous hissing, rumbling sounds associated with intestinal colic; probably the patient has not had any pain recently. What we are so anxious to know is—is the intestine paralysed? By listening intently and long, it may be that the clinician will hear the faint and fleeting sweet music of a tinkling runnel—proof indeed that peristaltic action, though feeble, is not completely stayed.

Intestinal peristalsis is abolished by the presence in the peritoneal cavity of intestinal contents, pus, bile, hæmorrhagic exudate from strangulated intestine, and exudate from an acutely inflamed pancreas. It is not abolished by the presence of blood or of urine in the peritoneal cavity (Rob).

## POST-OPERATIVE PERITONITIS

The salient signs of peritonitis are often lacking.  For instance distension is not a notable feature ;  there is usually some tenderness, but it is difficult to assess how much of this is due to the laparotomy wound ;  even pain is sometimes absent.  Vomiting, if present, is of the small ' mouthful ' variety.

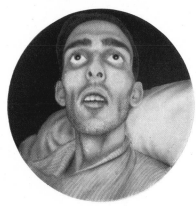

*Fig.* 548.—Hippocratic facies.   Streptococcal peritonitis.

A steadily increasing pulse-rate and perhaps an undue sharpness of the intellect with some excitability are signs that give an astute clinician a lead in this now fortunately uncommon, but very fatal, catastrophe.

The Hippocratic facies (*Fig.* 548), characterized by " a sharp nose, hollow eyes, collapsed temple, and the ears cold ", is seen comparatively early in the progress of the case.

CHARLES GEOFFREY ROB, *Contemporary Senior Assistant, Surgical Unit, St. Thomas's Hospital, London*
HIPPOCRATES, *regarded by common consent as the Father of Medicine, was born on the island of Cos about*
   460 B.C.

## CHAPTER XXVI

## THE SACRO-ILIAC JOINT

To those engaged in industrial medical practice, the differential diagnosis between sacro-iliac strain, torn lumbar muscle-fibres, fibrositis, and lumbago with sciatica, to which must be added ' malingerer's low-back pain ', constitute an everyday conundrum.

Before the possibility of a lesion of the sacro-iliac joint is entertained, it is usually wise to eliminate both the spine and the hip-joints as the seat of the trouble.

The patient should be stripped, at any rate to the gluteal clefts. While the routine examination must be modified to suit particular circumstances, a good method of procedure is as follows :

### a. EXAMINATION STANDING

Ask the patient to point to the place where he gets the pain (*Fig.* 549). All sufferers with persistent pain in the ' orthopædic triangle ' require an orthopædic investigation. Some require a genito-urinary examination in addition (*see* p. 331). Instruct the patient to bend forwards and endeavour to touch his toes ; in the type of case referred to in the introductory paragraph, this movement is usually performed reluctantly. If it is *pain* that prevents flexion of the back, again ask the patient to put his finger on the place that hurts him most.

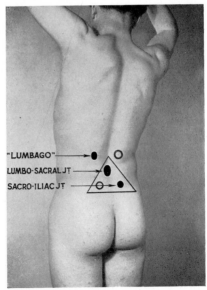

### b. EXAMINATION SITTING

When a low stool is not available, instruct the patient to sit sideways on a chair. The examiner should be seated.

*Fig.* 549.—The ' orthopædic triangle'. Note that ' lumbago ' is outside it.

1. Request the patient to bend forwards. In sacro-iliac lesions this movement is now comparatively free, because the pelvis is supported. In lumbosacral and muscular lesions the movement is just as limited as it was in (**a**).

2. Tenderness over the sacro-iliac joint and nowhere else strongly suggests a lesion of this joint. Usually the joint is located easily in females, for directly over it lies a dimple (*Fig.* 550). When the dimple is not present, it is best to follow the iliac crest medially until the

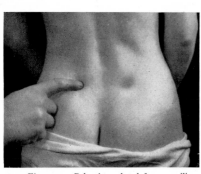

*Fig.* 550.—Palpating the left sacro-iliac joint. Note the dimple overlying the joint on the right.

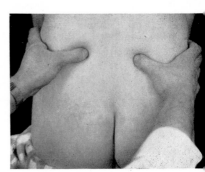

*Fig.* 551.—Deep comparative palpation of the sacro-iliac joints. Exercising considerable pressure, first one thumb and then the other passes over the joint. The left thumb is performing the movement at the time of the photograph.

joint is reached. The joint having been located accurately, it is examined by palpation. On deep palpation over the joint cleft (*Fig.* 551) sometimes a small bursa can be rolled under the thumb, and in pathological states of the joint this bursa is tender.

**Larrey's Sign** is occasionally useful in obscure cases, especially when the individual is thick-set. The patient sits in a wooden armchair. He raises himself in the chair by his arms, and then lets himself drop on to the seat. The jar causes pain in the affected joint.

### c. EXAMINATION ON A COUCH

### 1. On the Back.—

*The ' Straight-leg-raising ' Test.*—Carefully performed, this test often proves a mine of information. Ascertain that there is no compensatory lordosis by insinuating a hand beneath the lumbar spine (*see* p. 339). Keeping the knee quite straight, raise the leg from the couch (*Fig.* 552). When this manœuvre produces pain in the region of the sacro-iliac joint, it is significant.

A lesion of the lumbosacral joint is suggested when the pain is located higher up, and when it comes on only after the leg has reached

BARON DOMINIQUE LARREY, 1766–1842, *Surgeon-in-Chief to the Napoleonic Army.*

an angle of 90° or over. When pain is produced, but not so located, other pathological lesions are suggested (e.g., torn muscle-fibres).

Injury to the hamstring muscles will cause pain to be located near the gluteal fold, and usually during an early part of the test.

A sudden pull on the thigh flexed at about 45° and with the knee bent is a good test for sacro-iliac pain.

Sciatica can confuse the issue in any of the foregoing. By dorsiflexing the foot (*Fig.* 552, A B) the pain of sciatica is increased, whereas in other lesions this additional manœuvre is symptomless.

*The 'Pump-handle' Test.*— Commencing on the unsuspected side, grasp the limb just below the knee. In order to steady the trunk, with the free hand firmly grasp the

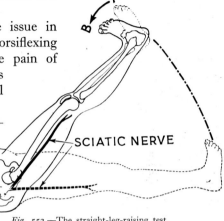

Fig. 552.—The straight-leg-raising test.

shoulder of the same side. Fully flex the hip and the knee on the hip, then push the thigh and the pelvis steadily towards the opposite shoulder (*Fig.* 553). Pain in the sacro-iliac joint is a positive sign.

Tenderness of the sacro-iliac joint, if affecting the anterior ligament, can be demonstrated by pressure from the corresponding iliac fossa. (Woodall.)

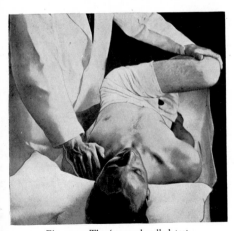

Fig. 553.—The 'pump-handle' test.

*The Compression and Distraction Tests.*—Excellent as are these tests in cases of suspected fracture of the pelvis (*see* p. 311), I have found them valueless in sacro-iliac joint conditions, except in cases of well-established tuberculosis of the joint.

*Gaenslen's test* is helpful for differentiating between sacro-iliac and lumbosacral lesions. While one hip and knee are held acutely flexed,

Lord Uvedale of North End, *formerly* Sir Ambrose Woodall, *Contemporary Senior Surgeon, Manor House Hospital, London.*
Frederick Gaenslen, *Contemporary Professor of Surgery, University of Wisconsin, U.S.A.*

which fixes the lumbar spine and the lumbosacral joint, the other hip is forcibly hyperextended as the limb hangs over the side of the couch

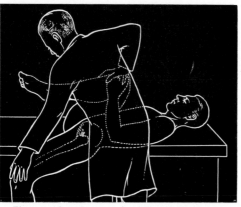

(*Fig.* 554). Pain is generally produced in sacro-iliac, but not in lumbosacral, lesions.

**2. On the Face.—**

*Yeoman's Test.—* Standing on the side to be tested, place the base of the palm firmly over the sacro-iliac joint in order to steady the pelvis. Grasping the leg near the ankle, extend the hip-joint (*Fig.* 555). In a normal person this

*Fig.* 554.—Gaenslen's test for differentiating between sacro-iliac and lumbosacral lesions.

action is painless, but as it stretches the anterior sacro-iliac ligament, pain is produced in lesions implicating the anterior part of the

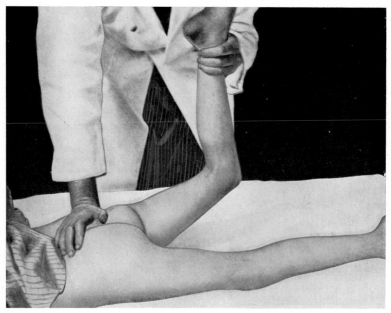

*Fig.* 555.—Yeoman's test.

WILLIAM YEOMAN, *Contemporary Physician, Royal Bath Hospital, Harrogate, England.*

sacro-iliac joint. (This test is precisely the same as that for extension of the hip-joint. (*See* p. 343.)

*          *          *          *          *

After other joints have been examined for crepitus, in many, if not in most, examples of low-back pain it is highly desirable to search for a focus of infection. The student and the practitioner are familiar with the teeth and the tonsils in this connexion. While not decrying these proven locations of possible toxic absorption, my own experience tends to coincide with that of Wesson, who found that the most expensive industrial lesion (Wesson's patients hailed from San Francisco's water-front) was ' strained back ', until the insurance companies realized that a large number of these patients did not require orthopædic, but urological, treatment. For this reason more attention should be directed to the prostate and seminal vesicles (*see* p. 259 et seq.) as a possible source of infection.

**Malingerer's Low-back Pain.**—In some communities this condition is a clinician's nightmare. A conscientious physical examination on the lines suggested above, together with a radiological examination, will do much to segregate the drones from the worker bees. When still perplexed, my only suggestion is to follow Magnuson's practice. He presses here and there over the whole of the lower back, and marks out areas of special tenderness. Between two examinations of this kind, Magnuson looks at the patient's throat, examines him per rectum, or performs any relevant examination of parts well away from the site of the alleged pain. By this expedient the patient's attention is diverted (from his back) for at least two or three minutes. The

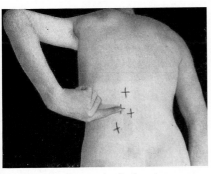

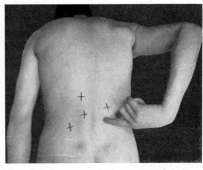

*Fig.* 556.—Constant localized tenderness ; probably a case of genuine pain.

*Fig.* 557.—Migratory tenderness ; probably malingering or possessed of a high degree of ' compensitis '.

MILEY B. WESSON, *Contemporary Urologist, San Francisco.*
PAUL B. MAGNUSON, *Contemporary Associate Professor of Surgery, North-western University, Chicago.*

examination of the back by pressure is then resumed. If the man experiences real local tenderness, assuredly its position will remain steadfast (*Fig.* 556). If he is malingering, he may not remember the exact place where he located the pain (*Fig.* 557).

## SCIATICA

The diagnosis of sciatica can be confirmed by the following signs :—

**Applying Tension to the Sciatic Nerve.**—The thigh is flexed fully on the abdomen. The knee is then extended slowly (*Fig.* 558). This causes stretching of the great sciatic nerve, and when the sign is positive great pain is experienced along the course of the nerve. (Lasègue.)

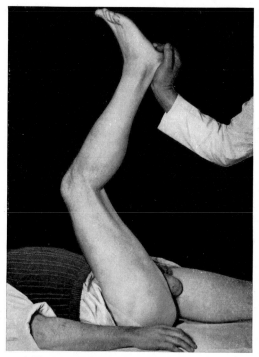

*Fig.* 558.—Applying tension to the sciatic nerve.

**Rolling the External Popliteal Nerve.**—The external popliteal nerve, as it winds round the neck of the fibula, is rolled under

CHARLES ERNEST LASÈGUE, 1816–1883, *Professor of Clinical Medicine, Paris.*

the thumb (*Fig.* 559). In sciatica the nerve is exceedingly tender.

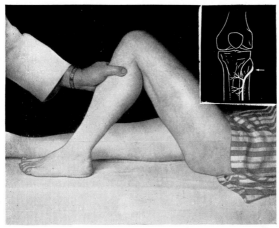

*Fig.* 559.—Rolling the external popliteal nerve.

## ENDEAVOURING TO ELUCIDATE THE CAUSE, AND DIFFERENTIAL DIAGNOSIS

Before making a diagnosis of idiopathic sciatica, always carry out an examination of the rectum in order to exclude the possibility of a *carcinoma of the rectum* pressing upon the sacral plexus. After this has been done, and before labelling sciatica idiopathic, examine the spine, sacro-iliac joint, and hip-joint for disease. Hare's method of making a differential diagnosis between sciatica and *arthritis of the hip-joint* is useful, and is shown in *Figs.* 560, 561. Even the foot

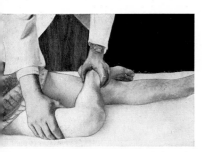

*Fig.* 560.—Differential diagnosis of sciatica and arthritis of the hip-joint. The affected limb can be [pla]ced in this position in both sciatica and arthritis [of] the hip-joint.

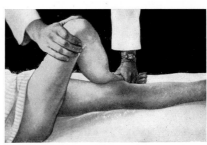

*Fig.* 561.—The limb can be placed in this position in sciatica, but not in arthritis of the hip-joint.

HOBART A. HARE, 1862–1931, *Professor of Therapeutics, Jefferson Medical College, Philadelphia, U.S.A.*

should be examined thoroughly, for extravagant *hallux valgus* associated with metatarsalgia has been known to be the starting-point of a great-sciatic neuritis.

It is also most advisable to eliminate contracture of the fascia lata and ilio-tibial band, for, when contracted, this fascial sheet can press upon the sciatic nerve and give rise to low-back pain combined with sciatica.

**Ober's Test.**—The patient lies on his side with the non-affected thigh in contact with the couch. The non-affected thigh is flexed sufficiently to obliterate any lumbar lordosis. The examiner grasps the affected leg at the ankle, flexes the knee-joint to a right angle with one hand, and steadies the pelvis with the other. The thigh is now abducted and at the same time extended so that the thigh is in a line with the trunk. If there is contraction of the ilio-tibial band, the limb will remain more or less passively abducted. The contracted band can be felt easily between the iliac crest and the anterior part of the great trochanter. When Ober's test is positive, division of the ilio-tibial band is indicated.

FRANK ROBERTS OBER, *Contemporary Professor of Orthopædic Surgery, Harvard Medical School, Boston, Mass.*

# CHAPTER XXVII

## THE HIP-JOINT

**Gait.**—If the patient is able to walk, watch his gait. Take note of a limp.

**Preparation of the Patient for the Examination.**—Except for a shirt, all clothing must be removed. In the case of a female, a nurse sees that the necessary clothing is removed, and the patient is provided with a pair of bathing triangles to wear during the examination.

**Mensuration** is the first step in the examination. It is necessary to compare the length and girth of the affected limb with its fellow. In the case of length, real shortening is what we want to know. Apparent shortening (measured from the umbilicus) causes much confusion. It is of academic interest, but of no clinical importance. Disregard it. The possibilities of error in carrying out necessary measurements are considerable; many of them can be eliminated by careful technique. So great is the percentage of inaccuracies in the measurement of length by Method I that Method II is recommended in every case where the patient is not confined to bed.

LENGTH.—

*Method I.*—The normal limb must be placed in an exactly similar position to the affected limb before the measurements are taken, i.e., if there is an abduction deformity, the normal limb must be abducted a similar amount. Find the tip of the medial malleolus on each side, and mark the point with a blue skin pencil. Define the anterior superior spine on both sides; an error in measurement frequently occurs because an identical point on the anterior superior spine is not chosen on each side. With one finger palpate Poupart's ligament, and follow this up until the first bony point is reached. If this is done on each side and the first bony part is marked, error from this cause is avoided. Measure the distance (from the anterior superior iliac spine to the tip of the medial malleolus) on each side (*Fig.* 562). Record the measurement of each limb.

FRANÇOIS POUPART, 1661–1708, *Surgeon, Hôtel-Dieu, Paris.*

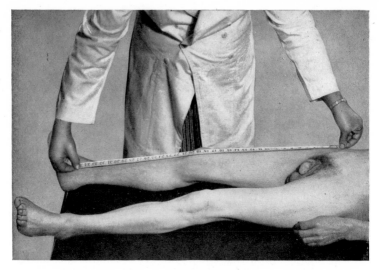

*Fig.* 562.—Measuring the length of the limb.   The distance between the anterior superior iliac spine and the tip of the medial malleolus is measured on each side.

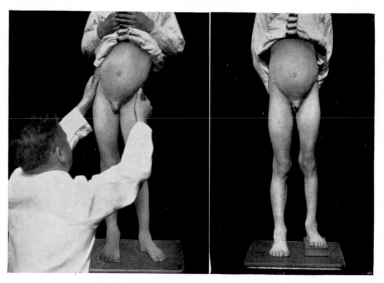

*Fig.* 563.—Measuring the amount of shortening by inserting blocks under the short limb to such a height as to make the pelvis absolutely level.   (*Alan Todd.*)

In watching relays of students carry out this measurement I have observed that differences in the lengths of the limbs are found where none exist. This is always due to one of two errors—the first is the fallacy in locating the anterior superior spine (which is guarded against by the above technique); the second is due to allowing the tape measure to get hitched up on the patella of one side. It should lie evenly along the inner border of the patella.

*Method II.*—Build blocks (or books) under the short limb to such a height as to make the pelvis absolutely level (*Fig. 563*). By measuring the height of the support the amount of real shortening is ascertained with an accuracy unobtainable by any other method. If the patient is not confined to bed, this is undoubtedly the method that should be employed.

GIRTH.—Minor degrees of wasting can be revealed by measuring and comparing the girth of the thigh and leg on each side.

*a.* From the anterior superior iliac spine, measure off a convenient distance down the thigh. Mark this point. Measure off the same on the other thigh, and mark it. At the points marked, measure the girth of the thighs (*Fig. 564*).

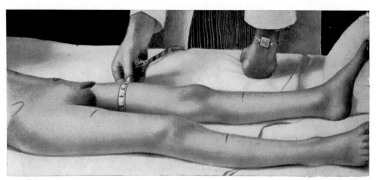

*Fig. 564.*—Mensuration for wasting. Both thighs and both calves are measured at exactly corresponding points. It is easier to avoid inaccuracies due to pulling on the tape if a metal tape-measure is used.

*b.* From the superior border of the patella, mark off identical points down each leg, and measure the girth of the calves. A possible source of error here is voluntary contraction of one quadriceps and consequent pulling up of the patella on that side. See that the quadriceps is relaxed whilst the measurement is taken.

METHODS OF DETERMINING SHORTENING IN THE HEAD OR NECK OF THE FEMUR.—If there is shortening of the leg, determine whether all or part of this shortening lies above the intertrochanteric line— that is to say, if this shortening is due to a deficiency in the head and/or neck of the femur.

22

There are several methods of obtaining this information. They are all based on the relative positions of three anatomical points, viz. : the anterior superior iliac spine, the tip of the great trochanter, and the centre of the tuber ischii (*Fig.* 565).

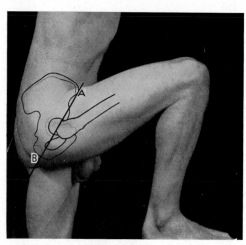

*Fig.* 565.—The relationship of the anterior superior iliac spine, the tuber ischii, and the tip of the great trochanter is the foundation of the various tests to determine if shortening is due to a deficiency in the head and neck of the femur.

*Schoemaker's Method.*—This is very simple, and clinically accurate. It consists in prolonging a line joining the anterior superior spine with the tip of the great trochanter on to the abdomen. This prolonged line normally meets the median plane at the level of the umbilicus, or above it. If the trochanter on one side is raised, the line intersects the median plane below the umbilicus.

*Nélaton's Line.*—The patient lies on his side, with his hip semiflexed, and a line is drawn from the anterior superior iliac spine to the tuber ischii. This line normally passes across the tip of the great trochanter. If there is shortening in the head or neck of the femur, the tip of the trochanter will lie above this line. The tuber ischii is difficult of precise definition ; moreover, this structure has quite considerable dimensions. The point of its greatest convexity should be chosen. Even so, this method is open to the objection of inaccuracy. No account should be taken of elevations of the trochanter up to half an inch.

*Bryant's Triangle.*—This method is more accurate than the foregoing, but as a triangle has to be erected on each side, it is time-consuming. The patient lies in the dorsal position. The anterior superior iliac spine is defined, and a plumb line is drawn towards the floor from this point. This is the base line of the triangle. Next, a line is drawn from the anterior superior spine to the tip of the great trochanter. The triangle is then completed by connecting the tip of the great trochanter to the base line by the shortest route, forming the horizontal side of the triangle. This horizontal line is measured on both sides, and if a difference exists, the amount of shortening can be determined by subtraction.

Alan Todd says : No orthopædic surgeon draws Bryant's triangle. It suffices to kneel facing the patient, and to put the thumbs on his anterior superior iliac spines, the middle fingers on the tips of the great trochanters and the ring and little fingers behind the great trochanters. Slight differences in the height of the trochanters are detected easily in this rapid way (*see Fig.* 563).

**Testing the Movements of the Hip-joint.**—Before testing the movements of the hip-joint, it is necessary to try for

Jan Schoemaker, 1871–1940, *Surgeon, The Hague, Holland.*
Auguste Nélaton, 1807–1873, *Professor of Surgery, University of Paris.*
Thomas Bryant, 1828–1914, *Surgeon, Guy's Hospital, London.*
Alan Herapath Todd, *Contemporary Consulting Orthopædic Surgeon, General Hospital, Croydon, England.*

Thomas's sign, and we must clearly understand the significance of this sign.

*Hugh Owen Thomas's Sign.*—Flexion of the hip-joint can be compensated by lordosis. As one looks at the patient lying down in *Fig.* 566, one would not dream that the hip is flexed, for the whole leg lies flat upon the couch. The sign is really to see if the examiner is being 'foxed' by the patient's posture. Hugh Owen Thomas's sign reveals the true position of the limb.

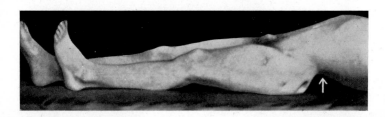

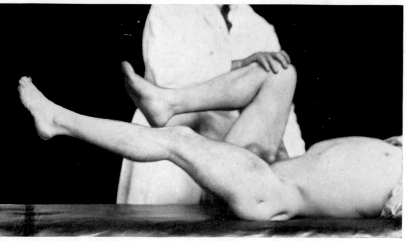

*Figs.* 566, 567.—Hugh Owen Thomas's sign. Note the result of flexing the normal thigh.

Pass the hand (palm upwards) under the lumbar spine, and with the other hand flex the *sound* hip. Flex the sound hip until the lumbar vertebræ can be felt hard against the hand. This means that all the lordosis has been corrected. Observe the affected limb. If flexion is present, estimate and record the angle (*Fig.* 567).

HUGH OWEN THOMAS, 1834–1891, *Orthopædic Surgeon, Liverpool.*

The movements may now be tested as follows :—

1. *Rotation.*—Lay the flat of the hand upon the thigh, and rock the leg (*Fig.* 568). This is a delicate test, and can be carried out with the utmost gentleness. This is why we do it first. If such a refined manipulation brings on pain (e.g., in acute arthritis), it is evident that the programme must be modified. If there is doubt as to the existence of limitation of movement, refer to the sound side.

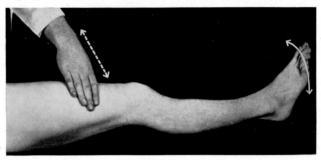

*Fig.* 568.—Rotation. Method I : ' Rocking ' the hip-joint. The most delicate test for rotation.

Rotation at the hip can also be carried out by flexing the thigh to a right angle and using the foot to lever the limb round (*Fig.* 569). Common sense will dictate that this violent method will be employed only in appropriate cases. Its zenith of usefulness is in the early diagnosis of coxa vara (due to a slipped epiphysis) in a child, where limitation of internal rotation is the leading, if not the only, physical sign.

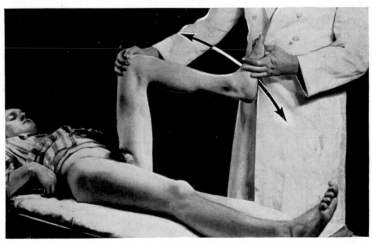

*Fig.* 569.—Rotation. Method II.

2. *Abduction.*—Steady the pelvis by placing a hand on the iliac crest. Grasp the ankle and slowly abduct, keeping the knees extended (*Fig.* 570). Record the angle.

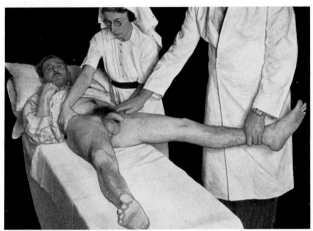

*Fig.* 570.—Abduction. The pelvis must be fixed efficiently or the test is valueless.

3. *Adduction.*—Again steady the pelvis, and carry the thigh over its fellow. Normally it should cross the middle third (*Fig.* 571). Record in terms of the opposite thigh—i.e., whether the lower, middle, or upper third of the opposite side can be crossed.

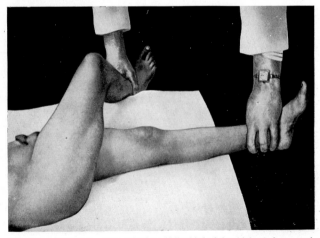

*Fig.* 571.—Adduction. Normally the middle third of the thigh can be crossed.

4. *Flexion.*—Flex the knee on the *affected side*, and then flex the hip as far as possible, proceeding cautiously (*Fig.* 572).

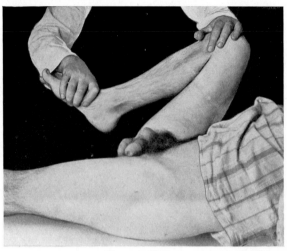

*Fig.* 572.—Flexion.

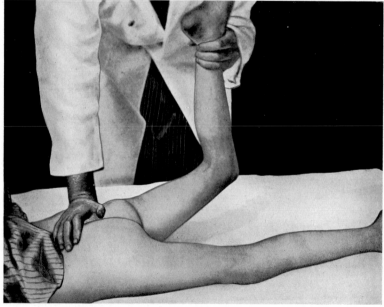

*Fig.* 573.—Extension.    Note that this test is also of considerable value for demonstrating spasm of the psoas muscle (*see* p. 285) and lesions of the anterior part of the sacro-iliac joint (*see* p. 330).

All these movements have been carried out with the patient on his back. Now ask him to turn over on to his abdomen. Observe the gluteal folds. A flattening of the fold is seen frequently in tuberculosis of the hip.

Lastly test—

5. *Extension.*—Steady the pelvis. Place the hand under the dorsum of the foot, and with the knee flexed lift the limb (*Fig.* 573). Normal extension is only 15°. It is limited early in tuberculous arthritis.

**Trendelenburg's Test.**—This test is not diagnostic of congenital hip disease.

The patient, stripped, stands with her back to the examiner and is told to lift first one foot and then the other from the ground. The position and movements of the gluteal folds are watched. When she stands on the normal leg, raising the other leg off the ground, the gluteal fold on this side rises slightly with the limb in a normal manner. When, however, she stands on the affected limb, the gluteal fold on the sound side does not rise, but falls (*Fig.* 574). This is because the glutei on the affected side are unable to support the pelvis properly.

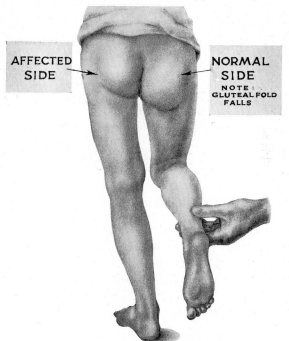

Fig. 574.—Trendelenburg's test positive.

FRIEDRICH TRENDELENBURG, 1844–1924, *Professor of Surgery, Leipzig.*

This indicates nothing more than a defect in the osseo-muscular mechanism between the pelvis and the femur. It is present in poliomyelitis when the glutei are affected, in ununited fracture of the femoral neck, in pathological dislocation, and the severer degrees of coxa vara, as well as in congenital dislocations. (Fairbank.)

The 'Anvil Test' (*Fig.* 575) is often a valuable method of ascertaining early hip-joint disease.

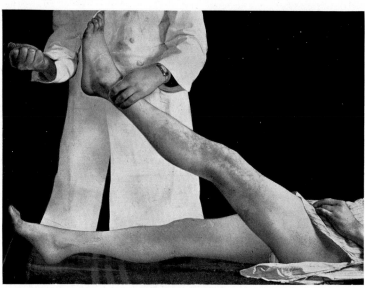

*Fig.* 575.—The ' anvil test ' for early hip disease. When positive, pain will be experienced in the hip-joint.

**Telescopic Movement.**—The pelvis is fixed, and the leg is grasped firmly. Traction is made. In congenital dislocation of the hip, especially in a young child, the characteristic sensation, which can be likened to that of pulling out a telescope, may be elicited.

## FRACTURE OF THE UPPER END OF THE FEMUR

That a fracture of the femur has occurred is sometimes perfectly obvious on inspection. *Fig.* 576 shows the leg rotated outwards, the typical deformity. When a fracture of the neck of the femur is impacted, the patient can lift the heel off the bed ; when it is not impacted, the patient is unable to do so.

Obscure injuries about the hip-joint require careful consideration. Attention is earnestly directed to impacted fracture of the neck of the

SIR HAROLD ARTHUR THOMAS FAIRBANK, *Consulting Orthopædic Surgeon, King's College Hospital, London.*

femur. The patient is often an old lady ; the accident is trivial—slipping on a polished floor ; the symptoms are few—she may even walk to seek advice. The penalties of failure to establish the diagnosis are gigantic. In such a patient, after such an accident, even the slightest degree of abduction deformity and the production of some pain on rotation of the hip by Method I provide sufficient data upon which to pass a confident diagnosis. In the absence of this evidence, by all means measure the limb and test the movement of the joint, but put not your trust in physical signs or, for that matter, in subperfect radiographs. Having seen conscientious practitioners perse-

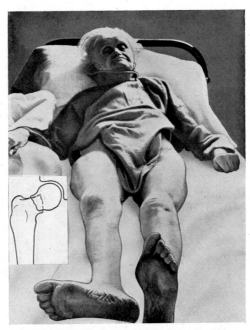

Fig. 576.—Inspection of a fractured femur (neck). Note the rotation of the limb.

cuted in the witness box for following the dictates of their training, I exhort the reader in relevant cases always to assume the diagnosis until it has been proved to be otherwise. This includes sharing the responsibility with a colleague.

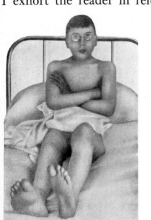

**The Sign of a Fractured Small Trochanter.**—The seated patient is unable to flex the affected thigh (*Fig.* 577). (Ludloff.)

The sign is more convincing when the patient is seated on a chair, and not in bed as shown in *Fig.* 577.

Fig. 577.—A sign of fracture of the small trochanter. Whilst the patient sits he is unable to lift the affected leg. The photograph was taken four days after the accident, and the patient is just able tremulously to move the leg in the sitting posture, but cannot get the foot off the bed.

KARL LUDLOFF, *Contemporary Professor of Orthopædic Surgery, Frankfurt, Germany.*

# CHAPTER XXVIII

## THE KNEE-JOINT

THE usual preparation for the examination of a male patient is to instruct him to roll up his trousers (*Fig.* 578). In a number of instances this procedure is rendered unsatisfactory because of tight trousers, and valuable points are missed in consequence.

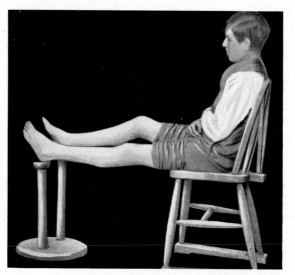

*Fig.* 578.—The usual posture for examination of the knee-joints in the out-patient department. Tight trousers considerably hinder a thorough examination.

Unless the patient is attired in very wide trousers, he should remove them. Excellent access to the joint can be obtained with the patient lying down.

**Inspection.**—Effusion into the joint can often be seen (*Fig.* 579). Look particularly for a fullness above and on either side of the patella. " If the surgeon, on passing his eyes critically over the natural hollows on each side of the patella, finds them abolished, he may be absolutely certain that he has to deal with an effusion into the knee-joint " (Whitelocke).

RICHARD HENRY ANGLIN WHITELOCKE, 1861–1927, *Surgeon, Radcliffe Infirmary, Oxford.*

Although it may be much in evidence (*Fig.* 580), in non-traumatic cases and in traumatic cases of long standing, minor degrees of swelling are not necessarily of such diagnostic significance ; indeed, apparent swelling is often due—at any rate in part—to wasting

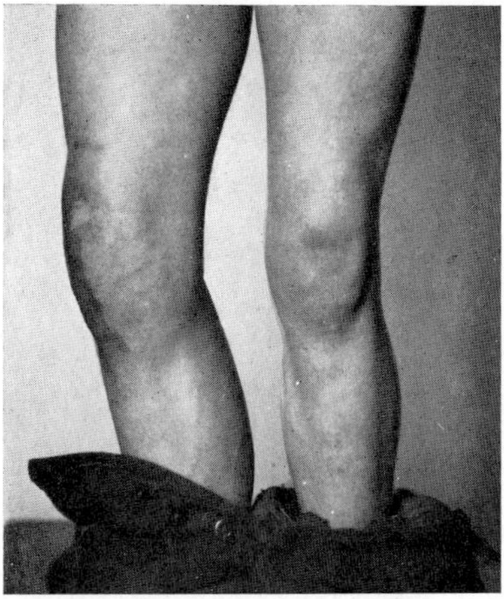

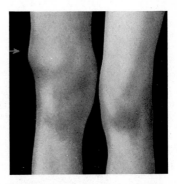

Fig. 580.—Large effusion into the knee-joint. Note the fullness caused by ballooning of the suprapatellar pouch.

*Fig.* 579.—Traumatic effusion into the knee-joint. Note the obliteration of the natural outline of the joint when compared with the other knee. The iodine was applied by a first-aid worker.

of the quadriceps (*see Fig.* 45, p. 30, and *Fig.* 504, p. 337). In such circumstances special physical signs are required to confirm the presence of an effusion into the joint, and measurement of the circumference of the limb at identical points three

*Fig.* 581.—The answer to the request, " Place your index finger on the exact spot you get pain ". Case of recurrent dislocation of the internal semilunar cartilage. The site of pain when the internal lateral ligament is torn is indicated also.

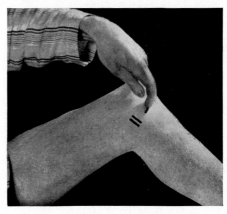

inches above each patella should be a routine to ascertain the amount, if any, of muscular wasting.

When pain in the knee is a leading symptom, ask the patient to point with one finger to the site of the pain (*Fig.* 581).

Constantly bear in mind that pain in the knee can be, and often is, referred from the hip-joint.

The swelling of prepatellar bursitis (housemaid's knee) (*Fig.* 582) is not likely to be confused with an effusion into the knee-joint, but I have found that an infra-patellar bursitis (clergyman's knee) (*Fig.* 583) often seems to give rise to perplexity.

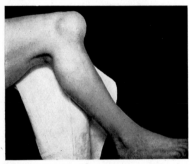

Fig. 582.—Prepatellar bursitis (housemaid's knee).

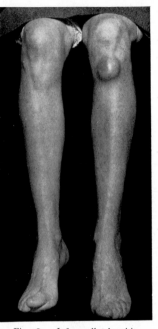

Fig. 583.—Infrapatellar bursitis (clergyman's knee).

When a clinician is aware that such a condition exists, because of its precise anatomical situation, a cyst connected with one of the semilunar cartilages is not a difficult condition to diagnose.

**Testing for the Presence of Fluid in the Knee-joint.**—As already noted, an effusion can often be seen because the natural hollows on each side of the patella are obliterated. If the amount of fluid is considerable, fluctuation can be elicited from above the patella to below, on one or other side of the ligamentum patellæ. An excellent sign, when it is positive, is the patellar tap.

*The Patellar Tap.*—In order to elicit the patellar tap, it is essential to realize that in the horizontal position a considerable amount of fluid gravitates into the suprapatellar pouch. With one hand above the patella, exert downward and backward pressure on this pouch, and drive fluid from that cavity into the knee-joint proper. Depress the patella with a sharp, jerky movement (*Fig.* 584). If the characteristic tap can be felt, it is proof positive of the existence of excessive fluid in the joint. Too much fluid can prevent the patella being pushed on to the condyles; too little fluid will not lift the patella free from them (Ovens). There must be a *moderate* amount of fluid in the knee-joint for this test to be positive.

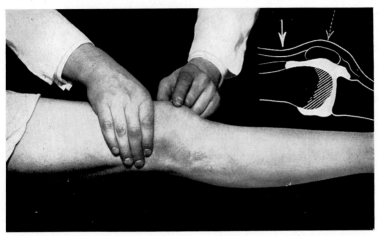

*Fig.* 584.—Testing for a patellar tap.

*Test for a Small Amount of Fluid in the Knee-joint.*—By compression, displace the fluid from one of the hollows on either side of the ligamentum patellæ into the knee-joint proper. In a good light, watch; the hollow slowly refills. Even a small effusion can be confirmed by this test.

*Subjective Movement.*—Ask the patient to bend his knee as fully as possible and observe the degree of flexion and extension he attains.

*Objective Movement.*—With the left hand laid upon the joint, grasp the ankle with the right; flex and extend the knee-joint several times, noting if there is joint crepitus or a ' click ' (*see* p. 13), which may prove significant (*see below*).

## EXAMINATION OF A CASE OF SUSPECTED INTERNAL DERANGEMENT OF THE KNEE

In order to arrive at a correct diagnosis, painstaking interrogation and intelligent examination are usually required in this frequently encountered type of case. From the formidable array of possible pathological conditions included under the heading of internal derangements, the student and practitioner will do well to confine

GERALD HUGH CAMPBELL OVENS, *Contemporary Surgeon, King Edward Hospital, Ealing, London.*

their attention to seeking for the following (as far as possible the conditions are arranged in order of frequency, the first two being by far the most common) :—

    1. Torn lateral ligament (usually the internal).
    2. Displaced (or split) internal semilunar cartilage.
    3. Displaced (or split) external semilunar cartilage.
    4. Ruptured crucial ligament.
    5. Loose body.
    6. Recurring dislocation of the patella.

In all cases of suspected internal derangement of the knee-joint the first sign to employ is the pointing test (*see Fig.* 581), which is frequently enlightening ; indeed, it often gives a lead to the conduct of further examination of the case.

### TORN LATERAL LIGAMENTS

The site of tenderness is over the internal lateral ligament, as is depicted in *Fig.* 581.

*Test for Lateral Movement.*—With the knee-joint fully extended, try to elicit lateral movement (*Fig.* 585).   If this is present, it usually means that the *internal lateral ligament* is ruptured—a fact that may settle the diagnosis.   This does not necessarily imply that the internal semilunar cartilage is not displaced in addition, because the deep fibres of the internal lateral ligament are attached to the cartilage.

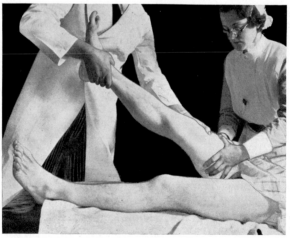

*Fig.* 585.—Testing lateral mobility.   Suspected torn internal lateral ligament.   The knee must be kept fully extended   In addition it is best to get an assistant to steady the thigh with both hands.

When it is suspected that the *external* lateral ligament is torn, the best method of testing lateral mobility is to place the straight leg (*see Fig.* 585) under your arm, and hold it gripped between your arm and your chest. With this grip it is possible to carry out in an *inward* direction the same manœuvre as is depicted in *Fig.* 585 for carrying out an outward movement.

### DISPLACED INTERNAL SEMILUNAR CARTILAGE

*Timbrell Fisher's Method.*—With the tip of the index finger, press firmly over the joint interval in front of the internal lateral ligament. While maintaining deep pressure with the finger, flex the knee-joint and at the same time rotate the foot inwards and then outwards; carry out this manœuvre several times. Suddenly one may feel a whipcord-like body (the torn semilunar cartilage) move under the finger and one may be enabled to trap it and roll it against the head of the tibia. In positive examples of this test an audible 'click' often accompanies the procedure.

*Kellogg Speed's Test for a Tear of the Anterior Horn of the Internal Semilunar Cartilage.*—While passive flexion and extension of the joint are carried out, tip-of-the-thumb pressure is made over the anterior horn of the internal semilunar carti-lage (*Fig.* 586) and then over the anterior end of the ex-ternal cartilage of both knees in succession. If tenderness is elicited in one particular location and is absent in the others, it is significant.

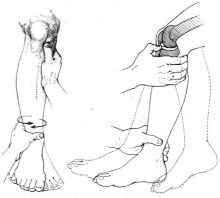

Fig. 586.—Method of testing the integrity of the anterior horn of the medial semilunar cartilage. (*After Kellogg Speed.*)

*McMurray's Test for a Tear in the Posterior Horn of the Internal Semilunar Carti-lage.*—The patient must lie *face downwards*. The foot is grasped and the knee-joint is flexed until the heel comes almost to the buttock. The foot is then rotated *outwards* to its extreme limit, and with the foot in this position, the knee-joint is steadily extended. When a 'click' can be felt during the manœuvre, it signifies that the posterior horn of the internal semilunar cartilage is torn.

ALFRED GEORGE TIMBRELL FISHER, *Contemporary Orthopædic Surgeon, St. John's Clinic, London.*
KELLOGG SPEED, *Contemporary Surgeon, Presbyterian Hospital, Chicago.*
THOMAS PORTER MCMURRAY, *Contemporary Professor of Orthopædic Surgery, University of Liverpool.*

### DISPLACED EXTERNAL SEMILUNAR CARTILAGE

*Kellogg Speed's Test* (*see above*) embraces this lesion.

*Timbrell Fisher's* method can be adapted as a confirmatory test.

*McMurray's Test for a Loose External Semilunar Cartilage.*—As in McMurray's other test, the patient lies face downwards. Again, the knee is flexed, but on this occasion the foot is rotated fully *inwards*. If, on extending the knee with the foot in this position, a distinct ' click ' is felt, the external cartilage is displaced.

### LOOSE BODY

If the patient has felt something " moving about in the joint ", ask him to try and find the joint ' mouse ' (loose body) himself.

### TORN CRUCIAL LIGAMENT

*Test for Anteroposterior Movement.*—The patient, who has been lying upon a couch, sits up and maintains his knee in flexion, as shown in *Fig.* 587. The surgeon grasps the leg below the knee with

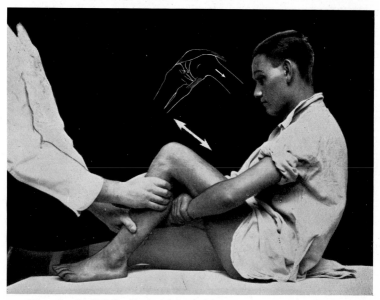

*Fig.* 587.—Method I. Testing the knee-joint for anteroposterior movement.

both hands. If there is movement of the tibia upon the femur when forcible *backward pressure* is exerted, it suggests that the posterior crucial ligament is ruptured. Similarly, if there is movement when the leg is *pulled forward*, the integrity of the anterior crucial ligament is open to question.

A good alternative method is as follows : The patient's knee is flexed, and the foot is placed firmly on the couch. The clinician's elbow rests on the dorsum of the foot, to steady it. A firm grasp is then taken with both hands around the calf (*Fig.* 588), and antero-posterior movement is attempted as before.

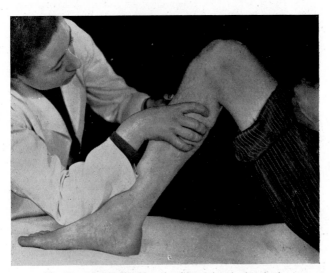

*Fig.* 588.—Method II. Note the elbow fixing the foot firmly.

## EXAMINATION OF THE PATELLA

If the patient lies at rest with the quadriceps absolutely relaxed, and the patella is grasped, it is possible to obtain slight lateral mobility, more in the female than in the male.

**Dislocation.**—Excessive mobility of the patella suggests the possibility of recurrent dislocation (*Fig.* 589), a condition that is liable to be confused with an internal derangement of the knee-joint.

**Fracture.**—Astounding to relate, a transverse patellar fracture (indirect violence) is amongst the lesions that are missed. Of course, if there is a great deal of separation, a layman knows what has happened. A useful method of examining a doubtful case is to pass the thumb-nail, held nearly horizontal with the surface, over the subcutaneous surface of the patella from above downwards (*Fig.* 590). When even the slightest separation is present, a sharp crevice will be felt.

23

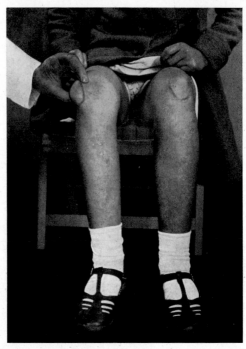

Fig. 589.—Sent up as a case of possible displaced internal semilunar cartilage, the patella could be manipulated into the position shown.   Case of recurrent dislocation.

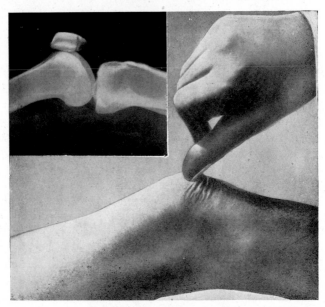

Fig. 590.—The thumb-nail test for fractured patella without separation.

## GENU VALGUM

The degree of deformity should be estimated in the following manner. The feet must be parallel, for outward rotation makes the separation of the knees greater. With his knees braced back, the patient grips a postcard between his condyles (Eric Lloyd). The distance between the internal malleoli is measured (*Fig.* 591). The patient is then examined lying down ; each knee is flexed. If the deformity disappears with flexion, the fault lies in the lower end of the femur.

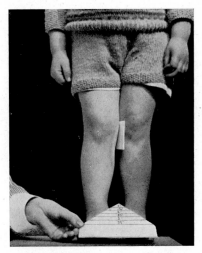

*Fig.* 591.—Genu valgum. The distance between the malleoli is being measured by a graduated wedge.

### EXAMINATION OF THE POPLITEAL SPACE

When the region of the knee is being examined the popliteal space is liable to be overlooked. It is worth while to make a routine of examining this sulcus. In obscure, deep-seated lesions the space is examined best with the patient lying face downwards (*Fig.* 592). A *popliteal abscess* is often deep-seated ; there is but slight fullness

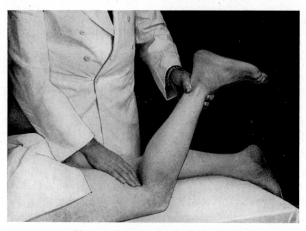

*Fig.* 592.—Palpating the popliteal space.

ERIC IVAN LLOYD, *Contemporary Orthopædic Surgeon, Royal Northern Hospital, London.*

in the space. The patient inclines to keep the knee-joint somewhat flexed ; full extension causes pain. When a popliteal abscess is suspected, the foot and leg must be scrutinized for an infected focus.

A patient is brought with an obvious swelling in the popliteal space.

Observe the region while he (or she) stands. If the patient is young, the commonest swelling in this recess is a semimembranosus

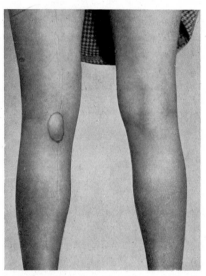

*Fig.* 593.—Semimembranosus bursa. Note that it is always situated towards the medial side of the space.

bursa (*Fig.* 593). When the patient is past 40 the swelling in question is likely to be a Morrant Baker cyst. After having confirmed that the swelling is cystic, demonstrate by compression whether a communication exists with the knee-joint, for a Baker's cyst (*Fig.* 594) originates as a pressure diverticulum of the synovial membrane. Test the knee-joint and other joints for signs of osteo-arthritis. I have concurred that a border-line candidate who omitted this step should be failed.

Although it is not within the confines of the popliteal space, this is a convenient place to draw attention to the existence of an enlargement of the bursa related to the insertion of the tendons gracilis and sartorius.

WILLIAM MORRANT BAKER, 1839–1896, *Surgeon, St. Bartholomew's Hospital, London.*

All the bursæ referred to above are practically painless ; they are never tender. When a patient is seen with what appears to be a typical enlarged bursa in the popliteal space, but it is tender and when pressed upon pain shoots down to the foot, the swelling is almost certainly a neurofibroma of either the internal or (if in relation to the deep aspect of the biceps tendon) the external popliteal nerve.

Aneurysms are far less common than they were 50 to 100 years ago, for three reasons : (1) Syphilis is treated more effectively, (2)

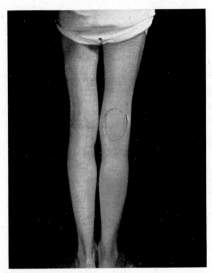

*Fig.* 594.—Baker's cyst. The swelling fills the popliteal space. The patient suffers from osteo-arthritis of the knee.

persons consume less alcohol, and (3) they do not perform such hard manual work. The candidate for distinction, cognisant that the popliteal space was, and is, the commonest site of a peripheral aneurysm, argues that the mature or elderly patient before him might have a strongly positive Wassermann, and is neither necessarily a supporter of prohibition nor a member of a trades' union. Consequently, such a candidate always tests a centrally placed cystic swelling of the popliteal space for an expansile impulse.

AUGUST VON WASSERMANN, 1866–1925, *Director of the Institute for Experimental Therapy, Berlin.*

358

# CHAPTER XXIX

## THE LEG AND FOOT

**Fractures of the Tibia and Fibula.**—Normally the inner side of the great toe, the internal malleolus, and the inner side of the patella

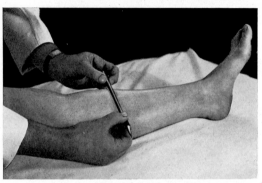

Fig. 595.—The pencil rolling test is useful for determining a point of localized tenderness of the tibia and other subcutaneous bones, and may prove useful is ascertaining the location of an obscure fracture or localized periostitis.

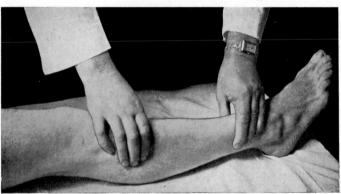

Fig. 596.—Springing the fibula.

are in a straight line. This relationship may be lost when both the tibia and fibula are fractured.

Fractures of the tibia are sought by running the fingers along its subcutaneous border. In obscure fractures without displacement the pencil rolling test (*Fig.* 595) is valuable. The integrity of the fibula is tested by 'springing'. Grasp the leg as shown in *Fig.* 596 ; in the case of the normal bone the fibula can be made to spring. This phenomenon is absent when the bone is fractured, and when attempted causes pain.

**Fractures about the Ankle.**—In the examination of fractures about the ankle the relationship of the two malleoli must receive special consideration. It should be remembered that Pott's fracture is usually a fracture-dislocation, and attention must be directed to the heel for that undue prominence which a backward dislocation of the ankle gives (*Fig.* 597).

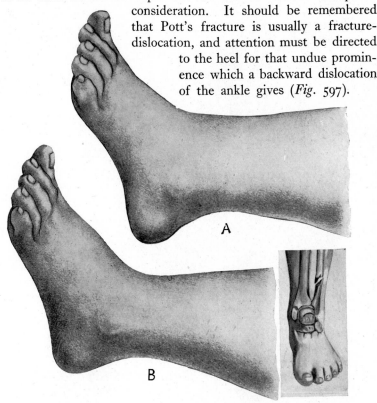

*Fig.* 597.—Pott's fracture-dislocation (inset). Note the prominence of the heel and the shortening of the dorsum of the foot (A) compared with the normal foot (B).

Obliteration of the normal hollow below the malleoli is a constant sign in fracture of the os calcis. Tenderness in fracture of this bone is inclined to be situated posteriorly near the insertion of the tendo Achillis, rather than upon the plantar aspect.

PERCIVAL POTT, 1713–1788, *Surgeon, St. Bartholomew's Hospital, London.*

## THE  FOOT

Shoes and socks are removed. If the patient is complaining of pain the cause may be obvious (*Fig.* 598). When there is no lead as to the cause, ask him to point to the place that hurts.

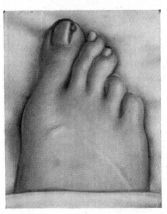

Fig. 598.—Ingrowing toenail. A small excrescence of granulation tissue in the situation shown is characteristic.

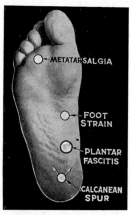

Fig. 599.—At these sites pain is felt on pressure in the conditions indicated. In atypical cases consider the possibility of gonorrhœa and also examine the great sciatic nerve (p. 332).

*Painful Feet.*—Some help in the diagnosis may be derived from *Fig.* 599. Methods of testing for a few common conditions will be referred to briefly.

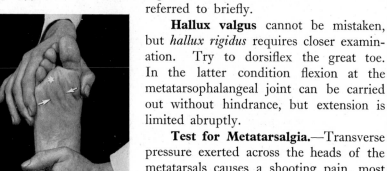

Fig. 600.—Testing for metatarsalgia. The star indicates where pain is usually located when the sign is positive.

**Hallux valgus** cannot be mistaken, but *hallux rigidus* requires closer examination. Try to dorsiflex the great toe. In the latter condition flexion at the metatarsophalangeal joint can be carried out without hindrance, but extension is limited abruptly.

**Test for Metatarsalgia.**—Transverse pressure exerted across the heads of the metatarsals causes a shooting pain, most marked between the second and third bones (*Fig.* 600).

This condition is attributed to a neuroma of a digital nerve. Test the area of sensation supplied by the affected nerve : in typical metatarsalgia there is often circumscribed, diminished sensation in this area.

**Freiberg's Disease** (Osteo-chrondritis of the Head of the Second and Third Metatarsal Bone).—There is pain somewhat similar to metatarsalgia, limitation of plantar flexion (*see Fig.* 606), and broadening of the affected foot.

**March Fracture.**—Occurs spontaneously especially in untrained soldiers after a fatiguing march. A crack in the neck of the 2nd, 3rd, or 4th metatarsal is the cause.

There is a ' puffy ' swelling of the adjacent interdigital web where pitting on pressure can usually be obtained. On deep palpation, thickening and tenderness of the affected bone is often in evidence.

**Calcanean Spur.**—There is localized, considerable tenderness of the bone in the position indicated in *Fig.* 599. Those whose occupation entails long hours of standing, e.g., policemen, are frequent sufferers.

**Tenosynovitis of the Tendo Achillis.**—Should be suspected when pain is experienced along the course of the tendon and tenderness

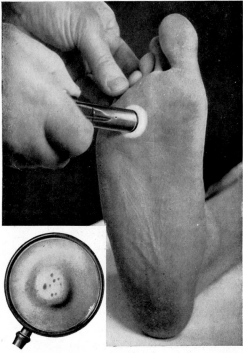

*Fig.* 601.—If on transillumination the hypertrophied dermis is homogeneous, the lesion is a callosity. The appearance of a plantar wart is shown in the inset.

ALBERT H. FREIBERG, 1868–1940, *American Surgeon.*
ACHILLES, *when an infant, was held by the heel and dipped into the river Styx to render him invulnerable. He remained vulnerable in the heel by which he was held (Greek mythology).*

localized about an inch above the os calcis. Swelling and crepitus are usually present, sometimes extending up to the muscle belly. The condition must not be confused with Achillis bursitis, in which the pain is nearer to the os calcis and there is no crepitus.

**Plantar Wart.**—Because the treatment of each condition is entirely different, this painful lesion must be distinguished from a callosity, for which it is frequently mistaken. Fitzgerald's transillumination test brings the differential diagnosis within the purview of every practitioner. The torch is placed to one side of the hypertrophied area (*Fig.* 601). If it be a plantar wart, dark dots (*Fig.* 601 inset) will become apparent ; if it be a callosity, it is homogeneous.

**Flat-foot.**—Look at the patient's boots. Unless they are new, or have been soled recently, information can be gleaned therefrom.

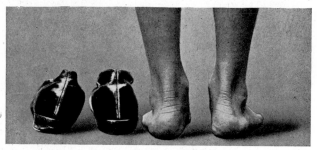

Fig. 602.—Flat-foot, especially left.

Hugh Owen Thomas wrote in 1890 : " There are three classes of feet—the excellent, the medium, and the bad. The first wear the outer side of the shoe heels more than the inner side ; the medium

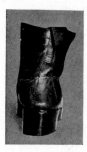

Fig. 603.—The boot of a child with flat-foot, showing tilting of the back seam. (*Alan Todd.*)

wear the heels level ; the bad ones wear down the inner edge and the posterior curve of the heels." In flat-footed patients it is the *inner* border of the sole that is inclined to be worn down. There is often treading over the waist of the boot or shoe (*Fig.* 602), and especially in the case of a child wearing boots, a tilting of the back seam (*Fig.* 603). In patients belonging to the last category, the tendines Achillis should always be examined for shortening that limits dorsiflexion of the ankle-joint.

*Searching for flattening of the arches of the foot.*—Ask the patient to stand. Cast the eye particularly along the inner border of the foot,

FREDERICK PATRICK FITZGERALD, *Contemporary Surgeon, Orthopædic Department, Royal Northern Hospital, London.*

HUGH OWEN THOMAS, 1834–1891, *Orthopædic Surgeon, Liverpool.*

and notice the inner arch, which is the first to be lost in flat-foot.

Footprints are useful in investigating the condition of the arches (*Fig.* 604). The easiest method of obtaining footprints is to dust the soles with powder and then get the patient to walk on linoleum.

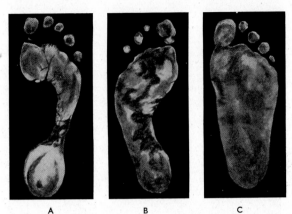

*Fig.* 604.—Footprints. A, Normal ; B, Early flat-foot ; C, Advanced flat-foot.
(*After De Quervain.*)

*Testing the movements of the foot.*—When examining the feet in cases of suspected flat-foot, the foot should be put through its four movements, up (*Fig.* 605), down (*Fig.* 606), in (*Fig.* 607), and out (*Fig.* 608). For instance, in spasmodic flat-foot only inversion is limited.

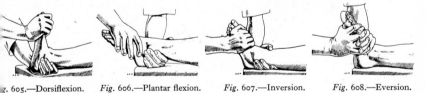

Fig. 605.—Dorsiflexion.  Fig. 606.—Plantar flexion.  Fig. 607.—Inversion.  Fig. 608.—Eversion.

In *spasmodic flat-foot* the peroneal muscles are contracted rigidly. When the condition, which occurs in adults, is suspected, the peronei should be palpated early in the examination of the case.

## CHAPTER XXX

## BONE

## EXAMINATION OF A CASE OF ACUTE OSTEOMYELITIS

*More sins of omission and commission occur in connexion with the diagnosis of acute osteomyelitis than in all the frequent diseases of surgery.* (*Hupp.*)

RADIOLOGY plays such an important part in the diagnosis of bone disease that students, and not a few practitioners, are astounded to learn that radiographs are quite valueless in the detection of early acute

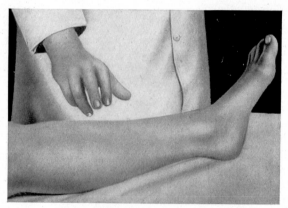

*Fig.* 609.—Percussing the tibia for tenderness. A useful sign in the diagnosis of osteomyelitis.

periosteomyelitis. This all-important diagnosis—the most important and urgent of all diagnoses connected with bone—must be made by clinical methods.

The classical description of the local findings in acute osteomyelitis is " a deep-seated brawny swelling situated near a joint " ; but if, before making the diagnosis, we relied upon the development of these signs, the mortality would be appalling.

If the patient is old enough, and not delirious, he will be able to signify which bone is painful (although he may refer the pain to the neighbouring joint). When the patient is too young

FRANK LE HAYNE HUPP, 1865–1929, *Surgeon, Ohio Valley General Hospital, Wheeling, West Virginia, U.S.A.*

or too toxic to give any information, the diagnosis is naturally more difficult.

**Methods of Examination.**—The following routine should be carried out :—

*Inspection.*—Compare carefully the two sides for minor degrees of swelling. Look for an abrasion or other superficial lesion where organisms might have entered.

*Test for Localized Heat* as described on p. 4.

*Bone Percussion* (*Fig.* 609) is exceedingly useful, especially when the affected bone is superficial, such as the tibia. Tenderness evoked by this method is characteristic. Bone percussion is also of the greatest service in determining which of two parallel bones (radius or ulna, tibia or fibula) is the seat of the disease.

*Pressure over the Bone* is often helpful, especially in early or mild cases of osteomyelitis. Commence by placing the pulp of the index finger over the bone at a distance from the suspected site of the disease. If pain is not complained of, exercise increasing pressure ; sometimes as the pressure increases the patient will

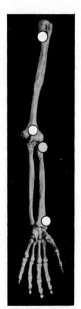
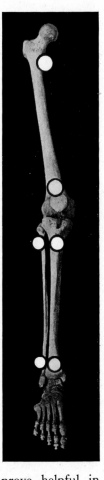

*Fig.* 610.—Points of maximum tenderness in acute osteomyelitis. The coloured circles are posterior. (*After Kennon.*)

cry out quite suddenly. Repeat the manœuvre nearer the suspected epiphysis, proceeding very gently, if pain has been caused by more remote pressure. By this means a point of maximum tenderness (*Fig.* 610) will be located. In mild, subacute cases the pencil rolling test (*see Fig.* 595) may prove helpful in superficial bones.

*Examine the Suspected Area for Evidence of Superficial Œdema.*— In cases of some standing, where there is a bone abscess, overlying edema is nearly always present.

*Examine Neighbouring Joints for Arthritis.*—It should be noted that in acute periosteomyelitis usually a secondary, so-called sympathetic, effusion occurs into the nearby joint, e.g., when the upper end of the tibia is infected, there is an effusion into the knee-joint.

*Palpate the Appropriate Lymphatic Glands*—for example, those of the groin—and compare with those of the opposite side.

The diagnosis of acute osteomyelitis in a patient too ill or too young to give any information is one of the most difficult tasks in clinical surgery.

Pressure over commonly affected bones may reveal that one bone is more tender than others ; because it is so thickly clothed with muscle the most obscure situation is the upper third of the femur.

**The Differentia Diagnosis between Acute Suppurative Arthritis and Acute Periosteomyelitis.**—It has just been pointed out that in periosteomyelitis a ' sympathetic ' effusion into the joint nearest the affected epiphysis is to be expected. In primary arthritis the infection is *in* the joint ; in osteomyelitis it is in the bone *near* the joint. Consequently, when it can be ascertained by percussion and/or pressure that the bone is tender, the joint signs (effusion) fade into insignificance in the assessment of the signs.

In the area of the hip-joint, for reasons stated already, the differential diagnosis is considerably complicated, if not impossible ; indeed both conditions may coexist. When the joint is rigidly maintained by the patient in the position of greatest ease (*see* p. 29) and even the gentlest attempts to rotate it cause exquisite pain, the diagnosis of purulent arthritis of the hip-joint should be favoured.

**The Differential Diagnosis between Acute Rheumatism and Acute Periosteomyelitis** is sometimes difficult. A point of considerable help is that in rheumatism the pain tends to flit from joint to joint, while in osteomyelitis it is stationary. The skin in rheumatism is moist—in early osteomyelitis it is dry. If there is any doubt whether the patient is perspiring, pass the hand into the axilla and note whether it is moist. With rheumatism, the disease is *in* the joint.

**The Differential Diagnosis between Acute Osteomyelitis and Erythema Nodosum** is easier than the foregoing, but must be mentioned, for I can remember at least three cases of erythema nodosum being admitted to surgical wards as osteomyelitis of the tibia. If the fingers are passed lightly over the plaques of erythema nodosum

(*Fig.* 611), it is at once evident that they are raised above the level of the surrounding skin. Each gives the impression of a miniature

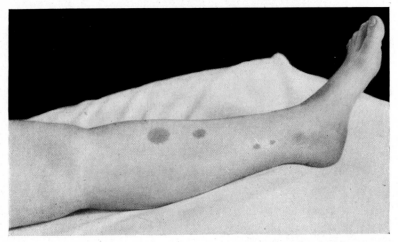

Fig. 611.—Erythema nodosum.

Table Mountain. Furthermore, if one of these areas is clasped gently between the finger and thumb, it will be found that it can be made to move on the bone.

**Chronic Osteomyelitis.**—Usually the diagnosis is not nearly so difficult as in the acute stage. When there has

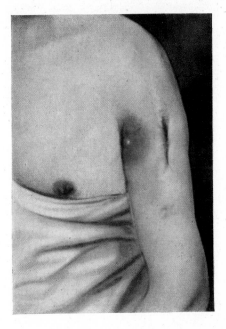

Fig. 612.—Chronic osteomyelitis. Recrudescence of the infection fifteen years after operation for acute osteomyelitis of the humerus.

been a previous operation for osteomyelitis, the diagnosis is self-evident (*Fig.* 612). Sometimes, when there is no such lead, the only physical sign is a deep-seated bony swelling situated near a joint (Brodie's abscess).

SIR BENJAMIN BRODIE, 1783–1862, *Surgeon, St. George's Hospital, London.*

## A SWELLING CONNECTED WITH A BONE

The ease with which the physical characteristics of a swelling connected with the bone are elicited depends upon whether or not the
bone is superficial.   The superficial aspects of the tibia, ulna, patella,
clavicle, and skull are readily palpable, but palpation of bones well
covered with muscles is extremely difficult.   In the latter situations
every effort should be made to get the muscles relaxed by attention
to the posture.

To illustrate an extreme instance :  *Fig.* 613 shows the position
adopted to relax the gluteus maximus in order that a swelling beneath
that muscle might be palpated.   Nothing could be made out until
this position was tried, when it became evident that the swelling
in question was attached to the tuber ischii.

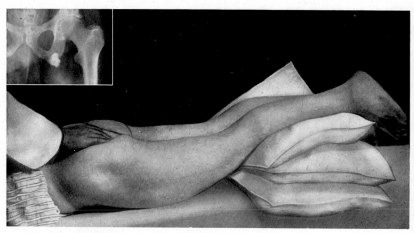

*Fig.* 613.—Palpating a lump beneath the gluteus maximus.  Position adopted in order
to ensure muscular relaxation.  Inset—Radiograph of the case.  Calcification in the bursa
overlying the tuber ischii.

In a case of localized swelling, obviously the first thing to do
is to make sure that it is attached intimately to the bone by trying
to move it on the bone.   Next, in the case of a long bone, try to
ascertain whether one aspect of the bone is involved alone, or whether
the whole of the circumference participates in the swelling.

*Subperiosteal nodes* occur, particularly on the tibia and the large
bones of the skull.   In the case of the tibia the bone feels thickened
over an area of two or three inches.   When the bones that make up

the calvarium are involved, a 'hot-cross bun' effect is produced (Parrot's nodes). Previous rickets or syphilis is responsible for the phenomenon.

**The Sign of Epiphysial Osteoma.**—Pass the fingers firmly down the side of the bone in such a way as to allow them to ride over the swelling. In the case of an epiphysial osteoma, the side farther away from the joint is overhanging (*Fig.* 614). Sometimes a bursa can be made out over the most prominent part of the osteoma.

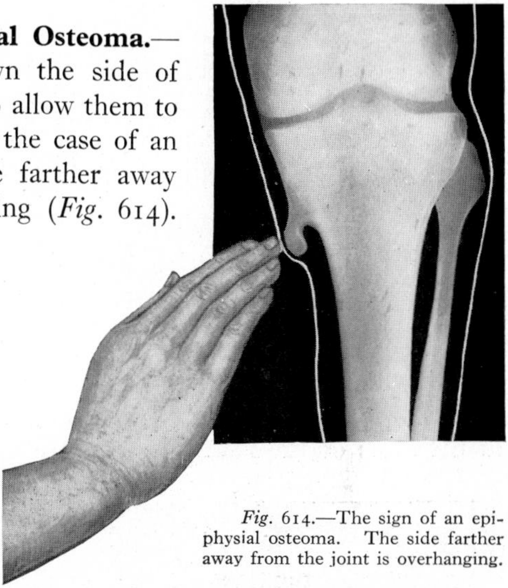

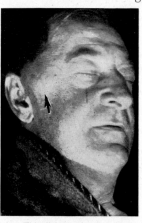

*Fig.* 614.—The sign of an epiphysial osteoma. The side farther away from the joint is overhanging.

**X-ray Examination.**—To-day the exact diagnosis of a swelling connected with a bone is mainly a matter of studying the X-ray films. The sign of egg-shell crackling in osteoclastomata (*Fig.* 615) and the pulsation of bone sarcomata in general are hardly ever noted, for radiography has rendered diagnosis possible long before these late signs develop. In this connexion

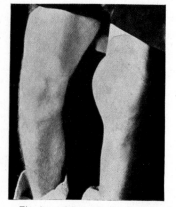

*Fig.* 615.—Advanced osteoclastoma of the lower end of the femur causing an expansion of the bone.

*Fig.* 616.—This slightly painful swelling connected with the zygomatic arch is the patient's only complaint. On examination it is intimately blended with the malar bone, and although it feels hard, there is an area of softening in the centre. On interrogation he admits to slight dysuria and some increased frequency of micturition. Rectal examination reveals a hard, grossly irregular prostatic enlargement. Diagnosis—secondary carcinoma from the prostate.



Joseph Marie Jules Parrot, 1829–1883, *Professor of Pædiatrics, Paris.*

it must be mentioned that when a neoplasm of a bone is considered to be a primary one, radiographs of the thorax should be examined for evidence of metastatic deposits.

*Is the Neoplasm Primary or Secondary ?*—From the purely clinical standpoint there yet remains one very important duty. When the diagnosis of a bone neoplasm has been made, it should be an unwavering rule to eliminate the possibility of this being a secondary carcinoma. Therefore examine the thyroid, the breast, the kidney (Grawitz's tumour), and, above all, the prostate, for a primary growth (*Fig.* 616).

## SOME PHYSICAL SIGNS CONNECTED WITH RARER BONE DISEASES

**Achondroplasia.**—In normal individuals the umbilicus is situated above the centre of a line extending from the top of the vertex to the soles of the feet. In achondroplasia alone the umbilicus is situated below this centre point (*Fig.* 617).

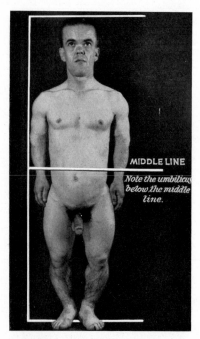

Fig. 617.—Achondroplasia (dystrophia chondrofœtalis). Normally the umbilicus lies above the middle line of the body. In achondroplasia it is regularly below the middle line.

MIDDLE LINE

*Note the umbilicus below the middle line.*

**Osteitis Deformans (Paget's Disease).**—" Begins in middle life or later, is very slow in progress, and may continue for many years without influence on the general health. It affects most frequently the long bones of the lower extremity and the skull, and is usually symmetrical. Even when the skull is hugely thickened and all its bones extensively altered in structure, the mind remains unaffected." So wrote Sir James Paget.

The condition is far from rare, and I am surprised how many examples I have seen in women during recent years. All the leading clinical features of osteitis deformans are summarized in the following diagram, which has helped a number of students to remember the essential features of

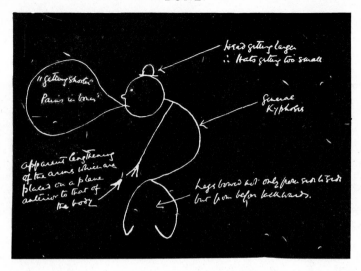

*Fig.* 618.—Diagram of the essential signs of osteitis deformans (Paget's disease).

the disease. This is my excuse for inserting the somewhat ridiculous caricature (*Fig.* 618).

So much for the generalized form of the disease. What is much more likely to be missed is the localized variety (*Fig.* 619). A single bone, usually the tibia or femur, but never the fibula, is alone affected—at least for many years.

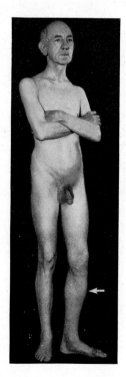

*Fig.* 619.—Osteitis deformans of the left tibia. Neither the other bones of the lower extremities nor the skull showed any clinical or radiological abnormality.

**Fragilitas Ossium.**—Examine the eyes of a patient who gives a history of repeated fractures. In fragilitas ossium the sclerotics are often blue (*Fig.* 620).

**Generalized Osteitis Fibrosa.**—Again, spontaneous fractures are frequent, but the bones are soft and therefore are inclined to exhibit deformities. Persistent benign tumours are prone to occur, especially in the long bones.

When a case exhibiting some of these features is presented, examine the thyroid gland with extreme care for the possible presence of a parathyroid tumour.

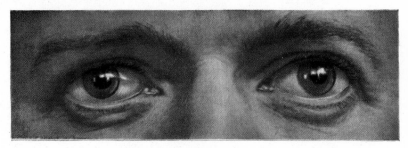

*Fig.* 620.—Blue sclerotics.  The patient was the subject of recurrent fractures of long bones.  He was 31 years of age when this photograph was taken, and since the age of 3 he had been in and out of hospital with broken bones.

**Scurvy Rickets.**—The diagnosis is often arrived at by the following sequence of thought : The mother says the child is losing weight and its bones are tender—you suspect rickets.  You next feel the bones ; the periosteum is thickened—you think of syphilis.  You now press the gums ; they bleed readily—you diagnose (correctly) scurvy rickets.

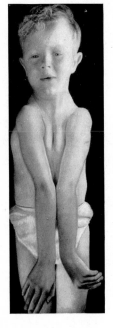

**Cranio-cleido-dysostosis.**—The arms can be folded across the chest in such a manner that the shoulders are almost touching one another (*Fig.* 621).  Owing to the sagging of the

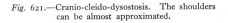

*Fig.* 621.—Cranio-cleido-dysostosis.  The shoulders can be almost approximated.

bones of the vault, the cranium presents an appearance which has been well likened to a ' Tam O' Shanter '.*

---

* *Tam O'Shanter.*—A round woollen cap having a flat, baggy top. Named after the hero of that name in Burns's poem.

## CHAPTER XXXI

## THE SPINE

### INJURY TO THE SPINAL COLUMN

IF possible, examine the back as the patient is being moved from the stretcher to the bed. This saves unnecessary movement. The important thing to look for is deformity ; incidentally, signs of local bruising should be noted. The most common deformity is an angular one, which signifies a fracture-dislocation.

**Motor Power.**—Ask the patient to move his legs. If he can draw up both legs, one can be certain that there is no serious damage of the spinal cord. If only one leg is drawn up, do not jump to the

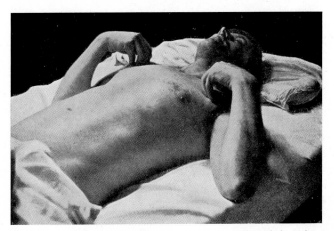

*Fig.* 622.—The attitude in a lesion at the level of the seventh cervical vertebra

conclusion that there is a unilateral lesion. Examine the immobile thigh and leg for local injury.

Test the movements of the arms. If the arms are paralysed, their position may be the key to the level of the lesion.

*Level of the 7th cervical.*—The half-closed hands with the elbows flexed assume the position shown in *Fig.* 622.

*Level of the 6th cervical.*—Arms held up above the head. Elbows flexed. Forearms supinated. Hands half-closed (*Fig.* 623).

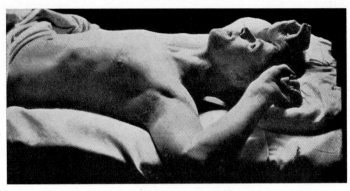

*Fig.* 623.—The attitude of a patient with a lesion at the level of the sixth cervical vertebra.

*Level of the 5th cervical.*—Arms completely immobile by the sides.

*Level above 5th cervical.*—A lesion here is fatal, for the phrenic nerves become implicated. It is from this cause that death results in judicial hanging.

The abdomen should be inspected. When respiration is purely *abdominal* (diaphragmatic) it implies that the intercostal muscles are paralysed. The lesion is situated, therefore, high in the cervical region.

Before completing the abdominal part of the examination percuss the bladder. Retention of urine is usual when the spinal cord is damaged ; priapism in addition makes the probability a certainty. In relevant cases consider the possibility of a fractured pelvis (*see* p. 311).

**Sensation** should be tested with a pin. A band of hyperæsthesia at the level of the lesion, with anæsthesia below, is indicative of a grave injury to the spinal cord.

**Reflexes.**—It is quite useless to make an elaborate examination of the reflexes soon after the injury. The patient will at this time be in a state of cerebrospinal shock, which masks much information that such an examination might otherwise reveal.

THE REFLEXES IN DIFFERENTIAL DIAGNOSIS BETWEEN A COMPLETE AND AN INCOMPLETE LESION OF THE SPINAL CORD.—

*A differential diagnosis between a complete and an incomplete lesion of the spinal cord cannot as a rule be made until between one and three weeks after the accident.*

1. *A Complete Lesion.*—Prick the inner side of the thigh with a pin. A flexor response is obtained—flexion of the toes, ankle, knee, and hip. Bear in mind that formerly, if a *flexor* response was obtained, it was considered to be a sign in favour of an incomplete lesion. It has now been shown that this is not true. A *flexor* response to the plantar reflex is in favour of a *complete* lesion.

*The mass reflex.* When the 'flexor state' (Riddoch) is at its height, a small stimulus such as pricking the inner side of the thigh, or drawing the prepuce over the erect penis, brings about not only flexion of all joints of the lower extremity, but an evacuation of the bladder and sometimes of the rectum also.

2. *An Incomplete Lesion.*—The stimulus (pin-prick) will bring on much less pronounced flexion, *and this is followed after a time by an extensor response.* A reaction of flexion followed by extension is therefore very much in favour of an incomplete lesion.

### ROUTINE EXAMINATION OF THE SPINE

The patient, stripped to the gluteal folds, stands in a good light with the back towards the surgeon and the arms hanging loosely by the sides. Inspection should not be hurried, for it takes some time for the patient to assume a natural attitude. If a deepened midline spinal sulcus is seen about the tenth dorsal vertebra you have noticed the first sign of Pott's disease in its earliest stages at the most frequent site. This deepened sulcus is due to increased muscular tonicity of the erector spinæ muscles ; it is nature's plaster cast (Jardine).

Note the symmetry of the body ; whether one half is more prominent than the other. This can be done by comparing the two sides of the trunk with reference

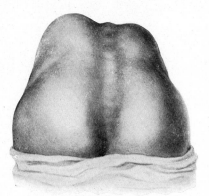

*Fig.* 624.—When a patient leans forward a spinal deformity becomes more evident. In this case compression of the right thorax due to scoliosis became obvious.

to an imaginary line prolonged upwards from the gluteal cleft (Tubby). In this way scoliosis is detected.

Direct the patient to lean forward and cross the arms over the chest so that the hands rest on opposite shoulders. It is remarkable how much greater any deformity appears in this position (*Fig.* 624).

GEORGE RIDDOCH, *Contemporary Neurological Physician, London Hospital.*

FRANCIS E. JARDINE, *Contemporary Surgeon, Edinburgh Royal Infirmary.*

ALFRED HERBERT TUBBY. 1862–1930, *Orthopædic Surgeon, Westminster Hospital, London.*

Sometimes the spinous processes of the vertebræ are not very prominent, and it may be difficult to detect scoliosis ; in such cases ask the patient to fold his arms and lean forward, and then run the finger firmly down the vertebræ without hurting the patient. A red line on the skin results, and the curve of the spine becomes evident. Next view the patient laterally, for in this position kyphosis is seen clearly. When kyphosis is present, pay particular attention to its type, whether it is a gentle curve or an angular deformity, having in mind the following aetiological table :—

*Angular deformity*
- Fracture-dislocation
- Tuberculosis (Pott's disease)
- Secondary carcinoma

*Gentle curve*
- Postural
- Osteochondritis deformans juvenilis dorsi (Scheuermann's disease)

## Testing the Mobility of the Spine.—(*See also* Low-back Pain, p. 327.)

*Flexion* is the principal movement to be tested.

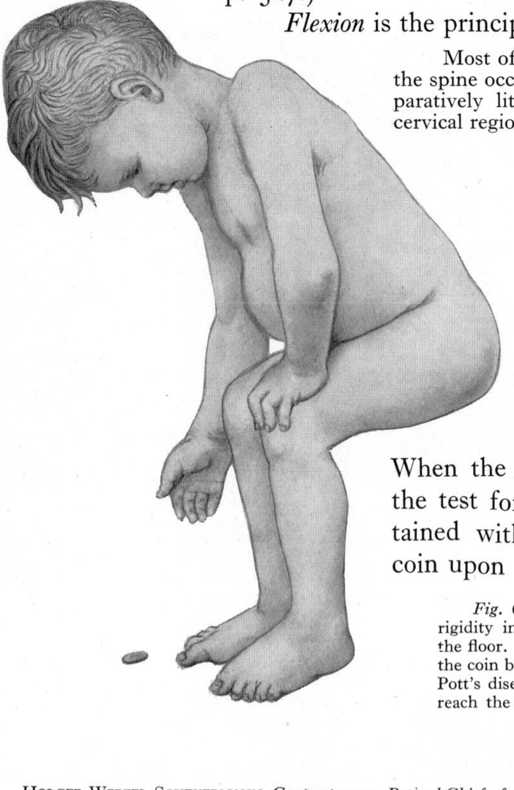

Most of the movement of true flexion of the spine occurs in the lumbar region ; comparatively little in the dorsal, while in the cervical region normal flexion merely consists of the obliteration of the anatomical backward curve. It is only after it has been pointed out that one realizes that flexion of the spine *per se* is largely apparent and much of this movement occurs at the occipito-atlantic and hip joints.

Ask the patient to bend forwards and endeavour to touch his toes, keeping the knees straight. When the patient is a young child, the test for flexion can often be obtained without tears by dropping a coin upon the floor and watching the

*Fig.* 625.—The coin test for spinal rigidity in a child. A coin is thrown on the floor. The normal child will reach for the coin by flexing the spine. A child with Pott's disease will keep the spine rigid and reach the coin by bending the knees.

HOLGER WERFEL SCHEUERMANN, *Contemporary, Retired Chief of the X-ray Department, Sundby Hospital, Copenhagen.*

child pick it up. A normal child will pick up the coin by flexing the spine, or, at least, the spine will be flexed to a considerable degree. On the other hand, should the child reach for the coin very cautiously by bending the knees (*Fig.* 625), it is obvious that spinal rigidity is present.

*Extension.*— The mobility of the spine can also be tested in young children by laying them on the face and lifting up the feet (*Fig.* 626). Rigidity is an early and constant feature of Pott's disease.

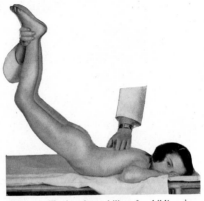

*Fig.* 626.—Testing the mobility of a child's spine.

**Vertebral Percussion.** — The spinous processes are struck with the percussing finger (*Fig.* 627) or a small percussion hammer.

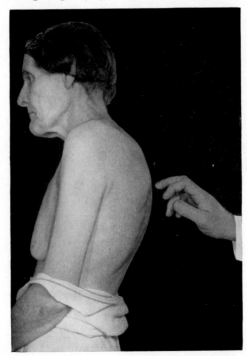

*Fig.* 627.—Percussing the spinous processes of the vertebræ.

Usually percussion is commenced at the vertebra prominens, and each spinous process down to the second sacral is percussed in turn. Tenderness over a particular vertebra is indicative of disease. The method is of particular value in the dorsal region.

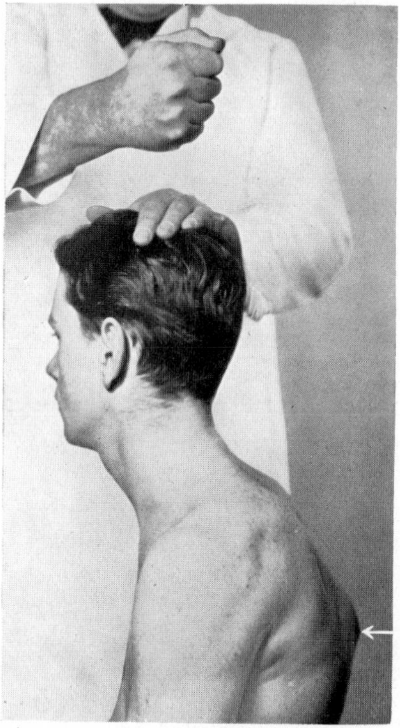

*Indirect Percussion (the 'Anvil Test').*—*Fig.* 628 is self-explanatory. The sign is positive when pain is experienced over a particular vertebra. This test has not much to recommend it.

Fig. 628.—The ' anvil test '. Pain was appreciated at the site of the deformity. This is not a test of great utility, and should be carried out only in exceptional cases.

**The Trapeze Test** may be employed to decide whether an obscure deformity of the spine is postural or structural. When the patient hangs from a trapeze a postural deformity disappears.

Early cases of psoas abscess (psoas irritation) can be revealed by performing the test of extension of the hip-joint (*see* p. 343). This manœuvre is both limited and painful when the psoas muscle is in spasm.

Except in cases of postural deformity, the examination of the spine should include an investigation of the integrity of the central nervous system.

A wise clinician remembers to examine the breasts of the female and the prostate of the male, and the thyroid and kidneys in both, for a primary growth when an angular deformity of the spine occurs during adult life.

## CHAPTER XXXII

## THE PERIPHERAL NERVES

## EXAMINATION OF PERIPHERAL NERVES

FOLLOWING Sherren's teaching, the examination of a peripheral
nerve injury consists essentially of three separate parts : (1) *The
general inspection of the injured member ;* (2) *The examination of
sensation ;* (3) *The examination of muscles.*

**1. General Inspection of the Injured Member.—**

*a.* The position of the limb may be characteristic—for instance,
the wrist-drop of the musculospiral (syn. radial) nerve lesion, or the
true claw-hand of an injury to the median and ulnar nerves.

*b.* If a wound or scar is present, its position in relationship to
underlying structures must be noted. Scars should be examined
for tenderness, adherence to deep structures, and bulbous
enlargements.

*c.* The condition of the skin should be investigated. Desquama-
tion is seen a few days after the injury. Often the skin is dry and
of a mottlish bluish appearance in an old nerve injury, or it may be
red, glossy, and perspiring (Weir Mitchell's skin) in the case of an
incomplete irritative division.

*d.* The nails should be inspected for curvature, ridging, change
in colour, absence of gloss, and growth of epithelium under their free
edges.

**2. The Examination of Sensation.—**The patient must be so
placed that no muscular effort is necessary to maintain the position of
the limb that is being examined. With his eyes closed, he is
told to say ' Yes ' whenever he feels *anything*, whether prick, touch,
or other sensation.

*Touch Sensation* is tested conveniently by stroking the skin
with cotton-wool (*Fig.* 629) or a soft camel-hair brush. The testing
of this sensation cannot be relied upon if the skin is clad with hair.

Touch sensibility also embraces acute localization of stimuli.
This is tested with a pair of callipers, the blunt points of which are

JAMES SHERREN, 1872–1945, *Surgeon, London Hospital.*
SILAS WEIR MITCHELL, 1829–1914, *Neurologist, Jefferson Medical College, Philadelphia, U.S.A.*

separated for a measured distance.  The skin is then touched, and
the patient is asked to say after each stimulation whether he has been

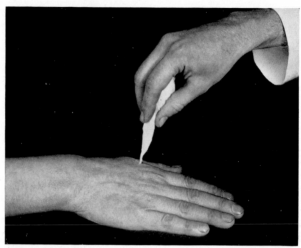

Fig. 629.—Testing for touch sensation with a wisp of cotton-wool.

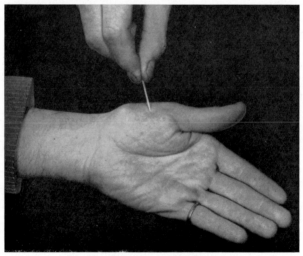

Fig. 630.—Testing for pain sensibility.

touched by one or two points.  Head and Sherren found that two
points could be recognized accurately over any part of the palm when
separated by 1 cm., and applied transversely.

*Pain Sensation.*—A sharp pin is used (*Fig.* 630), and care must be taken that the patient understands that he is to speak only when he feels the pain of a pin-prick, not when he feels pressure or touch. Unless this precaution is taken, the method is entirely inaccurate. Pain sensation also includes the appreciation of extremes of temperature. This can be tested readily by filling two test-tubes, one with hot and one with cold water, and applying them in turn to the skin of the affected part, at the same time noting the patient's remarks on what he feels.

(*The findings of touch and pain sensory loss in the various nerve lesions are not detailed, for they are depicted in standard text-books.*)

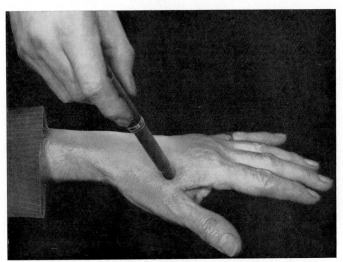

*Fig.* 631.—Testing for deep sensation.

*Deep Sensibility* should be tested by means of the pressure of a pencil or other blunt object (*Fig.* 631). The common practice of using the blunt end of a pin is not to be recommended, for a pressure of from 2 to 4 kilogrammes is necessary to call forth this sensation.

*Tinel's Sign* is designed to elucidate the question whether regeneration of a severed nerve is taking place. If, several months after a nerve has been divided, regeneration is proceeding, tapping over the course of the nerve-trunk *below* the lesion causes distal tingling. The tingling is produced by tapping on the growing end. If this place is marked at regular intervals, the rate of regeneration can be demonstrated. A negative Tinel's sign has no value (Rennie).

JULES TINEL, *Contemporary Physician, Hôpital de la Rochefoucauld, Paris.*
ALEX MILNE RENNIE, *Assistant in Department of Surgery, University of Aberdeen.*

**3. Examination of Muscles.**—Certain individual tests for muscular involvement due to common peripheral nerve lesions will now be described.

*Lesion of the Nerve of Bell* (syn. *Long Thoracic Nerve*).—Paralysis of the serratus magnus (syn. serratus anterior) is best demonstrated by getting the patient to push against the wall with his outstretched hand (*Fig.* 632).

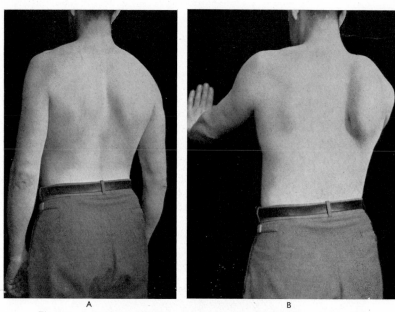

A                                             B

*Fig.* 632.—A, Paralysis of the right serratus magnus ; B, When the patient pushes against the wall, the scapula stands out like a wing.

*Lesion of the Circumflex* (syn. *Axillary*) *Nerve.*—Instruct the patient to lift the arm from the side at right angles to the body (deltoid).

*Lesion of the Spinal Accessory Nerve.*—Observe the patient from behind. In a case of some standing there is an alteration in the contour of the lower part of the neck and shoulder on the affected side (*Fig.* 633). Ask him to shrug his shoulders ; that the trapezius is wholly or partially paralysed now becomes obvious. The spinal accessory is one of the nerves most frequently injured during an operation for the removal of cervical glands.

*Lesion of the Musculospiral* (syn. *Radial*) *Nerve.*—There is the characteristic and unmistakable wrist-drop. Paralysis of the triceps

---

Sir Charles Bell, 1774–1842, *Surgeon, Middlesex Hospital, London ; later Professor of Surgery, Edinburgh.*

is unusual ; it can be tested easily by asking the patient to extend the forearm.

Below are given the clinical tests of some individual *muscles* not described already :—

*Latissimus Dorsi.* — The simplest method is to ask the patient to cough whilst the examiner has his fingers over this muscle, which forms part of the posterior axillary fold.

*Pectorals.*—" Press your hand into your side'' (*see* EXAMINATION OF THE BREAST, *Fig.* 236, p. 129).

*Biceps.*—Hold the elbow close to the side and get the patient to flex his arm against resistance.

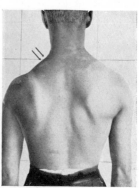

Fig. 633.—Characteristic flattening after a lesion of the spinal accessory nerve.

The diagnosis of lesions of the median and ulnar nerves being of such great clinical importance, the motor tests for the integrity of these nerves will be described more fully.

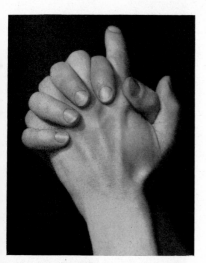

Fig. 634.—The clasping test in median paralysis ; the index finger fails to flex.

### MEDIAN NERVE

The median nerve is the nerve of grasp. It controls the coarse movements of the hand. A complete division of the median nerve *of some standing* gives the hand a characteristic appearance, due chiefly to the attenuated index finger, which sticks out as though in the act of pointing.

**Ochsner's Clasping Test** calls attention to this pointing index finger in cases where at first it is not evident (*Fig.* 634).

*In a recent division* of the median nerve, the following tests will be found the most reliable :—

*The Lesion is at the Wrist.*—Test the abductor pollicis. The action of this muscle is to take the thumb away from the index in a plane at right angles to the palm. To test for the integrity of the muscle, lay the hand flat upon the table, palm uppermost, and ask the patient to touch with his thumb a pencil held perpendicularly above it (*Fig.* 635).

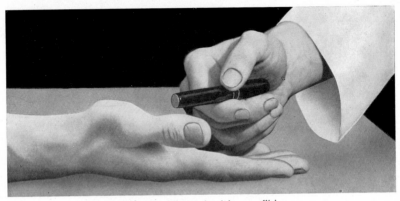

*Fig.* 635.—The test for abductor pollicis.

*The Lesion is at the Elbow.*—In addition to the above test, we ask ourselves the question, " Can the patient flex the terminal phalanx of his thumb ? " To test the integrity of the flexor pollicis longus, the thumb is held firmly at the metacarpo-phalangeal joint so that no movement can take place there ; then the patient is instructed to bend his thumb (*Fig.* 636).

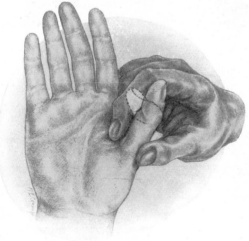

*Fig.* 636.—Lesion of median nerve at the elbow. Can the patient flex the terminal joint of his thumb ? The thumb is held at the metacarpo-phalangeal joint in order that no movement shall take place there.

### ULNAR NERVE

The ulnar nerve controls the fine movements of the hand, an example of which can be seen in the delicate fingering of the pianist. In a long-standing case of complete division of this nerve the hand is obviously wasted and the fingers are flexed.

It nearly approaches but is not quite, a true claw-hand. In contra-distinction to the median nerve, where the brunt of the deformity falls upon the index finger (*see* p. 383), it is the little finger that is characteristically thin and pointed. Often this deformed little finger is seen to be crooked, and the patient complains that it catches in everything.

A test of great utility in recent injury of the ulnar nerve is the test for paralysis of the interossei.

**The Card Test for the Integrity of the Interossei.**—Ask the patient to hold out his hand, keeping the fingers absolutely straight. Take a piece of stiff paper and insinuate it into an interdigital cleft.

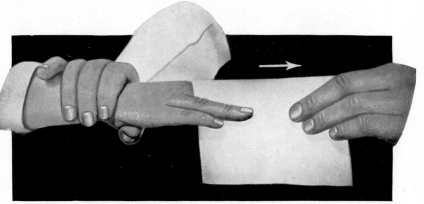

*Fig.* 637.—The card test. It is essential for the patient to keep the fingers quite straight.

Ask him to grip the paper between the fingers. It is essential to see that there is not even the slightest degree of flexion. Commence the test on the sound side, and notice the considerable resistance that the clasping fingers offer to your pull upon the paper. Now apply the test to the affected side. The grip is so feeble that the paper just slides out of the cleft (*Fig.* 637).

## KLUMPKE'S PARALYSIS

The result of an injury of the first dorsal nerve. It may follow a dislocation of the shoulder-joint or a violent upward pull of the arm, such as might be received by grabbing at a ledge while falling from a height. There is paralysis of all the intrinsic muscles of the hand, and a true claw-hand results eventually. It is necessary to look for paralysis of the cervical sympathetic (*see* p. 390), which is

25

MADAME AUGUSTE DEJERINE KLUMPKE, 1859–1927, *French Neurologist.*

sometimes implicated in this lesion. If the cervical sympathetic is involved, it indicates that the lesion of the first dorsal nerve is near its exit from the intervertebral foramen, and therefore in an inaccessible position.

## ERB'S PARALYSIS

Erb's paralysis is due to an injury of the fifth and sixth cervical nerves, and usually occurs in babies after a difficult labour. The arm is held in the characteristic ' policeman's tip ' position (*Fig.* 638).

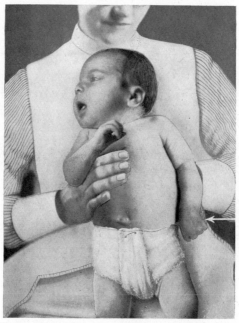

*Fig.* 638 —The left arm is held in the ' policeman's tip ' position. Erb's paralysis.

## CLAW-HAND

A true claw-hand (main-en-griffe) is found in several conditions, a list of which should be known. The cause can then be found by a process of elimination.

**Causes of Main-en-griffe.**—The following conditions give rise to true claw-hand :—

1. Lesion of median and ulnar nerves at the wrist.
2. Lesion of the inner cord of the brachial plexus.
3. Klumpke's paralysis.

WILHELM HEINRICH ERB, 1840–1921, *Professor of Medicine, Heidelberg.*

4. A late and severe Volkmann's ischæmic contracture (*see* p. 179).

5. An end-result of a neglected suppurative tenosynovitis of the ulnar bursa (*see* p. 176).

6. Syringomyelia.

7. Progressive muscular atrophy.

A complete lesion of the ulnar nerve of some standing (*Fig.* 639) results in a claw-like hand, but unless the median nerve is involved also it cannot be called a true claw-hand.

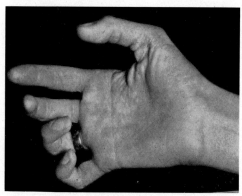

*Fig.* 639.—A claw-like hand resulting from complete division of the ulnar nerve.

## CERVICAL RIB

" Widows who take to washing " was Sir Henry Head's aphorism to describe the type of individual most commonly afflicted with a cervical rib that is *giving rise to symptoms*. This remark certainly aptly summarizes the fact that the condition is more common in females of middle age, and that the manifestation of symptoms is favoured by unaccustomed occupations. (*Fig.* 640.)

When a cervical rib is suspected, the neck should be palpated (*Fig.* 641). The transverse processes of the cervical vertebræ are located by deep palpation behind the sternomastoid, and these transverse processes are followed downwards as far as possible into the root of the neck. The head, of course, must be inclined well towards the side that is being examined, in order to relax the musculature.

A palpable cervical rib rarely gives rise to painful symptoms. Rather it is the unobtrusive variety that causes the tingling, numbness, and shooting pains down the ulnar side of the forearm. Raising

RICHARD VON VOLKMANN, 1830–1889, *Professor of Surgery, Halle.*

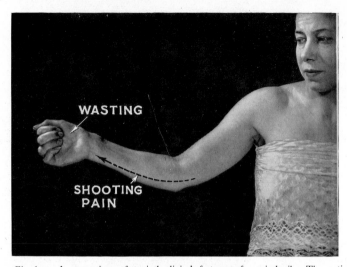

*Fig.* 640.—A symposium of typical clinical features of cervical rib. The patient was a woman aged 44 who had taken up war work in a factory. She mapped out the situation and direction of the pain along the ulnar side of the forearm, as depicted. A mere glance showed wasting of the thenar eminence.

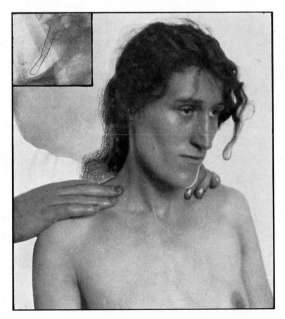

Fig. 641.—Palpating a cervical rib. The inset shows the radiograph of this case, with the cervical rib outlined.

the extremity tends to afford relief; pulling on the arm in a down-ward direction often intensifies the symptoms.

The hands are examined and compared, especial note being made of wasting of the thenar eminences (*Fig.* 642). When wasting is not obvious, test the abductor pollicis (*see Fig.* 635, p. 384), which is affected early in this condition. Sensation should be tested over the hand and arm. It tends to be lost over the ulnar aspect of the forearm. Another sign of value is what may be termed the 'piano stretch'. In a well-established case the patient finds difficulty in widely spreading the fingers and thumb.

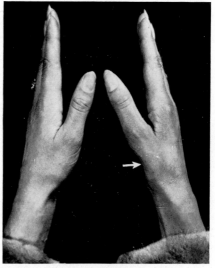

Fig. 642.—Obvious wasting of the thenar eminence in a case of cervical rib.

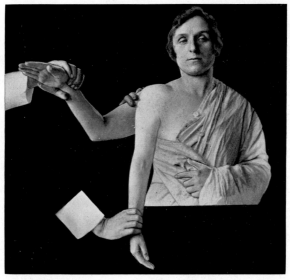

Fig. 643.—Testing for vascular involvement in cervical rib. The pulse is tested first with the arm moderately raised, and secondly with the arm fully depressed. If the rib is pressing on the subclavian artery, the pulse will become feeble when the arm is depressed.

**The Sign of Vascular Involvement.**—If signs of nerve involvement favour the diagnosis of cervical rib, the vascular system should be investigated also. Feel the pulse with the patient's arm slightly raised (*Fig.* 643). Then forcibly depress the arm. If the pulse is obliterated or weakened perceptibly, it signifies that the rib is compressing the subclavian artery.

**The Scalenus Anticus Syndrome.**—The signs and symptoms of cervical rib can exist without a cervical rib being present. What is known as the scalenus anticus syndrome is now well recognized ; the scalenus anticus compresses the lower cord of the brachial plexus and/or the subclavian artery and, in fact, it plays the part of a cervical rib.

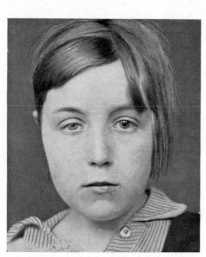

*Fig.* 644.—Paralysis of cervical sympathetic. Note the pseudo-ptosis, enophthalmos, and myosis. (Horner's syndrome.)

## PARALYSIS OF THE CERVICAL SYMPATHETIC

In surgical practice a lesion of the cervical sympathetic is found most frequently :—

1. In Klumpke's paralysis.

2. As a complication of wounds in the neck.

3. Where the nerve is involved in a malignant neoplasm.

Examine the eyes ; there is pseudo-ptosis (*Fig.* 644). The upper lid is only partially drooped, for the sympathetic nerve supplies only one-third of the levator palpebræ superioris. There is myosis—the pupil is contracted on the side of the lesion. There is enophthalmos —the opposite of exophthalmos—because of paralysis of Müller's muscle. Anhidrosis (absence of sweating) is present on the side of the lesion. This is difficult to demonstrate, but if the patient can be persuaded to eat a cayenne-pepper sandwich, it will be noted that sweating occurs only on the non-affected side of the face.

JOHANN FRIEDRICH HORNER, 1831–1886, *Professor of Ophthalmology, Zürich, Switzerland.*
JOHANNES PETER MÜLLER, 1801–1858, *Professor of Anatomy and Physiology, Berlin.*

## CHAPTER XXXIII

# EXAMINATION OF THE BLOOD-VESSELS OF THE EXTREMITIES ; THREATENED AND ESTABLISHED GANGRENE

## THROMBOPHLEBITIS DECUBITI

*The assumption that pulmonary embolus is an unavoidable accident is no longer tenable.* (J. Fine.)

THE temperature chart shows unexplained repeated slight elevations. Bearing in mind that the condition is more prone to occur past the meridian of life, and the highest incidence is between 50 and 60, if the patient has undergone an operation about a week previously, more particularly if that operation was one of herniotomy, hysterectomy, resection of the rectum, prostatectomy, cholecystectomy, or for perforated appendicitis, and decidedly if the patient has been nursed with a pillow placed beneath the knees, the well-trained clinician's thoughts should reflexly turn to the veins of the lower

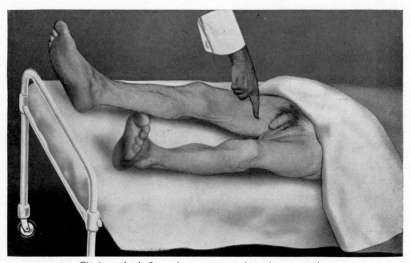

*Fig.* 645.—Apply finger-tip pressure over the saphenous opening.

JACOB FINE, *Contemporary Surgeon, Beth Israel Hospital, Boston, Mass.*

extremities.   While it is true that the fewer the symptoms caused by phlebothrombosis the greater the danger of pulmonary embolism, it is equally true that the majority of cases of phlebothrombosis decubiti remain undiagnosed until pulmonary embolism has occurred, *because the lower limbs have not been examined.*   When all those in attendance are alert to the dangers of clotting in the veins of the legs, when the nurse reports a slight pain in the calf, and, in relevant cases (especially between the third and seventh post-operative days) the clinician undertakes routine examinations to exclude phlebothrombosis, then, and then only, is real progress in the prevention of pulmonary embolism likely to occur.

Have the bedclothes turned up (not down) and display the whole of both lower extremities (*Fig.* 645).   Observe the limbs for swelling, which may be slight, fullness of the veins, and a cyanotic tinge.

In suspected early cases proceed as follows :—

1. Apply finger-tip pressure over each saphenous opening, and with a stroking motion, run the finger down the course of each femoral vein, seeking a segment of unilateral localized tenderness.

2. Let the patient draw up the knees, and lie quietly, relaxing the muscles.   Commence by palpating the feet for tenderness, especially the medial aspect and behind the internal malleolus (Payr).   Next, gently squeeze the calves, and thirdly (*Fig.* 646), palpate the whole of the thighs systematically, the object being to seek a localized area of muscular rigidity combined with deep tenderness (Frykholm).

Fig. 646.—Systematic palpation of the musculature of the lower limbs.
1, The feet ;   2, The calves ;   3, The thighs.

3. Palpate deeply in the popliteal spaces, noting if there is tenderness here, after which ask the patient to lower the legs on to the bed.

4. Homans' sign.   With the knee extended, dorsiflex the foot (*Fig.* 647).   Pain experienced in the calf is a positive sign of considerable significance.

5. Compare the femoral pulses.   When the femoral vein contains clot, the beat of the artery alongside it is usually perceptibly weaker.

If, as a result of this thorough examination, the diagnosis of femoral thrombosis is reasonably assured, the advisability of exposure of the sapheno-femoral junction should receive every consideration.

Erwyn Payr, *Contemporary, Director of the Surgical Clinic, Leipzig University.*
Ragnar Frykholm, *Contemporary, Assistant Surgeon, Seraphimer Hospital, Stockholm.*
John Homans, *Contemporary, Emeritus Professor of Clinical Surgery, Harvard University, Baltimore, U.S.A.*

Removal of clot and interruption of the femoral vein will forestall many pulmonary emboli.

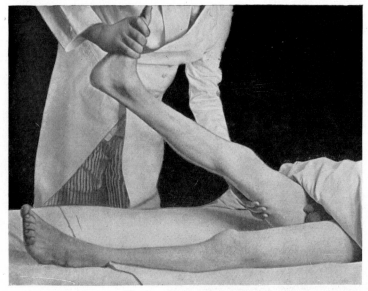

Fig. 647.—Eliciting Homans' sign.

## VARICOSE VEINS

It is necessary to observe the whole extent of both the lower limbs, and to note if a particular vein is mainly involved, e.g., the long (*Fig.* 648) or short saphenous vein.

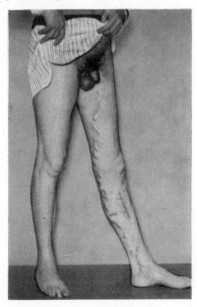

Fig. 648.—Varicose veins. Internal (long) saphenous vein mainly affected.

**Trendelenburg's Test.**—The patient lies down, and the limb is raised to allow the blood to drain out of the vein (*Fig.* 649, *a*). The thumb is placed firmly over the saphenous opening, which lies $1\frac{1}{4}$ in. below and lateral to the spine of the pubis. Still keeping firm

FRIEDRICH TRENDELENBURG, 1844–1924, *Professor of Surgery, Leipzig.*

pressure over this point, lower the limb and instruct the patient to stand (*Fig.* 649, *b*). The pressure is then removed suddenly. If the veins fill immediately, it is obvious that the valves in the saphenous vein are incompetent, and the sign is positive (*Fig.* 649, *c*). A positive Trendelenburg test is an indication for Trendelenburg's operation.

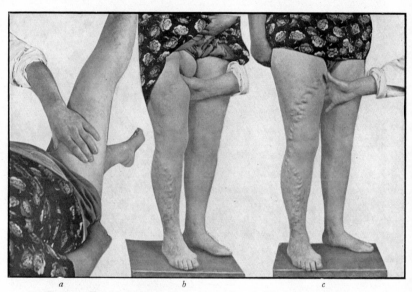

a       b       c

Fig. 649.—Trendelenburg's test in varicose veins. *a*. The limb is raised in order to empty the veins of blood, after which the thumb is placed over the saphenous opening ; *b*, The thumb is still kept over the saphenous opening whilst the patient stands upright ; *c*, The pressure over the saphenous opening has just been released, and the vein has filled from above downwards—the test is therefore positive.

**The Tourniquet Test** (Ochsner and Mahorner).—The varicose veins are inspected after the patient has walked about. A light rubber tourniquet is applied three inches below the fold of the groin, and just tight enough to constrict the superficial veins. The patient again walks about. (*a*) If, after exercise, the varicose veins are *less* prominent, it suggests that the valves of the internal saphenous vein are incompetent ; (*b*) If there is no change, it strongly suggests that these valves are competent ; (*c*) If the varicose veins are *more* prominent, it signifies that the deep veins are thrombosed. The tourniquet test can be repeated with the tourniquet around the middle, and then the lower part, of the thigh. If, after exercise, with the tourniquet in these positions, the varicosities are *less* evident, it suggests that the

EDWARD WILLIAM ALTON OCHSNER, *Contemporary Professor of Surgery, Tulane University of Lousiana, New Orleans.*

HOWARD RAYMOND MAHORNER, *Contemporary Assistant Professor of Clinical Surgery, Tulane University of Louisiana, New Orleans.*

communicating veins between the superficial and deep venous systems are incompetent.

The above tests are of considerable importance when the question of treatment of varicose veins is under consideration.    It should be noted that in all the above tests the condition of veins above the tourniquet is disregarded.

Varicose veins may be primary or secondary, and it behoves us, especially in bilateral cases, to exclude the possibility of a pelvic tumour, notably pregnancy.

## EXAMINATION OF PERIPHERAL ARTERIES

**Feeling the Pulse in the Lower Extremity.**—Taking the pulse in the lower extremity is of considerable importance to the surgeon.    The student is well advised to practise this accomplishment in the case of the smaller arteries in normal subjects.    Sooner or later the practice he gains thereby will stand him in good stead.    When in doubt as to whether a pulse in the distal part of the lower extremity is really being felt, or whether it is the examiner's own arterial beat that is being appreciated by the finger pulp, simultaneously palpate the patient's radial pulse ; if the latter synchronizes with the doubtful pulse, it must be the patient's!

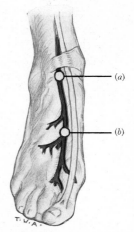

The pulse should not be regarded as absent until examination has failed to detect it in a thoroughly warm limb (Sir Thomas Lewis).

The *anterior tibial pulse* becomes superficial just above the level of the ankle-joint, and it can be felt midway between the two malleoli (*Fig.* 650).

*The Dorsalis Pedis Pulse.*—The dorsalis pedis is sometimes absent and therefore absence of its pulsation is valueless unless corroborated by other signs of obliterative arterial disease.

*Fig.* 650.—Points for seeking the pulsation of the anterior tibial (*a*) and dorsalis pedis (*b*) arteries.

The toes are grasped lightly in the left hand, so as to steady the foot.    A finger of the right hand is slid in the groove between the first and second metatarsal bones, upwards towards the ankle, the pulp of the finger being directed slightly towards the first metatarsal bone.    The pulse is usually felt just lateral to the tendon of the extensor hallucis longus at the proximal end of the groove (*Fig.* 650).

SIR THOMAS LEWIS, 1881–1945, *Physician, University College Hospital, London.*

The *posterior tibial pulse* should be accessible about half-way between the back of the internal malleolus and the inner side of the tendo Achillis, especially when the foot is dorsiflexed. This artery is sometimes difficult to feel and I do not place absolute reliance upon the absence of its pulsation.

The *popliteal pulse* can be detected satisfactorily only with the patient lying on his face and the leg in the position shown in *Fig.* 592, p. 355.

The *femoral pulse* is not always easy to feel in a well-covered individual. Palpate rather deeply below Poupart's ligament, midway between the anterior superior iliac spine and the symphysis pubis.

**Occlusion of a Main Peripheral Artery by an Embolus.**—Often, if the diagnosis is made within six to ten hours, it is possible to remove the embolus with considerable hope of success : hence the importance of examining the patient immediately. We will consider the case of an embolus arrested in the femoral artery.

Observe the limb. It is anæmic, but a patchy, mottled cyanosis is in evidence.

Test the local temperature (*see* p. 4).

If the pulsation of the femoral artery can be felt, obviously the embolus lies below this point. Feel for the dorsalis pedis and the posterior tibial pulses. In selected cases turn the patient on to his face and endeavour to elicit the popliteal pulsation. If it is obvious that the circulation is deficient below the knee, sterilize the dorsum of the foot with spirit and prick the skin with a sterile needle. If there is little or no bleeding, proceed at once to auscultate the femoral artery.

*The Auscultatory Test.*—Temporarily occlude the femoral (or brachial) artery at the root of the limb with the pressure of a sphygmomanometer cuff, if available. Alternatively, instruct an assistant to compress the artery with his thumb. A stethoscope is applied at various points along the course of the artery, from above downwards. After the pressure is released the booming of the returning arterial flow will be heard until the site of the embolus is reached, when there is an abrupt cessation of sound. (R. J. Last.)

*The Fork Test.*—Take a dinner fork, examine its prongs and see that they are level and blunt. With the patient in a good light draw the fork down the front of the limb towards the foot. Repeat the process on the inner and outer aspects of the limb. Ask the patient to roll over, and draw the fork down the back of the limb. Vasomotor stripes appear. These can be made plainer by rubbing the part with moist gauze. Stripes fading at a certain level indicate the site of failure of the circulation. Probably the embolus is arrested at the first bifurcation of the artery above this point.

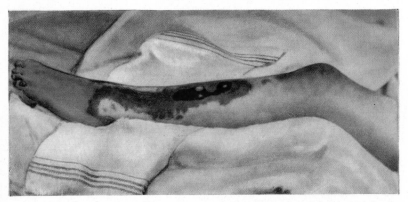

*Fig.* 651.—Too late for embolectomy! An embolus became lodged in the common femoral artery forty-eight hours before the patient's admission to hospital. The patient was a young woman with mitral stenosis.

If the patient has an embolus lodged in the main artery of a limb, to delay a few hours is to await inevitable local death (*Fig.* 651).

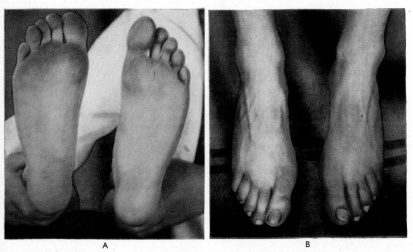

A                                    B

*Fig.* 652.—Buerger's test. A, Pallor of the involved foot in the elevated position ; B, Cyanosis of the same foot in the dependent position.

**Obliterative Arterial Disease.**—This is a frequent cause of defective peripheral circulation and threatened gangrene.

*The Buerger test* is a practical clinical test. It should be performed in broad daylight. The patient lies on his back, and lifts both legs high, keeping the knees straight. The legs are supported by the examiner, while the patient flexes and extends his ankles and toes to the point of mild fatigue. When there is a defective arterial blood-supply to the limb, the sole of the foot assumes a cadaveric

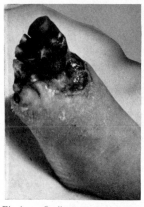

Fig. 653.—Senile gangrene showing a well-defined line of demarcation.

pallor. The feet are lowered, and the patient adopts a sitting posture. In two or three minutes a ruddy, cyanotic hue spreads over the affected foot (*Fig.* 652).

**Examination of a Case of Established Gangrene.**—A patient with gangrene of a portion of an extremity is presented. We wish to know the probable cause, and to ascertain the condition of the circulation above the gangrenous area. Inspect the limb. Note particularly the area between the living and dead tissue (*Fig.* 653). Decide if the process is infected or ' dry '.

Lay the hand upon the surface of the skin above the gangrenous area and observe whether it is colder than it should be.

An atheromatous temporal artery can often be seen ; feel the pulse at the wrist and at the temple and note the thickness of the arterial walls.

Return to the limb, palpate the main artery. In cases of doubt its pulsations can be compared with those of the corresponding artery of the opposite side.

Test the urine for sugar. Most cases of gangrene are due to arteriosclerosis (senile gangrene) or diabetes, or both. We will refer briefly to the examination of other varieties. When puzzled as to the cause of local death in a given case it may be helpful to ask oneself a few questions :—

*Is it Frost-bite ?* (*Fig.* 654). On one occasion during June I was confronted with a case of gangrene of two fingers in a man who described himself as a meat porter. Further inquiry brought to light the fact that he spent his working days in a refrigerator!

*Is it Carbolic Acid Gangrene ?* Even a weak solution of carbolic acid occasionally causes gangrene when applied locally for some time. Inquire whether the chemical has been used as a dressing. Examine the urine in a good light. In carbolic acid poisoning it is often smoky or distinctly dark brown.

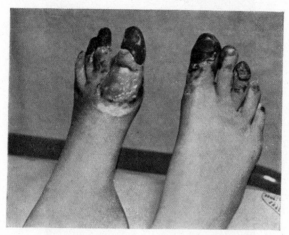

*Fig. 654.*—Gangrene developing after frost-bite in a Kentish farm labourer during the severe frost of January, 1940.

*Is it Thrombo-angiitis Obliterans ?* Such a condition is to be suspected when the patient is a man (95 per cent of sufferers are men) between 30 and 40, or even younger, whose arteries appear to be supple and in whom other causes of gangrene have been eliminated. Persistent paronychia of the great toe is a common precursor.

*Is it Raynaud's Disease?* (*Fig.* 655).—To diagnose Raynaud's disease the typical spasms must be observed. There are two varieties of this affection. In the first the digits become paroxysmally ashen white ; in the other they become blue. One may not be present when an arteriospasm is in progress ; ask the patient to put one hand (the comparatively normal one) into cold water. Sometimes the cold immersion will initiate an attack.

When the condition occurs in a working man (women are the usual sufferers) inquire whether he works with a road drill or other vibrating tools. (Agate.)

MAURICE RAYNAUD, 1834–1881, *Physician, Hôpital Lariboisière, Paris.*

JOHN NORMAN AGATE, *Contemporary, Assistant Physician, Department for Research in Industrial Medicine, Medical Research Council, London.*

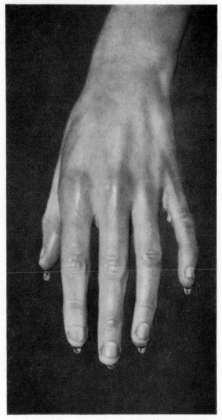

*Fig.* 655.—Raynaud's disease; spasm induced by the patient dipping her hands in ice-cold water.

## GAS GANGRENE

A wound is infected and angry; the infection is spreading. Observe the temperature chart; the pulse and temperature are both raised. In advanced cases the facies is somewhat characteristic. The expression is anxious; the complexion is muddy; the sclerotics are particularly white. There is often a peculiar smell, which has been described as sickly and sweetish. Gas gangrene spreads along the muscle planes. Test for crepitus over each group of muscles in the vicinity. The sign is usually not apparent until the condition is advanced.

## CHAPTER XXXIV

# SOME SIGNS TO CONFIRM A SUSPICION
# OF NEUROSIS

As in medicine, so in clinical surgery, it is sometimes necessary to confirm a suspicion that the patient is neurotic.

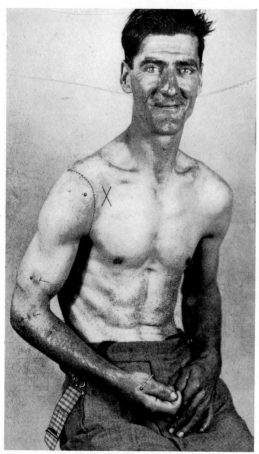

*Fig.* 656.—The patient had a recently healed superficial scar in the palm of the hand, for which he was claiming compensation. Actually he smiled while the five pins shown were thrust through the skin distal to the line marked by the pencil. Proximal to this line (X) a touch of the point of a pin caused him to cry out.

26

Among the most extraordinary purely functional phenomena is that known as glove and/or stocking anæsthesia. The patient says the limb is numb. That he is correct there can be no doubt, for one can transfix the skin with pins and the patient does not mind (*Fig.* 656). However, the area of anæsthesia ends abruptly at a certain level not in keeping with any anatomical distribution of nerve-supply.

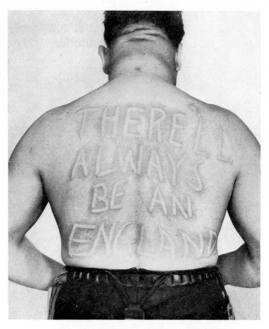

*Fig.* 657.—Dermatographia. (*B. S. Kent's case.*)

Usually, however, cases seen by the surgeon cannot be proved to be functional so easily. Indeed, it is wise to assume that the symptoms have an organic basis until it is proved irrefutably that this is not the case. As aids to arrival at this difficult conclusion the following tests are among the most helpful.

1. Test the knee-jerks. They are likely to be exaggerated.

2. Touch the soft palate with a blunt object. Normally, this will cause the patient to gag, but in advanced neurasthenia and other neuroses the reflex is entirely absent.

3. The corneal reflex may also be tried. Sometimes it is absent in this condition.

4. The handle of a knee-jerk hammer or other smooth blunt object is drawn evenly over the skin. Shortly afterwards, in a patient with an unstable vasomotor system, a red line appears which, in well-marked cases, may amount to a wheal. It is possible to write a word in this manner ; hence this phenomenon is called dermatographia (*Fig.* 657).

Perhaps the most difficult neurosis with which the surgeon has to contend is the hysterical joint. This usually takes the form of 'locking'. The joint is fixed in some degree of flexion. It is sometimes possible, by suddenly diverting the patient's attention, to release the joint and extend it.

" Clinical diagnosis is an art, and the mastery of an art has no end ; you can always be a better diagnostician."

(CLENDENING.)

LOGAN CLENDENING, 1884–1945, *Professor of Clinical Medicine, University of Kansas, U.S.A.*

# GLOSSARY OF ANATOMICAL TERMS

*Old Terminology*        *Birmingham Revision of the B.N.A.*

### LIGAMENTS, TENDONS, ETC.

| | |
|---|---|
| Poupart's ligament | Inguinal ligament |
| Anterior annular ligament | Flexor retinaculum |
| Intercolumnar fibres | Intercrural fibres |
| Internal lateral ligament of knee-joint | Medial ligament of knee-joint |
| Internal semilunar cartilage | Medial semilunar cartilage |
| External semilunar cartilage | Lateral semilunar cartilage |
| Anterior crucial ligament | Anterior cruciate ligament |
| Posterior crucial ligament | Posterior cruciate ligament |
| Tendo Achillis | Tendo calcaneus |

### MUSCLES

| | |
|---|---|
| Tibialis anticus | Tibialis anterior |
| Erector spinae | Sacrospinalis |
| Corrugator supercilii | Corrugator |
| Psoas magnus | Psoas |
| Serratus magnus | Serratus anterior |
| Scalenus anticus | Scalenus anterior |
| Müller's muscle | Deep lamella of levator palpebræ superioris |

### NEUROLOGY

| | |
|---|---|
| Pre-Rolandic area | Precentral gyrus |
| Fissure of Rolando | Central sulcus |
| Axillary nerve | Circumflex nerve |
| Genito-crural nerve | Genitofemoral nerve |
| Great sciatic nerve | Sciatic nerve |
| External popliteal nerve | Lateral popliteal nerve |
| Musculospiral nerve | Radial nerve |
| Long thoracic (Nerve of Bell) | Nerve to serratus anterior |
| Inner cord of brachial plexus | Medial cord of brachial plexus |
| Lower cord of brachial plexus | Posterior cord of brachial plexus |

### OSTEOLOGY

| | |
|---|---|
| Internal condyle of femur | Medial condyle of femur |
| Spheno-maxillary fossa | Pterygo-palatine fossa |
| Maxillary antrum | Maxillary sinus |
| Malar bone | Zygomatic bone |
| Ascending ramus of mandible | Superior ramus of mandible |
| Horizontal ramus of mandible | Body of mandible |
| Condylar process | Condyloid process |
| Meniscus | Articular disc |
| Eustachian tube | Pharyngo-tympanic tube |
| Mastoid antrum | Tympanic antrum |
| Sphenoidal fissure | Superior orbital fissure |
| Angle of Louis | Sternal angle |
| Semilunar bone | Lunate bone |
| Internal malleolus | Medial malleolus |

| *Old Terminology* | *Birmingham Revision of the B.N.A.* |
|---|---|

## OSTEOLOGY—*contd.*

| | |
|---|---|
| Tuber ischii | Ischial tuberosity |
| Great trochanter | Greater trochanter |
| Small trochanter | Lesser trochanter |
| Os calcis | Calcaneus |
| Vertebra prominens | Seventh cervical vertebra |

## GENITAL SYSTEM

| | |
|---|---|
| Mons veneris | Mons pubis |
| Fallopian tube | Uterine tube |
| Bartholin's glands | Greater vestibular glands |
| Cowper's glands | Bulbo-urethral glands |
| Globus major ⎱ of epididymis | Head ⎱ of epididymis |
| Globus minor ⎰ | Tail ⎰ |
| Hydatid of Morgagni | Appendix of epididymis |
| Bulbous urethra | Bulb of penis |

## LYMPHATIC SYSTEM

| | |
|---|---|
| Submaxillary lymph-glands | Submandibular lymph-glands |
| Post-auricular lymph-glands | Mastoid lymph-glands |
| Pre-auricular lymph-glands | Superficial parotid lymph-glands |

## DIGESTIVE SYSTEM

| | |
|---|---|
| Anterior pillar of fauces | Palatoglossal arch |
| Wharton's duct | Submandibular duct |
| Submaxillary gland | Submandibular gland |
| Stensen's duct | Parotid duct |
| Ampulla of Vater | Ampulla of bile-duct |
| Omphalomesenteric duct | Vitello-intestinal duct |

## SURGICAL MARKINGS, SPACES, ETC.

| | |
|---|---|
| Scarpa's triangle | Femoral triangle |
| Submaxillary triangle | Digastric triangle |
| Suprameatal triangle of Macewen | Suprameatal triangle |
| Costocoracoid membrane | Clavipectoral fascia |
| Angle of Louis | Sternal angle |
| External abdominal ring | Superficial abdominal ring |
| Internal abdominal ring | Deep abdominal ring |
| Hesselbach's triangle | Inguinal triangle |
| Pouch of Douglas | Recto-uterine pouch |
| Scarpa's fascia | Deep layer of superficial fascia of anterior abdominal wall |
| Genito-crural fold | Fold of groin |
| Colles's fascia | Deep layer of superficial perineal fascia |
| Triangular ligament | Perineal membrane |

## BLOOD-VASCULAR SYSTEM

| | |
|---|---|
| Superior longitudinal sinus | Superior sagittal sinus |
| Lateral sinus | Transverse sinus |
| Angular vein | Anterior facial vein |
| Deep epigastric artery | Inferior epigastric artery |
| Internal saphenous vein | Long saphenous vein |
| External saphenous vein | Short saphenous vein |

# INDEX

PRINTED IN GREAT BRITAIN BY JOHN WRIGHT AND SONS LTD., STONEBRIDGE PRESS, BRISTOL.